ISSUES IN KIDNEY DISEASE SERIES

ISSUES IN KIDNEY DISEASE

ACUTE KIDNEY INJURY

ISSUES IN KIDNEY DISEASE SERIES

Stephen Z. Fadem – Series Editor

SELZMAN INSTITUTE FOR KIDNEY HEALTH, SECTION OF NEPHROLOGY,
AND MICHAEL E. DEBAKEY VETERANS AFFAIRS MEDICAL CENTER,
BAYLOR COLLEGE OF MEDICINE, HOUSTON, TX, USA;
KIDNEY ASSOCIATES, HOUSTON, TX, USA

Issues in Kidney Disease – Transplantation
Bhamidipati V. R. Murthy and Stephen Z. Fadem (Editors)
2021. ISBN: 978-1-53619-960-4
(Hardcover)

Issues in Kidney Disease – Dialysis
Stephen Z. Fadem and José A. Moura-Neto (Editors)
2021. ISBN: 978-1-68507-000-7
(Hardcover)

Issues in Kidney Disease – Acute Kidney Injury
Stephen Z. Fadem and Ahmed Arslan Yousuf Awan (Editors)
2021. ISBN: 978-1-68507-002-1
(Hardcover)

Issues in Kidney Disease – Chronic Kidney Disease
Stephen Z. Fadem and Samaya Javed Anumudu (Editors)
2021. ISBN: 978-1-68507-001-4
(Hardcover)

ISSUES IN KIDNEY DISEASE SERIES

ISSUES IN KIDNEY DISEASE

ACUTE KIDNEY INJURY

STEPHEN Z. FADEM
AND
AHMED ARSLAN YOUSUF AWAN
EDITORS

nova
Medicine & Health
New York

https://doi.org/10.52305/OWCU8763

Library of Congress Cataloging-in-Publication Data

ISBN: 978-1-68507-002-1

Published by Nova Science Publishers, Inc. † New York

To my amazing parents - who encouraged me
to be a compassionate physician,
to my lovely wife Nida - whose support makes it possible, and to my beautiful kids Inaya and Abdullah – who give me hope for the future.

Ahmed Arslan Yousuf Awan

To my lovely wife, Joyce, who is my rock. I am nurtured by her constant support and encouragement.

Stephen Z. Fadem

CONTENTS

FOREWORD

Claudio Ronco, MD

Dipartimento di Medicina (DIMED) - University of Padova
Director Dept. Nephrology Dialysis & Transplantation
International Renal Research Institute (IRRIV)
San Bortolo Hospital - Vicenza, Italy

It is an honor and a privilege to write the introduction to *Issues in Kidney Disease – Acute Kidney Injury*, a book authored by Stephen Z. Fadem, MD and Ahmed Arsian Yousuf Awan, MD. This area of medicine has been neglected or marginally considered for too long, but it has emerged as a significant healthcare challenge in recent years thanks to the commitment of a small group of scientists and investigators. While acute kidney injury has been clinically diagnosed for decades and subsequently has relied mostly on changes in serum creatinine and urine output, today we have a consistent definition and classification that allows us to apply well-defined criteria for identification of the syndrome even in the very early phases thanks to new diagnostic tools such as biomarkers. Acute kidney injury was originally described as acute tubular necrosis and then later as acute renal failure. Thanks to the Acute Disease Quality Initiative (ADQI), the unifying term acute kidney injury (AKI) has been adopted and utilized in recent studies making possible comparative analyses and large observational and prospective studies. The observation of AKI in hospitalized patients was mostly common in renal wards before the last decades of the last century, but since the late seventies, AKI in hospitalized patients is mostly observed in critically ill patients admitted to intensive care units as a component of multiple organ dysfunction syndromes and sepsis. This change in case mix has led to the development of a new specialty called "Critical care Nephrology" whose origin lies in the very first and innovative collaboration between intensive care and nephrology departments of Vicenza hospital to the point that, for many years, this multidisciplinary approach has been defined "Vicenza Model". This authentic and effective collaboration has definitely contributed to the mutual need of expanding knowledge and information about the kidney patient suffering from critical illness, as well as the continuous evolution in the technology of renal replacement therapy and extracorporeal organ support. Specialists tend to focus their attention on one specific organ or apparatus forgetting that other organs may contribute to critical illness. Organ cross-talk is defined as the continuous interaction among different organs and is in fact responsible for many disorders due to one dysfunctioning organ affecting another organ or multiple organs simultaneously. Often this interaction is mediated by physical (pressures and flows), chemical (acid-base and electrolytes) or biological (cytokines and chemokines) signals. Such pathological conditions can be multidirectional and temporally regulated. This is the case of cardio-renal syndromes, hepato-renal syndromes, cardio-metabolic syndromes, brain-kidney, and lung-kidney interactions. Vascular endothelium and circulating blood can be significantly affected by a dysregulation of the immuno-system; this is what typically occurs in sepsis where the inevitable consequence is a multiple organ dysfunction syndrome mediated by an altered organ cross-talk. The effects of pregnancy on either the kidney or drugs or procedures represent typical cases that involve organ cross-talk. We have learned about physiological and pathological interactions between native organs, but now we face other challenges. Advancements in technology and application or extracorporeal therapies imposed today allow us to learn about another type of interaction: the artificial organ cross-talk. We must understand the effects of different extracorporeal organ support systems on various organs, and even possible interactions between various organ support therapies representing a new area of science defined artificial organ cross-talk. These and many other issues are debated in this interesting book in an effort to shed some light on still controversial issues in kidney diseases and Acute Kidney Injury.

PREFACE

Acute Kidney Injury (AKI) is one of the most common diagnoses in patients admitted to the hospital, also the top reason why a Nephrologist is consulted to see a patient. Understanding the factors that lead to development and progression of AKI is critical to the management of hospitalized patients. Timely diagnosis and appropriate treatment can prevent significant morbidity and mortality. This book is an effort to address the most common issues in patients with AKI using evidence-based and updated recommendations, written by experts in the subject across US and Canada.

Our target audience for this book remains the trainees in Internal Medicine and Nephrology, as well as the practicing clinicians who would like to update their knowledge of various facets of AKI. The chapters have been written with focus on issues encountered in clinical practice. Practical management strategies based on current guidelines and most recent evidence is discussed throughout the book, composed by authors who have a wealth of experience dealing with these clinical scenarios. Clinical pearls are distributed throughout this book, making it a valuable resource for teaching and learning on rounds, as well as preparation for exams. Readers will find this book easy to read and hence be able to assimilate the essential information. References at the end of each chapter are useful for readers who wish to gain in-depth knowledge of each subject.

Our book is divided into 19 chapters. The first 5 chapters discuss the approach to the diagnosis and management of AKI, including use of biomarkers and various imaging studies that facilitate the diagnosis. Chapters 6 to 10 discuss primary diseases of the kidney, including acute tubular injury, interstitial nephritis, glomerulonephritis, and obstructive uropathy. Chapters 11 to 16 discuss kidney injury secondary to other disorders such as viral infection, dysproteinemias, heart disease, liver disease, malignancy, and drug use. Chapter 17 discusses the principles of drug use in patients with AKI. Finally, the last two chapters address AKI in specialized patient populations including pregnant patients and patients with a kidney transplant.

This book is a valuable resource for internal medicine residents, renal fellows, nurse practitioners, practicing nephrologists, and all other physicians and allied professionals involved in the care of patients with acute kidney injury, and those interested in the evolution of this field. This book contains clinically relevant and updated information that can be used in rounds and can serve as a resource for exam preparation.

Finally, we hope that this book will help medical professionals make a difference in the lives of people they diagnose and treat. Ultimately, the center of our medical universe is our patients, and their health and well-being should always remain our top priority.

Ahmed Arslan Yousuf Awan
Stephen Z. Fadem
May 2021

ACKNOWLEDGMENTS

Transforming a manuscript into a readable and understandable format, yet with appropriate use of punctuation and grammar, takes a lot of time and effort. We are so grateful for Michelle (Misha) L. Nguyen, our Master Copy Editor, who read every word of each manuscript to make sure that the writing is clear and free of errors. She had a major impact on the quality of this work.

We are thankful to all the authors who contributed to this book and spent hours researching and refining their manuscripts, in addition to their clinical and administrative responsibilities. Writing a book chapter is a labor of love; hence, it is only taken up by people with a passion for teaching and education. We are indebted to all our authors for making it possible to get this book out in time and for helping us meet the deadlines.

We would also like to acknowledge our families. They provided us with the support and strength to dedicate innumerable hours to editing this book over the last two years.

Ahmed Arslan Yousuf Awan
Stephen Z. Fadem
May 2021

Editors' Contact Information

Stephen Z. Fadem, MD, FACP, FASN
Selzman Institute for Kidney Health, Section of Nephrology, Department of Medicine,
Baylor College of Medicine, Houston, TX, USA
Michael E. DeBakey VA Medical Center, Houston, TX, USA
Kidney Associates, Houston, TX, USA
Email: fadem@bcm.edu

Ahmed Arslan Yousuf Awan
Selzman Institute for Kidney Health, Section of Nephrology, Department of Medicine,
and Division of Abdominal transplantation, Department of Surgery,
Baylor College of Medicine, Houston, TX, USA
Email: ahmed.awan@bcm.edu

List of Contributors

Irfan A. Aghan, MD
Dallas Renal Group, PA, USA
Medical City Dallas Transplant Institute , Dallas, TX, USA

Joseph Alge, MD, PhD
Department of Pediatrics, Section of Renal, Baylor College of Medicine, Houston, TX, USA

Sehrish Ali, DO
Selzman Institute for Kidney Health, Section of Nephrology, Department of Medicine, Baylor College of Medicine, Houston, TX, USA
Michael E. DeBakey VA Medical Center, Houston, TX, USA

James Anaissie, MD
Baylor College of Medicine, Houston, TX, USA

Utsav K. Bansal, MD, MS
Baylor College of Medicine, Houston, TX, USA

Harini Bejjanki, MD
University of Texas, MD Anderson Cancer Center, Houston, TX, USA

Ira H. Blau, MD
Penn Medicine, Philadelphia, PA, USA

Kiran Chintam, MD
Geisenger Medical Center, Danville, PA, USA

Edward Clark, MD
University of Ottawa, Ottawa, Canada

Amanda Condon
Medical City Dallas Transplant Institute, Dallas, TX, USA

George M. Dolson, MD
Selzman Institute for Kidney Health, Section of Nephrology, Department of Medicine, Baylor College of Medicine, Houston, TX, USA

Sebastian Franco, MD
Duke University School of Medicine, Durham, NC, USA

Vidhi A. Gandhi, PharmD
Medstar Georgetown University Hospital, Department of Pharmacy, Washington DC, USA

Swapnil Hiremath, MD, MPH, FASN
University of Ottawa, Ottawa, Canada

Michael W. Holliday Jr., MD, PhD
Selzman Institute for Kidney Health, Section of Nephrology, Department of Medicine, Baylor College of Medicine, Houston, TX, USA
Michael E. DeBakey VA Medical Center, Houston, TX, USA

Ingrid Hougen, MD
University of Ottawa, Ottawa, Canada

Amna Ilahe, MD
Dallas Renal Group, PA, USA
Methodist Dallas Medical Center Transplant Center, Dallas, TX, USA

Luis A. Juncosm, MD
University of Arkansas for Medical Sciences and Central Arkansas VA Medical Center, Little Rock, AR, USA

Kartik Karla, MD
Geisenger Medical Center, Danville, PA, USA

Pascale Khairallah, MD
Selzman Institute for Kidney Health, Section of Nephrology, Department of Medicine, Baylor College of Medicine, Houston, TX, USA

Jacob L. Kraus
Baylor College of Medicine, Houston, TX, USA

Edgar V. Lerma, MD
University of Illinois at Chicago College of Medicine/
Advocate Christ Medical Center, IL, USA

Forrest F. Lindsay-Mcginn, MD
Penn Medicine, Philadelphia, PA, USA

Richard E. Link, MD, PhD
Baylor College of Medicine, Houston, TX, USA

Hector Madariaga, MD
Goodsamaritan Medical Center, Department of Medicine, Brockton, MA, USA

Omar Mamlouk, MD
University of Texas, MD Anderson Cancer Center, Houston, TX, USA

Wesley A. Mayer, MD
Baylor College of Medicine, Houston, TX, USA

David M. Mckelvey, DO
Penn Medicine, Philadelphia, PA, USA

Van N. Ngo
Medical City Dallas Transplant Institute, Dallas, TX, USA

Annelise Nolan, PharmD
Medstar Georgetown University Hospital, Department of Pharmacy, Washington DC, USA

Sayna Norouzi, MD
Loma Linda University Medical Center, Loma Linda, CA, USA

Jenny S. Pan, MD
Selzman Institute for Kidney Health, Section of Nephrology, Department of Medicine, Baylor College of Medicine, Houston, TX, USA
Michael E. DeBakey VA Medical Center, Houston, TX, USA

Vishnu Parvathareddy, MD
Selzman Institute for Kidney Health, Section of Nephrology, Department of Medicine, Baylor College of Medicine, Houston, TX, USA

Amir Abdi Pour, MD
Loma Linda University Medical Center, Loma Linda, CA, USA

Venkat Ramanathan, MD
Selzman Institute for Kidney Health, Section of Nephrology, Department of Medicine, Baylor College of Medicine, Houston, TX, USA
Michael E. DeBakey VA Medical Center, Houston, TX, USA

Kavitha Ramaswamy, MD
Wellspan Chambersburg Hospital, Department of Medicine, Chambersburg, PA, USA

Nathaniel C. Reisinger, MD
Penn Medicine, Philadelphia, PA, USA

Sohail Riaz, MD
Selzman Institute for Kidney Health, Section of Nephrology, Department of Medicine, Baylor College of Medicine, Houston, TX, USA

Solomiia Savedchuk, MD
Duke University School of Medicine, Durham, NC, USA

Micah Schub, MD
Duke University School of Medicine, Durham, NC, USA

Silvi Shah, MD, MS, FACP, FASN, FAST
University of Cincinnnati, Cincinnati, OH, USA

Matthew A. Sparks, MD
Duke University School of Medicine and Durham VA Healthcare System, Durham, NC, USA

Samuel Y. Suen, PharmD
Medstar Georgetown University Hospital, Department of Pharmacy, Washington DC, USA

Beje Thomas, MD
Medstar Georgetown University Hospital, Medstar Georgetown Transplant Institute, Washington DC, USA

Chandan Vangala, MD
Selzman Institute for Kidney Health, Section of Nephrology, Department of Medicine, Baylor College of Medicine, Houston, TX, USA
Michael E. DeBakey VA Medical Center, Houston, TX, USA

Juan Carlos Q. Velez, MD
Ochsner Clinic Foundation, New Orleans, LA, USA
Ochsner Clinical School, The University of Queensland, Brisbane, Australia

Biruh Workeneh, MD
University of Texas, MD Anderson Cancer Center, Houston, TX, USA

Carl P. Walther, MD
Selzman Institute for Kidney Health, Section of Nephrology, Department of Medicine, Baylor College of Medicine, Houston, TX, USA

James Yoon, MD
Loma Linda University Medical Center, Loma Linda, CA, USA

In: Issues in Kidney Disease – Acute Kidney Injury
Editors: S. Z. Fadem and A. Arslan Yousuf Awan

ISBN: 978-1-68507-002-1

Chapter 1

ACUTE KIDNEY INJURY: A PRIMER

Joseph Alge*[*], *MD, PhD
Department of Pediatrics, Section of Renal,
Baylor College of Medicine, Houston, TX, USA

ABSTRACT

Acute kidney injury (AKI) is a clinical syndrome that is characterized by an abrupt reduction in renal function and is common among hospitalized patients, particularly the critically ill. It has a tremendous negative impact on both acute and long-term morbidity and mortality. Unfortunately, there are no treatments available for this disease; therefore, clinicians must be vigilant in their efforts to prevent AKI and its complications. This chapter reviews expert recommendations for AKI diagnosis and staging; it also provides an overview of the epidemiology of AKI. The pathogenesis and pathophysiology of AKI are discussed, and basic concepts of AKI clinical management are introduced. This primer will provide the reader with a conceptual framework for understanding the AKI as a disease and a basic understanding of the tenets of its management.

Keywords: acute kidney injury, epidemiology, pathophysiology, biomarkers, renal replacement therapy

ACUTE KIDNEY INJURY: INTRODUCTION

Acute kidney injury (AKI) is a clinical syndrome that has been known by other names, including acute renal insufficiency, acute renal dysfunction, and acute renal failure. AKI has been recognized since the advent of medicine. Ancient Greek and Roman physicians noted that a decrease in urine output (oliguria) accompanied by anorexia, nausea, and vomiting often occurred after crush injuries, serpent bites, and poisonings, and they understood prolonged anuria to be a grave sign of impending death [1]. While urine output is still a useful diagnostic

[*] Corresponding Author's E-mail: joseph.alge@bcm.edu.

and prognostic indicator, much has changed regarding how the disease is defined [2]. Now there is an increase in use of objective measures of renal function, such as serum creatinine and blood urea nitrogen (BUN), which are filtered at the glomerulus and accumulate in the blood when renal function declines. Despite the long-standing availability of these conventional AKI biomarkers, there was not an agreed upon nomenclature or consensus definition of AKI until the early 21st century.

The lack of an accepted definition and classification scheme was recognized as a key barrier to progress in AKI research and clinical practice. In 2004, the Acute Dialysis Quality Initiative (ADQI) Group, an international consensus workgroup, proposed the RIFLE definition and classification system for acute renal failure, which allows for the diagnosis and staging of AKI based on changes in serum creatinine and urine output [3]. Over the next decade, the nomenclature would be changed from acute renal failure to acute kidney injury, thus the definition of AKI would be further refined. In 2012, the definition and staging of AKI was finally crystallized by the Kidney Disease Improving Global Outcomes Clinical Practice Guideline (KDIGO) for AKI, which is shown in Table 1 [4, 5]. Key features of the KDIGO AKI definition and classification system include its recognition that even modest changes in serum creatinine are clinically significant and that creatinine can rise slowly as AKI evolves over the time course of a week. An important caveat is that oliguria can be a normal physiologic response, such as in the setting of hypovolemia, and so urine output must be interpreted in the context of a patient's volume status. Nevertheless, the definition proposed by KDIGO is a significant step forward and has achieved widespread use.

Table 1. KDIGO Criteria for Diagnosis and Staging of AKI

Stage	Serum Creatinine Criteria	Urine Output Criteria
1	1.5 - 1.9 times baseline within 7 days or ≥0.3 mg/dL (26.5 μmol/L) within 48 hours	< 0.5 mL/kg/hr for 6-12 hrs
2	2 - 2.9 times baseline	<0.5 mL/kg/hr for ≥12 hrs
3	>3 times baseline	<0.3 mL/kg/hr for ≥24 hrs or anuria for ≥12 hrs
	or increase ≥4 mg/dL (335.36 μmol/L)	
	or initiation or renal replacement therapy	
	or, in patients < 18 years old, decrease in eGFR <35 mL/min/1.73m^2	

EPIDEMIOLOGY OF ACUTE KIDNEY INJURY

Acute kidney injury is a significant contributor to the morbidity and mortality of hospitalized patients. The incidence of AKI has increased in recent decades, and the prevalence of AKI among hospitalized adults is approximately 25% in the United States, with more than two-thirds of cases being present at the time of admission (i.e., community-acquired AKI) [6–9]. The critically ill population is disproportionately affected by AKI, with a large multinational cross-sectional study reporting AKI in 57% of patients admitted to the intensive care unit (ICU) [10]. The most common causes of AKI among these patients in the ICU are sepsis and hypovolemia, which account for 75% of cases [10]. While overall in-hospital mortality related to AKI has declined, most studies report rates of 10-20%[8]. Importantly, there is a stepwise increase in the risk of death as AKI severity increases, and severe AKI (KDIGO Stage 2 or 3) has been identified as an independent predictor of in-hospital death [10]. However, even less severe cases of AKI are associated with an increased risk of death, both in-hospital and in the long-term after hospital discharge [11, 12]. In addition to its association with mortality risk, AKI increases a patient's length of stay in the hospital and has a tremendous economic impact. In the United States, the economic burden of AKI is estimated to range from $5.4 to $24.0 billion per year, or $11,016 to $42,077 per hospitalization [13].

AKI significantly increases long-term morbidity and specifically increases the risk of renal and cardiovascular outcomes. AKI has been called a "springboard" for chronic kidney disease (CKD), and patients who develop AKI superimposed on pre-existing CKD, so-called acute-on-chronic kidney injury, are at risk for CKD progression [14]. However, even patients with normal renal function can develop CKD after incident AKI. For example, the Acute Kidney Injury-Epidemiological Prospective (AKI-EPI) study reported new CKD in 16% of patients who developed AKI during an admission to the intensive care unit (CKD was defined as an estimated glomerular filtration rate < 60 mL/min/1.73m2 at 6 months after hospital discharge) [10]. Of patients with severe AKI requiring renal replacement therapy, 20% will remain dialysis-dependent one year after discharge [15]. Additionally, AKI is associated with a heightened long-term risk of cardiovascular disease, including myocardial infarction, heart failure, and stroke [16].

Table 2. Risk Factors for AKI in Hospitalized Patients*

Demographic Variables • Older age • Male sex Comorbidities • Pre-existing chronic kidney disease • Diabetes mellitus • Heart failure • Advanced chronic liver disease • Sepsis Medications • Nonsteroidal anti-inflammatory drugs • Diuretics • Angiotensin-converting enzyme inhibitors

* Adapted from reference 8.

Epidemiological studies have identified a number of risk factors for AKI in the hospital, which are shown in Table 2 (adapted from REF [8]). Older age and male sex confer an increased risk of AKI and are positively correlated with AKI severity [8]. AKI is a common complication of sepsis, and the risk of AKI increases with sepsis severity [8]. A number of medical comorbidities also increase the risk of AKI, including pre-existing CKD, diabetes mellitus, heart failure, and advanced liver disease [8]. Chronic exposure to certain medications is associated with AKI, particularly non-steroidal anti-inflammatory drugs (NSAIDs), diuretics, and angiotensin-converting enzyme inhibitors (ACEIs), which can be a particularly dangerous combination in the setting of hypovolemia [8]. In many cases, the risk of AKI can be attributed to exposure to nephrotoxins, including intravenous iodinated radiocontrast media and aminoglycoside antibiotics. Finally, AKI is a well-described post-operative complication and is especially common after cardiac surgery, which is discussed subsequently in more detail.

CAUSES OF ACUTE KIDNEY INJURY

There are myriad potential causes of acute kidney injury, which have classically been organized into three general categories: pre-renal, intrinsic, and post-renal. Pre-renal AKI is a functional state of decreased renal perfusion that manifests with azotemia (elevated BUN with relatively mild changes in serum creatinine) and a reduction in urine output, whereas post-renal AKI occurs whenever there is obstruction of urine output. Obstruction creates pressure in the urinary space that opposes glomerular filtration and causes back leak, but severe obstruction causes dilation of the collecting system and can lead to irreversible damage to the renal parenchyma if uncorrected. Intrinsic AKI refers to impaired renal function due to renal parenchymal injury.

Pre-renal AKI is most often associated with hypovolemia, such as occurs with acute gastroenteritis; but it can be caused by other conditions that decrease effective circulating volume, including heart failure and cirrhotic liver disease (although these deserve special consideration). Nephrotic syndrome can also present with AKI due to intravascular volume depletion that may occur in children, but is uncommon in adults where the effective circulating volume (ECV) is typically normal [17]. Patients with significant atherosclerosis involving the renal arteries are at increased risk of pre-renal AKI due to reduced baseline renal perfusion, particularly elderly patients who are at risk for dehydration and frequently take diuretics and medications that alter renal hemodynamics, such as NSAIDs and angiotensin-converting enzyme inhibitors [18]. Calcineurin inhibitors (CNI) can also cause pre-renal AKI due to vasoconstriction of the afferent arteriole [19]. The risk of AKI is increased when these medications are used in combination, and they can be particularly dangerous when taken in the setting of a gastrointestinal illness. Importantly, pre-renal azotemia can lead to tubular injury and renal ischemia if prolonged and should be promptly corrected; therefore, counseling patients to hold these medications in the setting of an acute illness should be considered.

Clinical management of pre-renal AKI generally involves fluid resuscitation. Generally, a patient's volume status can be ascertained by history and clinical exam findings consistent with dehydration. However, it can be difficult to distinguish pre-renal from ischemic AKI; and in these cases, urine microscopy and urine biochemical studies can be helpful. Pre-renal AKI is a functional state characterized by avid renal reabsorption of sodium and water in an attempt to restore intravascular volume. Therefore, patients with pre-renal AKI will typically have a low fractional excretion of sodium *(FENa)* <1% [20]. However, it must be noted that FENa is unreliable in patients with significant chronic kidney disease or who are on diuretics [21]. In these cases, the fractional excretion of urea (FEUrea) <35% can be helpful [21]. Urine sediment will be bland or may contain hyaline casts, rather than granular casts typically seen with ischemic AKI [20].

Post-renal AKI is the result of urinary outflow obstruction. In general, both kidneys must be affected because the unaffected kidney is able to compensate in absence of bilateral disease. Therefore, patients with a solitary kidney are particularly susceptible to post-renal AKI. Important causes of post-renal AKI include benign prostatic hyperplasia, pelvic masses, neurogenic bladder, retroperitoneal masses or fibrosis, and more rarely, obstructing stones or clots [20]. Severe obstruction causes hydronephrosis, which can lead to irreversible parenchymal damage if prolonged [22]. Therefore, it is of paramount importance to quickly identify these conditions based on history and imaging; and to relieve the obstruction with placement of an indwelling bladder catheter, ureteral stent, or percutaneous nephrostomy as appropriate.

Intrinsic AKI can be the result of tubular, interstitial, glomerular, or vascular kidney diseases [20]. Renal ischemia is an important cause of intrinsic AKI and is the result of tubular injury caused by any condition that severely compromises renal perfusion. Irreversible cortical necrosis can ensue if renal perfusion is not restored. As noted earlier, prolonged pre-renal AKI will eventually progress to renal ischemia. Ischemic AKI often occurs in the setting of shock, of which sepsis is an important cause. Ischemic AKI is also a common post-operative complication, particularly if there is severe intraoperative blood loss or hypotension. Direct tubular injury can be caused by free hemoglobin and myoglobin from hemolysis and rhabdomyolysis, respectively, as well as many nephrotoxic medications, such as aminoglycosides, vancomycin, acyclovir, methotrexate, and amphotericin B. Acute interstitial nephritis causes intrinsic AKI due to a parenchymal inflammatory infiltrate. It is most often the result of an allergic reaction to a medication (most commonly NSAIDs) and usually resolves with discontinuation of the offending agent, although corticosteroids may also be used for treatment [23]. Finally, AKI is one of the cardinal features of nephritic syndrome and can be seen with any of the glomerulonephritides; it is also an important manifestation of the thrombotic microangiopathies, such as hemolytic uremic syndrome.

While the previously mentioned classification system for causes of AKI is useful, AKI is often multifactorial. Furthermore, there are several conditions with unique pathophysiology that merit discussion. These include contrast-induced AKI, post-cardiac surgery AKI, cardiorenal syndrome, and hepatorenal syndrome.

Contrast-Induced AKI

Parenteral administration of iodinated radiocontrast media for CT scan (intravenous) or angiography (intra-arterial) is an important cause of AKI. The incidence of contrast-induced AKI is variable based on the definition used, but large epidemiologic studies of patients undergoing percutaneous coronary intervention estimate the rate to be 2-13.3% [24, 25]. There is a higher risk associated with intra-arterial administration, exposure to larger volume of contrast media, and higher osmolar media [8]. Additionally, patients with pre-existing CKD, heart failure, liver disease, and concurrent hypovolemia or exposure to other nephrotoxins are at increased risk of contrast-induced AKI [8]. The mechanism of renal injury involves renal hemodynamic changes that promote medullary hypoxia and direct cytotoxicity and tubular injury. Prophylaxis with sodium bicarbonate and N-acetylcysteine has been recommended, but these treatments are no longer endorsed based on the results of the Prevention of Serious Adverse Events Following Angiography (PRESERVE) trial [26]. The current best practice for prevention of contrast-induced AKI is periprocedural volume expansion with isotonic fluids [5].

AKI after Cardiac Surgery

Post-operative AKI occurs in one-fourth of patients undergoing cardiac surgery [27, 28]. Approximately 2% of patients with AKI after cardiac surgery require renal replacement therapy; AKI in this population is an important determinant of mortality risk [28]. Perioperative risk factors for cardiac-surgery associated AKI include advanced age, elevated pre-operative serum creatinine, cardiopulmonary bypass time, aortic cross-clamp time, type of surgery and use of an intra-aortic balloon pump, concurrent infection, reduced cardiac output, and need for emergency or repeat surgery [8]. Cardiac surgery with cardiopulmonary bypass causes renal injury through multiple mechanisms, including ischemia-reperfusion injury, nephrotoxicity secondary to mechanical hemolysis, and a robust systemic inflammatory response [29].

Cardiorenal Syndrome

Cardiorenal syndrome (CRS) describes the complex pathophysiologic interactions between the heart and the kidneys in the setting of acute or chronic failure of one organ system. CRS can be divided into five sub-types, where types 1 and 2 refer to the renal effects of acute and chronic heart failure, respectively, and types 3 and 4 refer to the cardiac effects of acute kidney injury and chronic kidney disease, respectively (sometimes referred to as nephrocardiac syndrome). Type 5 CRS is diagnosed when there is concurrent cardiac and renal failure that is secondary to another disease process. The renal pathophysiology of type 1 CRS falls on the spectrum of pre-renal and ischemic AKI, and the classic rationale is that poor cardiac output compromises renal perfusion and induces upregulation of neurohormonal pathways, including the renin-angiotensin system, the sympathetic nervous system, and ADH, which leads to fluid retention, increased preload, and worsening heart failure [30]. However, many patients with CRS type 1 have preserved ejection fraction, and there is evidence that renal perfusion is compromised by elevated central venous pressures resulting in renal venous hypertension [31]. Additionally, there is experimental evidence that AKI can contribute to diastolic dysfunction [32]. Decongestive therapies are the cornerstone of CRS type 1 management with the goal of optimizing cardiac output and renal perfusion. Loop diuretics are first-line agents, and mechanical fluid removal via ultrafiltration can be used in severe or refractory cases [30].

Hepatorenal Syndrome

Cirrhotic liver disease can be associated with AKI (hepatorenal syndrome type 1; HRS-1) or CKD (hepatorenal syndrome type 2). Several mechanisms contribute to the pathogenesis of HRS-1, but it can be essentially regarded as the result of a severely perturbed hemodynamic state leading to reduced renal perfusion [33]. Cirrhosis leads to portal hypertension that is associated with the release of vasodilators, such as nitric oxide, that cause splanchnic vasodilation, which in turn reduces effective circulating volume and triggers activation of the sympathetic nervous system and renin-angiotensin system, ultimately reducing renal perfusion [33]. It can be clinically challenging to distinguish between HRS-1 and volume depletion, and current expert recommendations are to attempt a trial of volume repletion with intravenous albumin and withdrawal of diuretic therapy before initiating therapy for HRS-1 [34]. Albumin repletion is a mainstay of HRS-1 management and is often used in combination with vasoconstrictor therapy [33]. In the United States, norepinephrine and the combination of oral midodrine and octreotide are the most common treatments for HRS-1, but in other countries the vasopressin receptor agonist terlipressin is used [33, 35]. Additionally, paracentesis is sometimes performed to relieve intra-abdominal hypertension and treat abdominal compartment syndrome, which can develop in the setting of severe ascites and leads to AKI due to renal venous congestion [33].

AKI Pathophysiology

AKI is a multiphasic disease that begins with injury to the renal parenchyma (initiation phase) [36]. Following the initial renal insult is the extension phase, when there is potential to either mitigate or exacerbate the injury over the next 24-48 hours. Serum creatinine rises and peaks during this phase and afterward plateaus during the maintenance stage, then normalizes or reaches a new baseline in the recovery phase. Each of these clinical phases is characterized by distinct cellular and molecular processes that will be discussed in this section.

The pathophysiology of AKI has been largely elucidated by experimental animal models and has been best described in the context of renal ischemia-reperfusion injury [36, 37]. First, a reduction in renal perfusion leads to a decrease in the glomerular filtration rate (GFR) and causes renal ischemia. This initial phase of AKI is characterized by ATP depletion in the epithelial cells of proximal tubule that is accompanied by cytoskeletal rearrangement and loss of apical-basolateral polarity. Injured cells and bystander immune cells in the renal interstitium upregulate production of inflammatory mediators creating a pronounced pro-inflammatory microenvironment. Ultimately, epithelial cell death occurs by necrosis and apoptosis. Epithelial cells slough off the tubular basement membrane, creating granular casts that occlude the tubular lumen. Next, in the "extension phase", persistent hypoxia leads to microvascular endothelial injury, causing severe hemodynamic alterations that compromise perfusion to the corticomedullary junction and the outer medulla. There is ongoing inflammation, epithelial cell injury, and death during this phase, while the GFR continues to decline. Additionally, there is back leakage of glomerular filtrate across the damaged tubular epithelium, resulting in further impaired solute clearance. The next phase of AKI is "maintenance", during which renal function stabilizes, and there is a plateau in serum creatinine. During this phase, surviving epithelial cells dedifferentiate and acquire a proliferative and phagocytic phenotype. These cells clear the tubular lumen of apoptotic and necrotic cellular debris and repopulate the denuded tubular epithelium. In the recovery phase, tubular epithelial cell polarity and function are restored. There is also some evidence for the role of kidney-specific stem cells during tubular regeneration, but the relative contribution of these cells during AKI recovery is unclear [38].

As described previously, recovery from AKI is a multistep process, and maladaptive repair leads to incomplete resolution of the injury and progression from AKI to CKD. Cell cycle arrest, a cytoprotective response to tubular injury, has been identified as a hallmark of severe AKI and leads to early senescence, maladaptive repair, and the development of renal fibrosis [39, 40]. Additionally, tubular regeneration is a highly energy-dependent process; and mitochondrial dysfunction, a prominent feature of AKI, leads to impaired renal recovery and contributes to progression to CKD if prolonged [41, 42]. Finally, it is noteworthy that the regeneration phase is characterized by transition to an anti-inflammatory state, and prolonged inflammation has also been implicated in non-recovery of renal function and progression from AKI to CKD [43, 44]. Studies are ongoing to identify important pathways of renal injury and regeneration and develop novel interventions that can attenuate the severity of renal injury or enhance recovery from AKI.

Clinical Management of Acute Kidney Injury

Unfortunately, AKI is a disease without a treatment; therefore, its clinical management is best understood with the aphorism that "an ounce of prevention is worth a pound of cure". Murray et al. proposed a conceptual framework for AKI that envisages a patient progressing through successive stages of AKI beginning with risk and culminating in renal failure. The model is useful because it frames AKI in terms of its antecedents, complications, and outcomes [45]. Antecedents are conditions or events that put a patient at risk of developing AKI, such as pre-existing chronic kidney disease, admission to the intensive care unit for septic shock, or the need for cardiac surgery. Complications from AKI include fluid overload and metabolic derangements, including hyperkalemia, metabolic acidosis, and uremia. Recognition of the antecedents of AKI allows the clinical agility to modify that, which is modifiable, such as nephrotoxin exposure, in order to reduce a patient's risk of AKI and maximize the chances of renal recovery. Vigilance for the complications of AKI facilitates preventative strategies such as fluid and potassium restriction or diuretic use, which can delay or obviate the need for renal replacement therapy. To guide clinical decision-making, the 2012 KDIGO AKI Clinical Practice Guideline proposed a stage-based management strategy for AKI, which is summarized in Figure 1 [5].

Timely recognition of AKI is essential, and early diagnosis of AKI is a major barrier to improving clinical outcomes. Most cases are diagnosed based on serum creatinine criteria. However, creatinine is an index of renal function, rather than a marker of kidney injury, and changes in serum creatinine lag behind the timing of renal injury. Thus, clinicians miss a critical window for intervention; this has served as the impetus for the discovery of novel AKI biomarkers in the search for a so-called "renal troponin". Intensive research efforts in this area led to the discovery of several promising candidate biomarkers of renal injury over the last two decades. While it is beyond the scope of this work to provide an exhaustive review of novel AKI biomarkers, several are worth mentioning: cystatin C, neutrophil gelatinase-associated lipocalin (NGAL), kidney injury molecule-1 (KIM-1), interleukin-18 (IL-18), and liver-type fatty acid binding protein (L-FABP). With the exception of cystatin C which, like creatinine, is a marker of GFR, these biomarkers have provided unique mechanistic insights into the pathophysiology of AKI in the areas of iron metabolism (NGAL), inflammation (IL-18), oxidative stress (L-FABP), and efferocytosis (KIM-1) [46, 47]. Each of these four biomarkers initially demonstrated great promise for early diagnosis of AKI, but none has demonstrated the predictive power to justify widespread clinical use [48, 49].

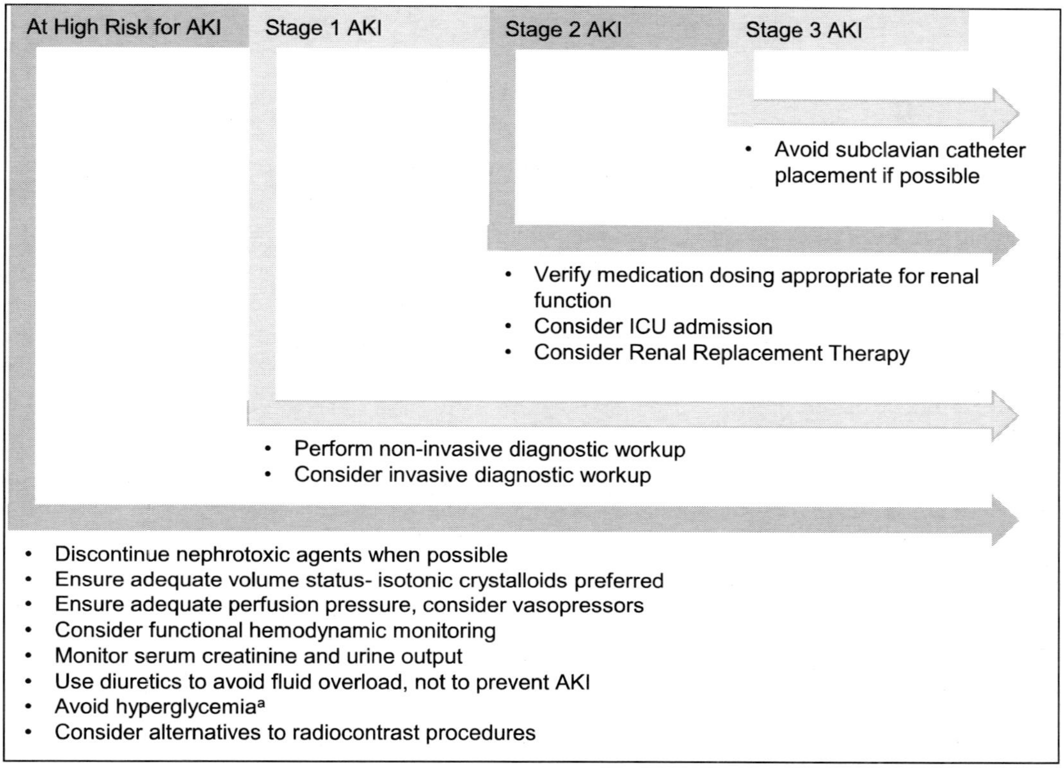

Figure 1. KDIGO Recommendations for Stage-based Management of Acute Kidney Injury. Suggested interventions are shown by stage, and interventions for lower stages are also generally applicable for higher stages. The KDIGO guideline suggests [a]using insulin therapy to target plasma glucose 110 – 149 mg/dL (6.1 – 8.3 mmol/L) and [b]administering 0.8 -1 g/kg/day of protein in noncatabolic AKI patients without the need for dialysis, 1.0 – 1.5 g/kg/day in patients with AKI on RRT, and up to 1.7 g/kg/day in patients on continuous RRT and in hypercatabolic patients. Adapted from reference 5.

Despite the disappointing performance of the aforementioned novel AKI biomarkers, there is reason to believe that two novel biomarkers of cell cycle arrest, TIMP-2 and IGFBP7, will be adopted in clinical practice. These biomarkers were identified in the two-stage, multicenter Sapphire study, which evaluated 340 candidate AKI biomarkers in over 1,200 critically ill adults [39]. Individually, TIMP-2 and IGFBP-7 outperformed NGAL, KIM-1, IL-18, L-FABP, and Cystatin C in head-to-head analysis for prediction of KDIGO Stage 2 or 3 AKI [39]. The accuracy was even higher when the biomarkers were used in combination. TIMP-2 and IGFBP7 have now been investigated in several studies, and a recent meta-analysis found that TIMP-2*IGFBP7 is a strong predictor for early diagnosis of AKI in adults (AUC = 0.85 by summary ROC curve analysis). Clinical testing for TIMP-2*IGFBP7 is now available through the NephroCheck assay [50]. More recently, the Prevention of Cardiac Surgery Associated-AKI (PREV-AKI) study has demonstrated the clinical utility of TIMP-2*IGFBP7 in early diagnosis of AKI. This study found that early initiation of the KDIGO AKI bundle using TIMP-2*IGFBP7 reduced the incidence of AKI after cardiac surgery by almost 25% and decreased the rate of severe AKI by one-third [51]. This study also demonstrates the utility of early diagnosis of AKI and timely implementation of best practices.

Renal Replacement Therapy

Renal replacement therapy *(RRT)* is a mainstay of AKI management that encompasses a broad range of modalities, a detailed analysis of which is beyond the scope of this chapter. Generally, renal replacement therapy modalities can be divided based on duration (intermittent vs. continuous) and the method of clearance (hemodialysis vs. hemofiltration vs. hemodiafiltration). In general, continuous renal replacement therapy *(CRRT)* is used for patients who are more hemodynamically unstable and require slower fluid removal. Both continuous and intermittent renal replacement therapy require anticoagulation, either systemically with heparin (or less commonly, another anticoagulant such as a direct thrombin inhibitor) or regionally with citrate. In the latter case, citrate is infused into the CRRT circuit at the arterial port of the dialysis catheter, where it functions as an anticoagulant by chelating calcium, while a calcium drip is infused at the venous return port in order to maintain the patient's ionized calcium within physiologic parameters [52]. Citrate is recommended over heparin due to a lower risk of hemorrhage. Importantly, it is metabolized by the liver and can bioaccumulate in patients with liver disease, leading to citrate accumulation and life threatening citrate toxicity [5, 52]. Most clinical trials have shown that early initiation of renal replacement therapy does not provide a mortality benefit for patients with AKI, but it may actually increase the risk of non-recovery of renal function [53–56]. Therefore, RRT is typically reserved for patients with AKI who have failed medical management.

Conclusion

AKI is a clinical syndrome that is a major driver of poor acute and long-term outcomes, including mortality among hospitalized patients. The clinical definition and staging of AKI relies upon changes in serum creatinine and urine output, which are reflections of renal function. Although many different types of insults can result in AKI, each with unique aspects to its pathogenesis and pathophysiology, AKI is often multifactorial. AKI is associated with a number of acute complications, including fluid overload, as well as electrolyte derangements, such as hyperkalemia, and metabolic disturbances, including metabolic acidosis and uremia. Diuretics are useful for preventing and treating fluid overload. Electrolyte and metabolic disturbances can often be medically managed. In severe cases, renal replacement therapy can provide metabolic support and fluid removal; it also serves as a bridge to recovery of renal function. However, the mortality rate associated with AKI remains unacceptably high. AKI survivors remain at risk of long-term sequelae, including chronic kidney disease and cardiovascular disease. Early initiation of RRT does not appear to provide a mortality benefit and could impair recovery of renal function. Therefore, much of the clinical management of AKI consists of measures to prevent causing or exacerbating renal injury, such as avoiding nephrotoxin exposure and hyperglycemia, as well as optimization of factors that maximize the chances of renal recovery, such as improving renal perfusion and provision of adequate nutrition. While AKI outcomes have improved in recent years, there remains much room for improvement in terms of both short-term outcomes such as in-hospital mortality and long-term outcomes such as the development of chronic kidney disease.

REFERENCES

[1] Marketos SG, Eftychiadis AG, Diamandopoulos A. Acute renal failure according to ancient Greek and Byzantine medical writers. *J R Soc Med.* 1993;86(5):290–3.

[2] Morgan DJR, Ho KM. A comparison of nonoliguric and oliguric severe acute kidney injury according to the risk injury failure loss end-stage (RIFLE) criteria. *Nephron Clin Pract.* 2010;115(1):c59-65.

[3] Bellomo R, Ronco C, Kellum JA, Mehta RL, Palevsky P. Acute renal failure - definition, outcome measures, animal models, fluid therapy and information technology needs: the Second International Consensus Conference of the Acute Dialysis Quality Initiative (ADQI) Group. *Crit Care.* 2004;8(4):R204-212.

[4] Mehta RL, Kellum JA, Shah SV, Molitoris BA, Ronco C, Warnock DG, et al. Acute Kidney Injury Network: report of an initiative to improve outcomes in acute kidney injury. *Crit Care.* 2007;11(2):R31.

[5] KDIGO AKI Work Group. KDIGO clinical practice guideline for acute kidney injury. *Kidney International Supplements.* 2012;(17):1–138.

[6] Waikar SS, Curhan GC, Wald R, McCarthy EP, Chertow GM. Declining mortality in patients with acute renal failure, 1988 to 2002. *J Am Soc Nephrol.* 2006;17(4):1143–50.

[7] Susantitaphong P, Cruz DN, Cerda J, Abulfaraj M, Alqahtani F, Koulouridis I, et al. World incidence of AKI: a meta-analysis. *Clin J Am Soc Nephrol.* 2013;8(9):1482–93.

[8] Hoste EAJ, Kellum JA, Selby NM, Zarbock A, Palevsky PM, Bagshaw SM, et al. Global epidemiology and outcomes of acute kidney injury. *Nat Rev Nephrol.* 2018;14(10):607–25.

[9] Mesropian PD, Othersen J, Mason D, Wang J, Asif A, Mathew RO. Community-acquired acute kidney injury: A challenge and opportunity for primary care in kidney health. *Nephrology (Carlton).* 2016;21(9):729–35.

[10] Hoste EAJ, Bagshaw SM, Bellomo R, Cely CM, Colman R, Cruz DN, et al. Epidemiology of acute kidney injury in critically ill patients: the multinational AKI-EPI study. *Intensive Care Med.* 2015;41(8):1411–23.

[11] Chertow GM, Burdick E, Honour M, Bonventre JV, Bates DW. Acute kidney injury, mortality, length of stay, and costs in hospitalized patients. *J Am Soc Nephrol.* 2005;16(11):3365–70.

[12] Lafrance J-P, Miller DR. Acute kidney injury associates with increased long-term mortality. *J Am Soc Nephrol.* 2010;21(2):345–52.

[13] Silver SA, Chertow GM. The Economic Consequences of Acute Kidney Injury. *Nephron.* 2017;137(4):297–301.

[14] Venkatachalam MA, Griffin KA, Lan R, Geng H, Saikumar P, Bidani AK. Acute kidney injury: a springboard for progression in chronic kidney disease. *Am J Physiol Renal Physiol.* 2010;298(5):F1078-1094.

[15] Oeyen S, De Corte W, Benoit D, Annemans L, Dhondt A, Vanholder R, et al. Long-term quality of life in critically ill patients with acute kidney injury treated with renal replacement therapy: a matched cohort study. *Crit Care.* 2015;19(1):289.

[16] Odutayo A, Wong CX, Farkouh M, Altman DG, Hopewell S, Emdin CA, et al. AKI and Long-Term Risk for Cardiovascular Events and Mortality. *J Am Soc Nephrol.* 2017;28(1):377–87.

[17] Maas RJ, Deegens JK, Beukhof JR, Reichert LJ, Ten Dam MA, Beutler JJ, et al. The Clinical Course of Minimal Change Nephrotic Syndrome With Onset in Adulthood or Late Adolescence: A Case Series. *Am J Kidney Dis.* 2017;69(5):637–46.

[18] Pascual J, Liaño F, Ortuño J. The elderly patient with acute renal failure. *J Am Soc Nephrol.* 1995;6(2):144–53.

[19] Naesens M, Kuypers DRJ, Sarwal M. Calcineurin inhibitor nephrotoxicity. *Clin J Am Soc Nephrol.* 2009;4(2):481–508.

[20] Thadhani R, Pascual M, Bonventre JV. Acute renal failure. *N Engl J Med.* 1996;334(22):1448–60.

[21] Pépin M-N, Bouchard J, Legault L, Ethier J. Diagnostic performance of fractional excretion of urea and fractional excretion of sodium in the evaluations of patients with acute kidney injury with or without diuretic treatment. *Am J Kidney Dis.* 2007;50(4):566–73.

[22] Lucarelli G, Ditonno P, Bettocchi C, Grandaliano G, Gesualdo L, Selvaggi FP, et al. Delayed relief of ureteral obstruction is implicated in the long-term development of renal damage and arterial hypertension in patients with unilateral ureteral injury. *J Urol.* 2013;189(3):960–5.

[23] Fernandez-Juarez G, Perez JV, Caravaca-Fontán F, Quintana L, Shabaka A, Rodriguez E, et al. Duration of Treatment with Corticosteroids and Recovery of Kidney Function in Acute Interstitial Nephritis. *Clin J Am Soc Nephrol.* 2018;13(12):1851–8.

[24] Bartholomew BA, Harjai KJ, Dukkipati S, Boura JA, Yerkey MW, Glazier S, et al. Impact of nephropathy after percutaneous coronary intervention and a method for risk stratification. *Am J Cardiol.* 2004;93(12):1515–9.

[25] Mehran R, Aymong ED, Nikolsky E, Lasic Z, Iakovou I, Fahy M, et al. A simple risk score for prediction of contrast-induced nephropathy after percutaneous coronary intervention: development and initial validation. *J Am Coll Cardiol.* 2004;44(7):1393–9.

[26] Weisbord SD, Gallagher M, Jneid H, Garcia S, Cass A, Thwin S-S, et al. Outcomes after Angiography with Sodium Bicarbonate and Acetylcysteine. *N Engl J Med.* 2018;378(7):603–14.

[27] Hu J, Chen R, Liu S, Yu X, Zou J, Ding X. Global Incidence and Outcomes of Adult Patients With Acute Kidney Injury After Cardiac Surgery: A Systematic Review and Meta-Analysis. *J Cardiothorac Vasc Anesth.* 2016;30(1):82–9.

[28] Vandenberghe W, Gevaert S, Kellum JA, Bagshaw SM, Peperstraete H, Herck I, et al. Acute Kidney Injury in Cardiorenal Syndrome Type 1 Patients: A Systematic Review and Meta-Analysis. *Cardiorenal Med.* 2016;6(2):116–28.

[29] Rosner MH, Okusa MD. Acute kidney injury associated with cardiac surgery. *Clin J Am Soc Nephrol.* 2006;1(1):19–32.

[30] Rangaswami J, Bhalla V, Blair JEA, Chang TI, Costa S, Lentine KL, et al. Cardiorenal Syndrome: Classification, Pathophysiology, Diagnosis, and Treatment Strategies: A Scientific Statement From the American Heart Association. *Circulation.* 2019;139(16):e840–78.

[31] Agrawal A, Naranjo M, Kanjanahattakij N, Rangaswami J, Gupta S. Cardiorenal syndrome in heart failure with preserved ejection fraction-an under-recognized clinical entity. *Heart Fail Rev.* 2019;24(4):421–37.

[32] Soranno DE, Kirkbride-Romeo L, Wennersten SA, Ding K, Cavasin MA, Baker P, et al. Acute Kidney Injury Results in Long-Term Diastolic Dysfunction That Is Prevented by Histone Deacetylase Inhibition. *JACC Basic Transl Sci.* 2021;6(2):119–33.

[33] Velez JCQ, Therapondos G, Juncos LA. Reappraising the spectrum of AKI and hepatorenal syndrome in patients with cirrhosis. *Nat Rev Nephrol.* 2020; 16(3):137–55.

[34] Angeli P, Ginès P, Wong F, Bernardi M, Boyer TD, Gerbes A, et al. Diagnosis and management of acute kidney injury in patients with cirrhosis: revised consensus recommendations of the International Club of Ascites. *J Hepatol.* 2015;62(4):968–74.

[35] EASL Clinical Practice Guidelines for the management of patients with decompensated cirrhosis. *J Hepatol.* 2018;69(2):406–60.

[36] Sutton TA, Fisher CJ, Molitoris BA. Microvascular endothelial injury and dysfunction during ischemic acute renal failure. *Kidney Int.* 2002;62(5):1539–49.

[37] Devarajan P. Update on mechanisms of ischemic acute kidney injury. *J Am Soc Nephrol.* 2006;17(6):1503–20.

[38] Bussolati B, Bruno S, Grange C, Buttiglieri S, Deregibus MC, Cantino D, et al. Isolation of renal progenitor cells from adult human kidney. *Am J Pathol.* 2005;166(2):545–55.

[39] Kashani K, Al-Khafaji A, Ardiles T, Artigas A, Bagshaw SM, Bell M, et al. Discovery and validation of cell cycle arrest biomarkers in human acute kidney injury. *Crit Care.* 2013;17(1):R25.

[40] Yang L, Besschetnova TY, Brooks CR, Shah JV, Bonventre JV. Epithelial cell cycle arrest in G2/M mediates kidney fibrosis after injury. *Nat Med.* 2010;16(5):535–43, 1p following 143.

[41] Jiang M, Bai M, Lei J, Xie Y, Xu S, Jia Z, et al. Mitochondrial dysfunction and the AKI-to-CKD transition. *Am J Physiol Renal Physiol.* 2020;319(6):F1105–16.

[42] Tang C, Cai J, Yin X-M, Weinberg JM, Venkatachalam MA, Dong Z. Mitochondrial quality control in kidney injury and repair. *Nat Rev Nephrol.* 2020;

[43] Black LM, Lever JM, Agarwal A. Renal Inflammation and Fibrosis: A Double-edged Sword. *J Histochem Cytochem.* 2019;67(9):663–81.

[44] Jang HR, Rabb H. Immune cells in experimental acute kidney injury. *Nat Rev Nephrol.* 2015;11(2):88–101.

[45] Murray PT, Devarajan P, Levey AS, Eckardt KU, Bonventre JV, Lombardi R, et al. A framework and key research questions in AKI diagnosis and staging in different environments. *Clin J Am Soc Nephrol.* 2008;3(3):864–8.

[46] Charlton JR, Portilla D, Okusa MD. A basic science view of acute kidney injury biomarkers. Nephrol Dial Transplant. 2014;29(7):1301–11.

[47] Alge JL, Arthur JM. Biomarkers of AKI: a review of mechanistic relevance and potential therapeutic implications. *Clin J Am Soc Nephrol.* 2015;10(1):147–55.

[48] Parikh CR, Devarajan P, Zappitelli M, Sint K, Thiessen-Philbrook H, Li S, et al. Postoperative biomarkers predict acute kidney injury and poor outcomes after pediatric cardiac surgery. *J Am Soc Nephrol.* 2011;22(9):1737–47.

[49] Parikh CR, Thiessen-Philbrook H, Garg AX, Kadiyala D, Shlipak MG, Koyner JL, et al. Performance of kidney injury molecule-1 and liver fatty acid-binding protein and combined biomarkers of AKI after cardiac surgery. *Clin J Am Soc Nephrol.* 2013;8(7):1079–88.

[50] Jia H-M, Huang L-F, Zheng Y, Li W-X. Diagnostic value of urinary tissue inhibitor of metalloproteinase-2 and insulin-like growth factor binding protein 7 for acute kidney injury: a meta-analysis. *Crit Care.* 2017;21(1):77.

[51] Meersch M, Schmidt C, Hoffmeier A, Van Aken H, Wempe C, Gerss J, et al. Prevention of cardiac surgery-associated AKI by implementing the KDIGO guidelines in high risk patients identified by biomarkers: the PrevAKI randomized controlled trial. *Intensive Care Med.* 2017;43(11):1551–61.

[52] Davenport A, Tolwani A. Citrate anticoagulation for continuous renal replacement therapy (CRRT) in patients with acute kidney injury admitted to the intensive care unit. *NDT Plus.* 2009;2(6):439–47.

[53] Bagshaw SM, Wald R, Adhikari NKJ, Bellomo R, da Costa BR, Dreyfuss D, et al. Timing of Initiation of Renal-Replacement Therapy in Acute Kidney Injury. *N Engl J Med.* 2020;383(3):240–51.

[54] Barbar SD, Clere-Jehl R, Bourredjem A, Hernu R, Montini F, Bruyère R, et al. Timing of Renal-Replacement Therapy in Patients with Acute Kidney Injury and Sepsis. *N Engl J Med.* 2018;379(15):1431–42.

[55] Gaudry S, Hajage D, Schortgen F, Martin-Lefevre L, Pons B, Boulet E, et al. Initiation Strategies for Renal-Replacement Therapy in the Intensive Care Unit. *N Engl J Med.* 2016;375(2):122–33.

[56] Zarbock A, Kellum JA, Schmidt C, Van Aken H, Wempe C, Pavenstädt H, et al. Effect of Early vs Delayed Initiation of Renal Replacement Therapy on Mortality in Critically Ill Patients With Acute Kidney Injury: The ELAIN Randomized Clinical Trial. *JAMA.* 2016;315(20):2190–9.

In: Issues in Kidney Disease – Acute Kidney Injury
Editors: S. Z. Fadem and A. Arslan Yousuf Awan

ISBN: 978-1-68507-002-1

Chapter 2

Approach to the Diagnosis of Acute Kidney Injury

Vishnu Parvathareddy*[1]*, MD and Jenny S. Pan*[1,2,*]*, MD

[1]Selzman Institute for Kidney Health, Section of Nephrology,
Department of Medicine, Baylor College of Medicine, Houston, TX, USA
[2]Michael E. DeBakey VA Medical Center, Houston, TX, USA

Abstract

Acute kidney injury (AKI) is a common clinical complication in patients admitted to the hospital. AKI is not a single disease, but a heterogeneous collection of clinical syndromes characterized by the sudden loss of kidney function measured by a rapid increase in serum creatinine, decrease in urine output or both. The diverse etiologies of AKI include volume depletion, sepsis, cardiorenal syndrome, a multitude of medications, urinary tract obstruction and more. The condition is associated with serious sequelae, including increased mortality and irreversible loss of kidney function. Thus, early recognition of AKI and timely diagnosis of the underlying etiology are critical for guiding therapy and improving outcomes. In this chapter, we discuss several classification systems and diagnostic frameworks that can aid in the timely diagnosis of AKI and identification of the underlying cause(s). The traditional anatomic (pre-, intrinsic-, post-renal) framework, and the new functional versus injury framework provide systematic approaches to the evaluation of a patient with AKI. Careful review of the patient's history, physical examination, select laboratory tests, imaging of the urinary tract, and microscopic examination of the urine are key in the diagnostic evaluation of AKI. Recent advances, including the discovery of novel AKI biomarkers, show promise in improving the diagnostic approach to and management of patients with AKI.

Keywords: acute kidney injury, nomenclature and staging, etiologies, diagnostic framework, cystatin C, biomarkers

[*] Corresponding Author's E-mail: jenny.pan@bcm.edu.

Introduction

Acute kidney injury (AKI) is a heterogeneous disorder defined by the sudden loss of kidney function measured by a rapid increase in serum creatinine, decrease in urine output or both. AKI is a global public health problem that continues to be a significant cause of morbidity, mortality and increasing healthcare costs [1, 2]. It is a frequent clinical complication in patients admitted to the hospital, which occurs in 10 to 15% of all hospitalizations, and up to 50% of patients in the intensive care unit [3]. Even relatively small changes in kidney function are associated with adverse outcomes in hospitalized patients, including increased mortality [4]. Furthermore, recent studies indicate that AKI is associated with serious sequelae, including irreversible loss of kidney function, accelerated progression to end-stage kidney disease (ESKD), and cardiac dysfunction via organ-to-organ crosstalk [5, 6]. Thus, early recognition of AKI and timely diagnosis of the underlying etiology are critical for guiding therapy and improving outcomes.

In recent years, there have been changing paradigms in AKI, including use of the term "acute kidney injury (AKI)" instead of "acute tubular necrosis (ATN)" or "acute renal failure (ARF)." Advances have been made in understanding the mechanisms and pathways of AKI, and new concepts encompassing many aspects of AKI from diagnosis to treatment and outcome have evolved. In this chapter, we provide a review of 1) the development of a consensus diagnostic criteria and staging nomenclature for AKI; 2) different clinical frameworks that can be used to systematically approach diagnosis of AKI etiologies; and 3) recent advances in AKI diagnosis and prognostication including novel biomarkers.

Diagnostic Criteria and Nomenclature for Staging

A survey published in 2002 found more than 35 separate definitions of AKI or ARF in the literature [7]. The absence of a common definition of AKI resulted in wide variation in reported incidence and clinical significance, which made assessments of new interventions for AKI difficult to interpret. Several AKI expert panels proposed that consensus for a well-defined diagnostic criteria and severity classification was mandatory for the advancement of clinical research in the prevention and treatment of AKI. In 2004, the Acute Dialysis Quality Initiative (ADQI) group of experts developed a landmark consensus definition of AKI in adults. The RIFLE criteria classified patients with kidney dysfunction according to the degree of impairment – patients at risk (R), with injury (I), with failure (F), with sustained loss (L) and with end-stage kidney disease (E) [8]. In recent years, additional standardized AKI diagnostic criteria have been developed and validated including the Acute Kidney Injury Network (AKIN) criteria [9], and a modified RIFLE criteria for pediatric patients (pRIFLE) [10]. In 2012, the Kidney Disease Improving Global Outcomes (KDIGO) AKI consensus work group merged the RIFLE and AKIN criteria to provide a single definition of AKI for use in practice, research, and public health [11]. The different diagnostic systems all use increasing relative or absolute changes in serum creatinine concentration and increasing duration of oliguria in their staging classification.

Table 1. KDIGO definition and staging of AKI

Stage	Serum creatinine	Urine output
1	1.5-1.9 times baseline or ≥0.3 mg/dL increase in 48h	<0.5 ml/kg/h for 6-12 hrs
2	2-2.9 times baseline	<0.5 ml/kg/h for ≥ 12 hrs
3	≥3 times baseline or ≥4.0 mg/dL or initiation of renal replacement therapy	<0.3 ml/kg/h for ≥ 24 hrs or anuria for ≥ 12 hrs

Currently, the KDIGO AKI criteria (Table 1) is considered the standard diagnostic system; each component has been validated in both the pediatric and adult patient populations. When applying the KDIGO AKI definition and staging for clinical diagnosis and management, the initial diagnosis of AKI is based on a patient meeting any of the criteria for stage 1. Once a diagnosis of AKI has been made, the next step is to stage it. Staging determines the maximum severity of AKI and is carried out retrospectively at the end of the episode. Patients should be staged according to the criteria (serum creatinine rise or urine output) that give them the highest stage [11, 12]. Staging of AKI is important because it conveys prognostic information; with increasing stage of AKI, the risk of death and need for kidney replacement therapy (KRT) increases [13, 14].

FRAMEWORKS FOR DIAGNOSIS OF AKI ETIOLOGIES

AKI is not a single disease, but rather a loose collection of clinical syndromes with diverse etiologies. Determining the underlying cause of AKI is essential for management, but can be difficult as there are frequently multifactorial mechanisms. Traditionally, AKI is seen as a single disease and classified according to semi-anatomical categories (e.g., pre-renal, intrinsic renal, and post-renal). Recent evidence has shown that an anatomic classification of AKI is insufficient as differing etiologies lead to distinctive phenotypes with unique pathophysiological mechanisms, which require specific treatments and confer different outcomes. For example, pre-renal AKI encompasses a collection of syndromes as diverse as renal hypoperfusion from hypovolemia, cardiorenal syndrome, intra-abdominal hypertension, and drug-induced intrarenal vasoconstriction. The simplistic classification of all these syndromes as "pre-renal AKI," which is often equated with "hypovolemia" can lead to indiscriminate fluid administration when in fact, careful assessment of the patient's hemodynamic status and fluid balance is critical in the management of these conditions. Thus, emerging AKI classification systems attempt to reflect the underlying disease etiology and pathophysiology in order to better inform our therapeutic approach. Below, we discuss different frameworks for identifying and classifying the causes of AKI, including the traditional anatomic approach, classification of AKI syndromes based on functional and injury criteria, and classification according to the dominant etiology [3, 15].

ANATOMIC FRAMEWORK: PRE-, INTRINSIC-, AND POST-RENAL

The traditional diagnostic framework classifies AKI into three categories based on the primary kidney site affected: pre-renal, intrinsic renal, and post-renal. Although this classification does not reflect the complexity of AKI and unique pathophysiology of the different etiologies, it does provide a useful systematic approach to narrow the differential diagnosis of the underlying cause. Evaluation of AKI includes careful review of the patient's history, physical examination, select serum and urine chemistries, and imaging of the urinary tract. Urine microscopic examination is one of the most important noninvasive tests in the diagnostic evaluation of AKI to guide the differential diagnosis and direct further work-up (Figure 1). Management should be tailored to the underlying etiology once identified.

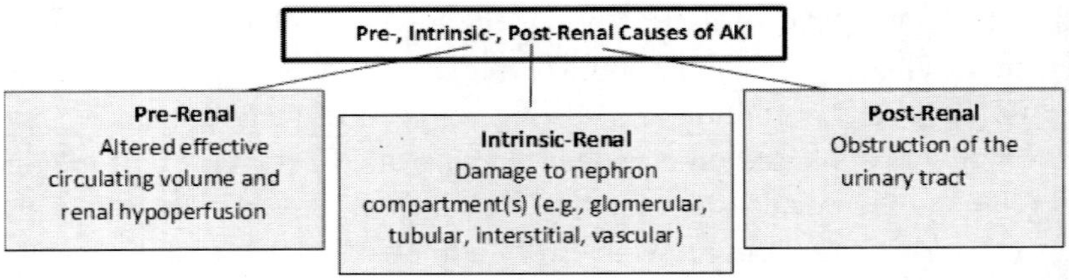

Etiology	Evaluation		
	History/Physical Exam	**Diagnostic Tests**	**Urine Sediment**
Pre-Renal • Volume loss • Cardiorenal syndrome • Hepatorenal syndrome • Intra-abdominal hypertension/Abdominal compartment syndrome • Nephrotic syndrome w/hypoalbuminemia • Drugs (e.g., ACE-I, ARB, NSAIDs, CNI)	• Renal volume loss: diuretics; osmotic diuresis • Extrarenal volume loss: GI loss; blood loss; burns • Heart failure • Cirrhosis • Abdominal surgery • Hypotension	• BUN/Cr > 20:1 • UNa < 20 mEq/L • FENa < 1% • FEUN < 35% • FEUA < 10% • Intra-abdominal pressure > 12 mmHg or abdominal perfusion pressure < 60 mmHg (IAH)	• Bland • Few squamous epithelial cells • Hyaline casts
Intrinsic-Renal: Glomerular • *Rapidly Progressive GN* – ANCA-associated GN – IgA nephropathy – Post infectious GN – Lupus nephritis – Anti-GBM GN • *Nephrotic Syndrome* – Minimal change disease – Membranous nephropathy	• *RPGN* – Hematuria – Rash – Hemoptysis • *Nephrotic syndrome* – Anasarca – Foamy urine • Glomerular disease specific	• Serologic tests for specific glomerular disease • Thrombo-embolic complications on imaging • Kidney biopsy	• *RPGN*: Hematuria; dysmorphic RBC; RBC casts • *Nephrotic syndrome*: Lipid droplet; granular casts
Intrinsic-Renal: Tubular • Sepsis • Ischemic: prolonged hypotension; procedure-related ischemia-reperfusion • Nephrotoxin exposure (e.g., sulfonamides, acyclovir, myoglobin, uric acid, CNI)	• Infections • Recent surgery • Hypotension • Exposure to nephrotoxic agent(s)	• FENa > 2% • FEUN > 50% • FEUN > 20% • Elevated CK • UA with (+) blood, no RBC • Elevated serum and urine uric acid	• Renal tubular epithelial cells or casts • Muddy brown, granular casts
Intrinsic-Renal: Interstitial • Drugs (e.g., penicillin, cephalosporin, NSAIDs, PPI, allopurinol) • Infections • Systemic disease – Sarcoidosis – Lupus	• Medication history • Fever, rash, eosinophilia (10% of patients) 7-10 days after drug exposure • Infections (viral, fungal)	• Eosinophilia • (+) urine eosinophils • FENa > 1% • Large kidneys on USG • Kidney biopsy	• WBCs, eosinophils • WBC casts

Figure 1. (Continued).

Etiology	Evaluation		
	History/Physical Exam	**Diagnostic Tests**	**Urine Sediment**
Intrinsic-Renal: Vascular • Renal vein compression or thrombosis • Renal artery stenosis/thrombosis/ • dissection • Renal atheroembolic disease • *Microvascular causes*: TMA, TTP/HUS	• Flank pain • Nephrotic syndrome • Vessel catheterization or vascular surgery • Abdominal bruit • Livedo reticularis	• Diagnostic imaging • Eosinophilia, elevated ESR, low serum complement (atheroembolic disease) • Schistocytes, ↑LDH, ↓haptoglobin	• Bland or RBCs • WBCs, eosinophils (athero-embolic disease)
Post-Renal • *Extrarenal* – Prostate hypertrophy – Neurogenic bladder – Retroperitoneal fibrosis or adenopathy – Bladder mass • *Intrarenal* – Kidney stones – Blood clots – Crystals	• Urinary retention or hesitancy • Bladder distension • Pelvic mass • Large prostate • Cancer history (cervical, prostate, bladder) • Hematuria • Passing stone	• Hydro-nephrosis on USG – Develops ~3 days after obstruction – May not see with retro-peritoneal fibrosis • Hyperkalemia and/or metabolic acidosis	• Bland or RBCs (extrarenal) • Crystals (intrarenal)

ACE-I, angiotensin-converting-enzyme inhibitor; ARB, angiotensin II receptor blocker; CNI, calcineurin inhibitor; NSAIDs, non-steroidal anti-inflammatory drugs; PPI, proton pump inhibitor; BUN, blood urea nitrogen; Cr, creatinine; UNa, urine sodium; FENa, fractional excretion of sodium; FEUN, fractional excretion of urea nitrogen; FEUA, fractional excretion of uric acid; IAH, intra-abdominal hypertension; CK, creatine kinase; UA, urinalysis; RBC, red blood cells; WBC, white blood cells; TMA, thrombotic microangiopathy; TTP, thrombotic thrombocytopenic purpura; HUS, acute hemolytic uremic syndrome; USG, ultrasonogram.

Figure 1. Diagnostic Framework of AKI with pre-renal, intrinsic-renal or post-renal causes.

Pre-Renal AKI

The kidneys receive up to 25% of the cardiac output, and renal perfusion can be altered by any significant reduction in cardiac performance, dysfunction of the general circulation or isolated dysfunction of the intrarenal circulation (16). Pre-renal AKI, characterized by a decrease in glomerular filtration rate (GFR) due to a reduction in renal perfusion pressure without evidence of parenchymal damage, is the major cause of community-acquired AKI (17). Causes of decreased renal perfusion include hypovolemia (e.g., from vomiting or diarrhea, hemorrhage, burns, aggressive diuresis), "third spacing" due to significant hypoalbuminemia or capillary leak in severe pancreatitis, impaired cardiac output from congestive heart failure (cardiorenal syndrome), systemic vasodilation (e.g., from sepsis, anaphylaxis, vasodilator drugs), and renal vasoconstriction (e.g., from abdominal compartment syndrome, vasoconstrictive drugs). Renal hypoperfusion activates adaptive mechanisms, including autoregulation mechanisms and the renin-angiotensin-aldosterone system (RAAS), to concentrate urine maximally and avidly reabsorb sodium in order to increase intravascular volume and normalize renal perfusion. Thus, common laboratory findings in pre-renal AKI include low urinary sodium (<20 mEq/L) and fractional excretion of sodium <1%; in the setting of diuretic use when renal handling of sodium is altered, low fractional excretion of urea nitrogen and fractional excretion of uric acid may be useful for the diagnosis of pre-renal AKI (18). When the adaptive response is inadequate, GFR is initially decreased without kidney parenchymal injury; at this stage, urine microscopic examination reveals a bland urine sediment. Prompt institution of therapy aimed at rapidly restoring renal perfusion will improve kidney function. However, if adequate renal perfusion is not restored, organ damage can result from ischemic injury; in this case, urine microscopic examination reveals many renal tubular epithelial cells or muddy brown, granular casts consistent with tubular injury/necrosis.

Intrinsic Renal AKI

In the approach to intrinsic AKI, it is helpful to group the etiologies by the primary site of nephron pathology: glomeruli, tubules, interstitium or vasculature (Figure 1). The spectrum of clinical presentation that occurs with glomerular diseases varies from asymptomatic hematuria, to heavy proteinuria, to chronic kidney disease, to rapidly progressive glomerulonephritis (RPGN). AKI from acute glomerulonephritis (AGN) can be due to a primary kidney disease (such as primary membranoproliferative glomerulonephritis) or can manifest as part of a systemic disease. Careful review of the history and physical exam may reveal an underlying systemic illness, such as a prior throat or skin infection with post-infectious glomerulonephritis, hemoptysis and sinusitis with ANCA-associated glomerulonephritis, or a rash with lupus nephritis. AGN is typically characterized by new-onset or accelerating hypertension and edema. Urinalysis shows an active sediment with abnormal proteinuria (typically in the non-nephrotic range, <3.5 g/day) and hematuria; microscopic urine examination may reveal dysmorphic RBC and RBC casts. Another group of glomerular diseases, such as membranous nephropathy and minimal change disease, commonly cause AKI due to massive proteinuria and the related complications. These may include hypovolemia due to aggressive diuresis, acute renal vasoconstriction that leads to ischemic tubular injury, direct tubular toxicity from reabsorption of proteins filtered at the glomerulus [19], and thromboembolic events. Urine microscopic examination may reveal hyaline casts, lipid droplets, granular casts or red blood cells depending on the underlying complication. Specific serologic tests may be available to aid in diagnosis, including ANCA-antibodies, anti-nuclear antibody (ANA), anti-glomerular basement membrane (anti-GBM) antibody, and complements C3 and C4. The pattern of C3 and C4 levels can give a clue to the specific glomerular disease. Both complement C3 and C4 are low in lupus nephritis. However, C3 is decreased but C4 is normal in post-infectious glomerulonephritis and membranoproliferative glomerulonephritis because the alternative complement pathway is activated more so than the classical pathway. In AKI associated with glomerular diseases, kidney biopsy is often required for definitive diagnosis [20].

Intrinsic-renal causes of in-hospital AKI most commonly result in tubular damage. The most common pathophysiology include ischemic injury to the tubules (from prolonged hypotension in sepsis- or surgery-associated AKI), and exposure to exogenous or endogenous nephrotoxic agents (Table 2). In most cases, the etiology is multifactorial in nature. Again, a diagnosis of the underlying etiology can be made with thorough review of the patient's history (including medication use), physical examination, and select serum and urine chemistries. For example, history of recent trauma with muscle injury, and laboratory evaluation demonstrating elevated creatine kinase and urinalysis positive for blood but negative for red blood cells suggests a diagnosis of rhabdomyolysis. A combination of hyperkalemia, hyperphosphatemia, hypocalcemia, and hyperuricemia, is frequently seen in tumor lysis syndrome; urate crystals may also be present on microscopic examination of the urine [21]. Other common laboratory findings in intrinsic-renal AKI due to tubular injury include fractional excretion of sodium >2% or fractional excretion of urea nitrogen >50% due to impaired reabsorption by the damaged tubules. Microscopic urine examination may reveal many tubular epithelial cells and muddy brown, coarse granular casts.

Table 2. Common Nephrotoxic Agents: A through Z

Nephrotoxic Agent	Mechanism(s) of Kidney Injury
Acyclovir	AIN; Distal RTA
Allopurinol	AIN
Aminoglycosides	Tubular cell toxicity with Fanconi-like syndrome; Activation of CaSR in the TAL; Polyuria
Amphotericin B	ATN; Distal RTA
Bactrim	Inhibition of tubular secretion of creatinine; AIN; Crystal nephropathy; ATN
Calceneurin inhibitors (e.g., tacrolimus, cyclosporine)	Renal vasoconstriction; Thrombotic microangiopathy; Toxic tubulopathy
Cephalosporin	AIN
Check point inhibitors • CTLA-4 (e.g., pilimumab) • PD-1 (e.g., nivolumab)	AIN; ATN; Thrombotic microangiopathy; Glomerulopathies (e.g., membranous nephropathy, minimal change disease)
Cisplatin	ATN; CTIN
Colistin	ATN (due to increased permeability of the tubular epithelium and mitochondrial ROS); Rhabdomyolysis
Foscarnet	Crystal nephropathy; Electrolyte abnormalities (hypocalcemia, hypomagnesemia)
Gadolinium (rare)	ATN
HAART	Tenofovir, Cidofovir: PT damage (Fanconi syndrome) Indinavir: Crystal nephropathy
Interferon α	Proteinuria/Minimal change disease
Iodinated contrast	Vasoconstriction; ATN (non-ionic low osmolar agents are preferred)
Methotrexate	Crystal nephropathy
NSAIDS	Hemodynamic alteration; AIN; Minimal change disease
Penicillin	AIN
Phenytoin	AIN
PPI	AIN
Rifampin	AIN
Vancomycin	ATN; AIN

AIN, acute interstitial nephritis; CaSR, calcium sensing receptor; TAL, thick ascending limb; RTA, renal tubular acidosis; ATN, acute tubular necrosis; ROS, reactive oxygen species; CTIN, chronic tubulointerstitial nephritis; CTLA-4, IgG1 monoclonal antibody against cytotoxic T-lymphocyte antigen 4; PD-1, IgG4 monoclonal antibody against programmed cell death 1; PT, proximal tubule; HAART, highly active anti-retroviral therapy; PPI, proton pump inhibitors.

Drug-induced acute interstitial nephritis (AIN) is the most common cause of intrinsic-renal AKI related to interstitial pathology, accounting for >75% of biopsy-proven cases. The most frequent offending agents include penicillin, cephalosporins, other antibiotics, NSAIDs, proton pump inhibitors and allopurinol [22]. A diagnostic feature of AIN is large kidneys on ultrasound, as AIN is characterized by significant inflammatory infiltrates and edema within the interstitium. The drug-induced allergic-type reaction can also manifest with fever, a maculopapular skin rash, arthralgia, eosinophilia or eosinophiluria. The classic triad of maculopapular rash, fever and eosinophilia is seen in only a minority of patients (<10-15%) [23]; eosinophilia and eosinophiluria are even less common in NSAID-related AIN than in other types of drug-induced AIN. When present, these clinical manifestations typically occur 7-10 days after exposure to the offending drug. High clinical suspicion and thorough review of the patient's medication history are key to making a prompt diagnosis, identification and removal of the causative agent. Other cases of AIN are caused by infections (such as cytomegalovirus, Epstein-Barr virus, Leptospira) and systemic diseases (such as Sjogren syndrome, sarcoidosis, systemic lupus erythematosus, tubulointerstitial nephritis with uveitis).

Vascular causes of intrinsic-renal AKI can be divided into those that affect large vessels (renal artery obstruction from stenosis/thrombosis/dissection, renal vein thrombosis), and those that affect small vessels (thrombotic thrombocytopenic purpura (TTP), hemolytic uremic syndrome (HUS), and atherosclerotic or thrombotic emboli). Injury to extra-renal or intra-renal vessels decreases kidney perfusion and diminishes GFR. Vascular causes of AKI that affect large vessels may present with sudden-onset flank pain and hematuria, and usually require imaging to confirm the diagnosis. In TTP, HUS and other microvascular causes, laboratory data may reveal findings consistent with microangiopathic hemolytic anemia (presence of schistocytosis on peripheral blood smear, elevated LDH, and reduced haptoglobin). Atheroembolic disease should be suspected in patients with a recent history of arterial catheterization or vascular surgery, and eosinophilia, elevated ESR and low serum complement on laboratory finding.

Post-Renal AKI

Obstruction of the urinary tract causes a retrograde increase in tubular pressure, which in turn reduces GFR resulting in post-renal AKI. Extra-renal urinary tract obstruction can occur along the ureters (due to kidney stone, tumor, and retroperitoneal fibrosis), bladder (due to prostate enlargement, urologic/gynecologic tumors or neurogenic bladder), and urethra (due to strictures or phimosis in men). History that suggests post-renal AKI may include passing of a stone, prior pelvic surgery or radiation, and recent urinary catheterization. Common symptoms include gross hematuria and flank pain with kidney stone or papillary necrosis, urinary frequency and hesitancy with benign prostatic enlargement, and bladder fullness on exam. A bladder scan with high post-void residual can unmask partial obstruction. Post-renal AKI can also be caused by intra-tubular obstruction due to crystal nephropathy from medications like acyclovir and sulfonamide.

In post-renal AKI, a rise in serum creatinine may not be apparent if the obstruction is unilateral due to function of the contralateral normal kidney. However, if the obstruction is not relieved, progressive loss of GFR can result. Routine labs may also demonstrate a syndrome of hyperkalemic distal renal tubular acidosis with hyperkalemia and metabolic acidosis out-of-proportion to the reduction in GFR. This results from decreased sodium delivery to and absorption in the distal nephron, which leads to a defect in hydrogen and potassium secretion. Urine microscopic examination can be bland, or show red blood cells with extra-renal etiologies; with etiologies that cause intra-tubular obstruction, urine analysis may reveal crystals. Imaging of the urinary system may demonstrate hydroureter or hydronephrosis. However, with acute obstruction imaging may not show any abnormalities as hydronephrosis usually takes 2-3 days after the obstruction to develop. In addition, hydroureter and hydronephrosis are often not readily apparent in retroperitoneal fibrosis.

ALTERNATIVE FRAMEWORK: FUNCTIONAL AND INJURY CRITERIA

A new conceptual framework for classifying AKI proposes distinguishing between conditions that cause kidney dysfunction (those that reduce glomerular function), conditions that result in kidney parenchymal injury, or conditions that do both (Figure 2) [3]. Kidney function markers include serum creatinine, cystatin C, and direct measurement of GFR by use of exogenous filtration markers. Kidney injury markers include abnormalities on microscopic examination of the urine and novel biomarkers. An example of a condition that causes kidney dysfunction alone is volume depletion from diarrhea, which can reduce renal perfusion and GFR without injuring the kidney. In contrast, initial exposure to nephrotoxic drugs can lead to mild kidney injury without dysfunction. With AKI in these two categories, prompt implementation of mitigation or intervention strategies, such as volume optimization or removal of nephrotoxic drugs can lead to recovery. However, prolonged renal hypoperfusion or exposure to the nephrotoxic agent may result in the condition causing both kidney dysfunction and injury.

The functional and injury criteria framework is a useful tool that enables clinicians to diagnose and stratify patients across the clinical spectrum of AKI. During the initial evaluation, patients are classified into one of the four categories, which can guide differential diagnosis and management plan. Subsequently, sequential assessment of functional and injury markers can allow clinicians to track patient's transitions across the categories, providing information for modification of the management plan and prognostication. This framework is a novel approach to assessing patients with AKI for diagnosis and staging, identifying the underlying etiologies, and providing prognosis [24].

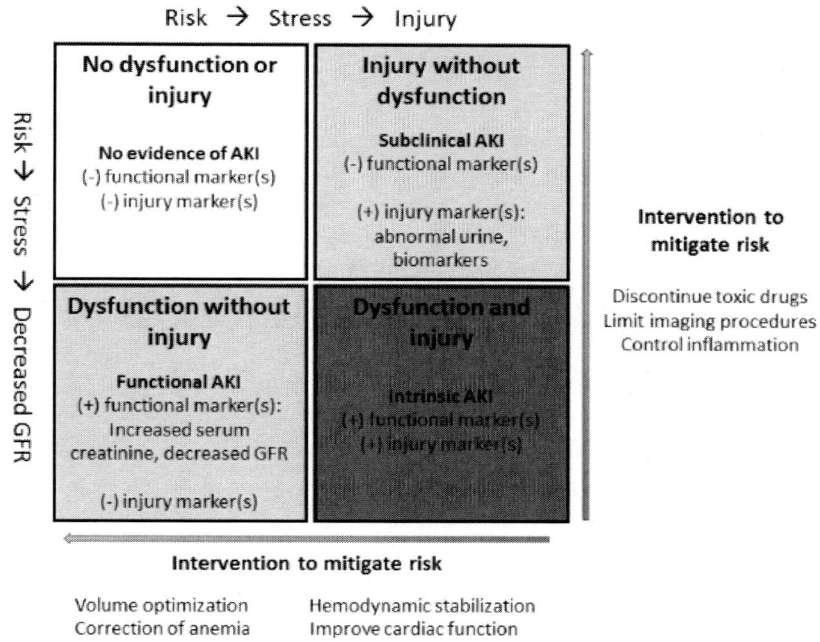

Figure 2. AKI Framework Based on Functional and Injury Criteria.

ALTERNATIVE FRAMEWORK: CLASSIFICATION ACCORDING TO DOMINANT ETIOLOGY

Given the wide range of etiologies and heterogeneous pathophysiological mechanisms, some authors have proposed approaching AKI according to the dominant etiology and usual clinical context rather than attempt to classify them into a few broad categories. As an example, surgery-associated AKI is a common cause of kidney injury in hospitalized patients. Multiple factors contribute to the development of perioperative AKI: hemodynamic alterations; activation of neurohormonal responses to hypotension and tissue injury (such as the sympathetic nervous system and the renin-angiotensin-aldosterone system); and upregulation of a systemic immune and inflammatory response [15]. Hemodynamic instability during surgery can result from blood and fluid losses, the vasodilatory properties of anesthetic agents, and poor cardiovascular reserve in patients with multiple comorbidities; this, then leads to altered renal perfusion (a pre-renal etiology) and kidney injury if prolonged. Tissue injury during surgery results in the generation of damage-associated molecular patterns (DAMPs), inflammatory mediators and reactive oxygen species, which trigger kidney endothelial and tubular cell stress and injury (an intrinsic-renal etiology). Furthermore, surgical patients are frequently exposed to potential nephrotoxic agents (e.g., antibiotics, contrast). Thus, a comprehensive approach to the prevention and treatment of surgery-associated AKI would need to include: appropriate management of intraoperative and perioperative hemodynamic changes and optimization of intravascular volume; control of inflammation; and proactive management of nephrotoxic drug use and dosing.

As discussed above, many drugs and diagnostic agents are associated with kidney injury or dysfunction (Table 2). These nephrotoxic agents are frequently used in the outpatient and hospital settings, and nephrotoxic AKI is a common cause of pre-renal and intrinsic-renal AKI. Some drugs affect kidney function through a systemic or renal/glomerular hemodynamic effect. For example, angiotensin-converting-enzyme inhibitors (ACE-I) cause efferent arteriole dilation while non-steroidal anti-inflammatory drugs (NSAIDs) reduce afferent arteriole dilation by inhibiting prostaglandin production [25]. Both can reduce renal perfusion pressure, which if sustained or severe can lead to ischemic kidney injury. Recent literature has shown that certain drug combinations, including the "triple whammy" of RAAS-inhibitors, diuretics and NSAIDs, are associated with increased AKI risk [26]. Other drugs cause kidney cell injury through mechanisms that include: 1) direct cytotoxic effects on renal tubular epithelial cells (e.g., cisplatin); 2) precipitation of crystals (e.g., acyclovir); or 3) triggering an allergic reaction (e.g., cephalosporin). Drug stewardship and proactive management of nephrotoxic drug use/dosing are key to preventing or mitigating drug-associated AKI. To achieve this, clinicians and patients need appropriate and effective education as to the potential for kidney injury and dysfunction from different nephrotoxic agents [26].

Another example of an etiology that can cause AKI due to several mechanisms, and thus does not fall under any one diagnostic category is the novel coronavirus SARS-CoV-2. Kidney involvement has been reported to be frequent in COVID-19, with >40% of patients demonstrating abnormal proteinuria at hospital admission [27]. According to recent studies, average incidence of AKI in all hospitalized patients with SARS-CoV-2 infection is 11% (range 8-17%), and approximately 25% (range 14-35%) in critically ill patients [28]. Multiple mechanisms have been proposed in the pathogenesis of AKI in COVID-19, including factors that impair kidney perfusion such as hypovolemia secondary to febrile illness and gastrointestinal fluid losses, hemodynamic instability from sepsis, and cardiorenal physiology from right ventricular failure secondary to COVID-19 pneumonia. In addition, autopsy data indicate that SARS-CoV-2 can directly infect the kidney endothelial cells, tubular epithelium, and podocytes leading to tubular damage or podocytopathy. Other potential mechanisms include imbalanced RAAS activation caused by SARS-CoV-2-mediated down-regulation of membrane-bound ACE2 that promotes angiotensin II accumulation, a cytokine release syndrome, and the microvascular thrombosis that has been observed in patients with COVID-19 [28]. Common laboratory abnormalities that have been reported include proteinuria (varying from mild to severe depending on the degree and site of damage from the virus), hematuria, leukocyturia and hypokalemia (due to increased kaliuresis or diarrhea). AKI appears to be a marker of COVID-19 infection severity and the mortality rate is higher for patients with kidney involvement. In the absence of SARS-CoV-2-specific treatment, early detection and a comprehensive approach to treatment aimed at hemodynamic support, avoidance of nephrotoxic agents, anticoagulation, control of inflammation, and prompt initiation of kidney replacement therapy may help improve clinical outcome.

Advances in AKI Diagnosis and Prognostication

Currently, clinical detection and diagnosis of AKI is based upon serum creatinine elevation or reduction in urine output. There are fundamental limitations with these measures. First, serum creatinine is an indirect marker for renal glomerular filtration. It lacks specificity for injury to kidney tissue, and does not distinguish between conditions that cause decline in GFR due to a reduction in renal perfusion via hemodynamic effects versus conditions that cause direct cytotoxic damage to kidney cells. Second, rise in serum creatinine and oliguria are relatively late responses to an acute decline in GFR and kidney injury. Due to the functional renal reserve, changes in serum creatinine and urine output do not occur until significant kidney function loss has occurred (~20-40% damage to healthy kidneys). This precludes early detection of AKI where mitigation strategies can still reverse or prevent further kidney injury [25]. Third, serum creatinine levels depend on factors other than urinary clearance, including the volume of distribution and rate of production of creatinine. Aggressive fluid administration and fluid overload alter the volume of distribution of serum creatinine and may result in lower concentrations, delaying recognition of AKI and underestimation of the severity [29]. Creatinine production is dependent on factors such as muscle mass, diet and physical activity, which are typically affected during hospitalization. In critically ill patients, significant muscle loss, fasting and bedrest may decrease creatinine production, leading to underdiagnoses of AKI.

An additional challenge in diagnosing AKI using rise in serum creatinine level as the foundational criteria is establishing baseline creatinine. Frequently, prior baseline, steady-state serum creatinine measurements are not available. Lack of an accurate baseline serum creatinine impedes AKI diagnosis, staging and prognostication. Recent advances have the potential to improve evaluation and management of patients with AKI. We will discuss two of these advances below, cystatin C and novel biomarkers. Other research tools being evaluated for clinical use include real-time GFR measurement, assessment of tubular reserve (furosemide stress test), and the use of information technology (IT) to develop algorithms for e-alert systems or AKI recognition and monitoring [3].

Cystatin C

Cystatin C, a small endogenous molecule produced by all human nucleated cells, is a relatively new filtration marker that has been suggested as an alternative or complement to serum creatinine. Cystatin C is filtered from the blood through the glomerulus and is cleared by reabsorption/catabolism by the proximal tubular cells and excretion in urine [30]. Properties that make Cystatin C a good biomarker of decreased kidney function include: 1) production and release into plasma at a relatively constant rate; 2) >99% filtration by glomeruli; and 3) no significant protein binding [31]. Furthermore, serum Cystatin C has been shown to be less affected by factors such as gender, muscle mass, and diet compare to serum creatinine. Recent studies found that serum Cystatin C performs comparably or superior to the diagnostic accuracy of serum creatinine in discriminating normal from impaired kidney function in patients at risk for or with CKD [31, 32]. The 2012 KDIGO guidelines for the evaluation and management of CKD incorporated use of Cystatin C based estimated GFR equations (e.g., CKD-EPI$_{cys}$ or CKD-EPI$_{creat\text{-}cys}$) in the CKD diagnostic criteria [33].

More recently, Cystatin C has been evaluated for the purpose of diagnosis, staging and prognostication in AKI. Studies utilizing serum Cystatin C for detection of AKI have shown mixed results. Although an earlier single-center study found that Cystatin C detected AKI 1-2 days earlier than creatinine in critically ill patients [34], a study from the multicenter TRIBE-AKI cohort demonstrated that Cystatin C was less sensitive for AKI detection [35]. However, the two filtration markers alone did not differ in their ability to predict dialysis or mortality outcomes, while combination of serum creatinine and Cystatin C provided better risk prediction for mortality and dialysis requirement [36]. Limitations of Cystatin C include high cost of the assay compared to serum creatinine measurement [30], and it cannot distinguish between conditions that cause kidney dysfunction and those that result in kidney parenchymal injury. Additional studies are required to inform clinical translation of serum Cystatin C in the evaluation and management of AKI.

Biomarkers

In the past decade, several novel biomarkers have been identified as potential candidates for the early detection of kidney injury before serum creatinine rises. Several have been evaluated in clinical trials, including kidney injury molecule-1 (KIM1), neutrophil gelatinase-associated lipocalin (NGAL), and liver-type fatty acid-binding protein (L-FABP) (25). Nephrocheck™, the first biomarker diagnostic test for AKI approved by the U.S. Food and Drug Administration, incorporates two markers of cell cycle arrest, urinary tissue inhibitor of metalloproteinases 2 (TIMP-2) and insulin-like growth factor binding protein 7 (IGFBP7). Studies have shown benefit associated with use of Nephrocheck™ in early detection of kidney injury in patients after surgery. Patients with a positive Nephrocheck™ received a care bundle that included early optimization of fluids and hemodynamics, and discontinuation of nephrotoxic drugs that led to decreased rates of moderate or severe AKI [37, 38]. In contrast to serum creatinine, the novel biomarkers may be able to distinguish between conditions that cause kidney dysfunction and those that result in kidney parenchymal injury. In 2013, the 10th Acute Dialysis Quality Initiative (ADQI 10) workgroup proposed incorporation of biomarkers into the "functional and injury/damage" framework for AKI classification (Figure 2), and a staging criteria for severity of AKI [24]. Kidney injury biomarkers may also provide insight into the location, severity and etiology of AKI, and additional research is needed in this area.

Clinical Pearls

- AKI is a global public health problem associated with serious sequelae, including mortality, accelerated progression to ESKD, and cardiac dysfunction via organ-to-organ crosstalk.
- AKI is not a single disease, but rather a heterogeneous disorder with diverse etiologies that presents with an abrupt increase in serum creatinine, decrease in urine output or both.
- Classification of AKI into three categories based on the primary kidney site affected (pre-renal, intrinsic renal, and post-renal) provides a useful systematic approach to diagnosis of the underlying cause (Figure 1).
- AKI classification based on anatomical categories is insufficient as it provides limited information on the pathophysiology to guide therapy; diagnostic frameworks based on functional and injury criteria (Figure 2) or the dominant etiology may be more useful.
- Microscopic examination of the urine is one of the most important noninvasive test in the diagnostic evaluation of AKI to guide the differential diagnosis and direct further work-up.
- In 2012, KDIGO proposed a unified diagnostic criteria and nomenclature for the staging of AKI based on changes in serum creatinine and duration of oliguria (Table 1).
- Advances in AKI diagnosis include Nephrocheck (TIMP-2 x IGFBP7), the first biomarker diagnostic test approved by the U.S. FDA. Other potential functional (e.g., Cystatin C) and injury (e.g., NGAL, KIM-1) novel biomarkers require additional research and validation prior to clinical use.

Conclusion

AKI is the leading reason for nephrology consultation and is associated with serious short- and long-term sequelae. It is a collection of syndromes defined by an abrupt increase in serum creatinine and/or fall in urine output that can be caused by a myriad of etiologies with different pathophysiology. Thus, rapid diagnosis and appropriate diagnostic evaluation to determine the underlying etiology is essential to guide timely institution of interventions that can prevent and/or reverse kidney injury. Recently, the field of AKI has undergone significant evolution in terms of definition and staging, understanding of pathophysiological mechanisms, and characterization of the disease across its full clinical spectrum. During the last few decades, KDIGO introduced standard diagnostic criteria for AKI; the ADQI workgroup proposed a new conceptual framework for diagnosis based on functional and injury biomarkers; and emerging causes of AKI including check point inhibitors and SARS-CoV-2 infection have been identified. Recent advances such as the discovery of novel AKI biomarkers and the use of health information technology for early detection show promise in improving the diagnostic approach to and management of patients with AKI.

REFERENCES

[1] Lameire NH, Bagga A, Cruz D, De Maeseneer J, Endre Z, Kellum JA, et al. Acute kidney injury: an increasing global concern. *Lancet*. 2013;382(9887):170-9.

[2] Rewa O, Bagshaw SM. Acute kidney injury-epidemiology, outcomes and economics. *Nat Rev Nephrol*. 2014;10(4):193-207.

[3] Ronco C, Bellomo R, Kellum JA. Acute kidney injury. *Lancet*. 2019;394(10212):1949-64.

[4] Chertow GM, Burdick E, Honour M, Bonventre JV, Bates DW. Acute kidney injury, mortality, length of stay, and costs in hospitalized patients. *J Am Soc Nephrol*. 2005;16 (11):3365-70.

[5] Coca SG, Singanamala S, Parikh CR. Chronic kidney disease after acute kidney injury: a systematic review and meta-analysis. *Kidney Int*. 2012;81(5):442-8.

[6] Fox BM, Gil HW, Kirkbride-Romeo L, Bagchi RA, Wennersten SA, Haefner KR, et al. Metabolomics assessment reveals oxidative stress and altered energy production in the heart after ischemic acute kidney injury in mice. *Kidney Int*. 2019;95(3):590-610.

[7] Kellum JA, Levin N, Bouman C, Lameire N. Developing a consensus classification system for acute renal failure. *Curr Opin Crit Care*. 2002;8(6):509-14.

[8] Bellomo R, Ronco C, Kellum JA, Mehta RL, Palevsky P, Acute Dialysis Quality Initiative w. Acute renal failure - definition, outcome measures, animal models, fluid therapy and information technology needs: the Second International Consensus Conference of the Acute Dialysis Quality Initiative (ADQI) Group. *Crit Care*. 2004; 8(4):R204-12.

[9] Mehta RL, Kellum JA, Shah SV, Molitoris BA, Ronco C, Warnock DG, et al. Acute Kidney Injury Network: report of an initiative to improve outcomes in acute kidney injury. *Crit Care*. 2007;11(2):R31.

[10] Akcan-Arikan A, Zappitelli M, Loftis LL, Washburn KK, Jefferson LS, Goldstein SL. Modified RIFLE criteria in critically ill children with acute kidney injury. *Kidney Int*. 2007;71(10):1028-35.

[11] Section 2: AKI Definition. *Kidney Int Suppl* (2011). 2012;2(1):19-36.

[12] Thomas ME, Blaine C, Dawnay A, Devonald MA, Ftouh S, Laing C, et al. The definition of acute kidney injury and its use in practice. *Kidney Int*. 2015;87(1):62-73.

[13] Hoste EA, Clermont G, Kersten A, Venkataraman R, Angus DC, De Bacquer D, et al. RIFLE criteria for acute kidney injury are associated with hospital mortality in critically ill patients: a cohort analysis. *Crit Care*. 2006;10(3):R73.

[14] Thakar CV, Christianson A, Freyberg R, Almenoff P, Render ML. Incidence and outcomes of acute kidney injury in intensive care units: a Veterans Administration study. *Crit Care Med*. 2009;37(9):2552-8.

[15] Kellum JA, Prowle JR. Paradigms of acute kidney injury in the intensive care setting. *Nat Rev Nephrol*. 2018;14(4):217-30.

[16] Basile DP, Anderson MD, Sutton TA. Pathophysiology of acute kidney injury. *Compr Physiol*. 2012;2(2):1303-53.

[17] Kaufman J, Dhakal M, Patel B, Hamburger R. Community-acquired acute renal failure. *Am J Kidney Dis*. 1991;17(2):191-8.

[18] Kosmadakis G, Viskaduraki M, Michail S. The validity of fractional excretion of uric acid in the diagnosis of acute kidney injury due to decreased kidney perfusion. *Am J Kidney Dis*. 2009;54(6):1186-7.

[19] Meyrier A, Niaudet P. Acute kidney injury complicating nephrotic syndrome of minimal change disease. *Kidney Int*. 2018;94(5):861-9.

[20] Hertzberg D, Ryden L, Pickering JW, Sartipy U, Holzmann MJ. Acute kidney injury-an overview of diagnostic methods and clinical management. *Clin Kidney J*. 2017;10(3): 323-31.

[21] Pession A, Masetti R, Gaidano G, Tosi P, Rosti G, Aglietta M, et al. Risk evaluation, prophylaxis, and treatment of tumor lysis syndrome: consensus of an Italian expert panel. *Adv Ther*. 2011;28(8):684-97.

[22] Perazella MA, Markowitz GS. Drug-induced acute interstitial nephritis. *Nat Rev Nephrol*. 2010;6(8):461-70.

[23] Praga M, Gonzalez E. Acute interstitial nephritis. *Kidney Int*. 2010;77(11):956-61.

[24] Murray PT, Mehta RL, Shaw A, Ronco C, Endre Z, Kellum JA, et al. Potential use of biomarkers in acute kidney injury: report and summary of recommendations from the 10th Acute Dialysis Quality Initiative consensus conference. *Kidney Int*. 2014;85(3): 513-21.

[25] van Duijl TT, Ruhaak LR, de Fijter JW, Cobbaert CM. Kidney Injury Biomarkers in an Academic Hospital Setting: Where Are We Now? *Clin Biochem Rev*. 2019;40(2):79-97.

[26] Ostermann M, Bellomo R, Burdmann EA, Doi K, Endre ZH, Goldstein SL, et al. Controversies in acute kidney injury: conclusions from a Kidney Disease: Improving Global Outcomes (KDIGO) Conference. *Kidney Int*. 2020;98(2):294-309.

[27] Ronco C, Reis T, Husain-Syed F. Management of acute kidney injury in patients with COVID-19. *Lancet Respir Med*. 2020;8(7):738-42.

[28] Gabarre P, Dumas G, Dupont T, Darmon M, Azoulay E, Zafrani L. Acute kidney injury in critically ill patients with COVID-19. *Intensive Care Med*. 2020;46(7):1339-48.

[29] Makris K, Spanou L. Acute Kidney Injury: Diagnostic Approaches and Controversies. *Clin Biochem Rev*. 2016;37(4):153-75.

[30] Ferguson TW, Komenda P, Tangri N. Cystatin C as a biomarker for estimating glomerular filtration rate. *Curr Opin Nephrol Hypertens*. 2015;24(3):295-300.

[31] Zhang Z, Lu B, Sheng X, Jin N. Cystatin C in prediction of acute kidney injury: a systemic review and meta-analysis. *Am J Kidney Dis*. 2011;58(3):356-65.

[32] Roos JF, Doust J, Tett SE, Kirkpatrick CM. Diagnostic accuracy of cystatin C compared to serum creatinine for the estimation of renal dysfunction in adults and children--a meta-analysis. *Clin Biochem*. 2007;40(5-6):383-91.

[33] Kidney Disease: Improving Global Outcomes (KDIGO) CKD Work Group. KDIGO 2012 Clinical Practice Guideline for the evaluation and management of chronic kidney disease. *Kidney Int Suppl*. 2013;3:1-150.

[34] Herget-Rosenthal S, Marggraf G, Husing J, Goring F, Pietruck F, Janssen O, et al. Early detection of acute renal failure by serum cystatin C. *Kidney Int*. 2004;66(3):1115-22.

[35] Spahillari A, Parikh CR, Sint K, Koyner JL, Patel UD, Edelstein CL, et al. Serum cystatin C- versus creatinine-based definitions of acute kidney injury following cardiac surgery: a prospective cohort study. *Am J Kidney Dis*. 2012;60(6):922-9.

[36] Park M, Shlipak MG, Thiessen-Philbrook H, Garg AX, Koyner JL, Coca SG, et al. Association of Peak Changes in Plasma Cystatin C and Creatinine With Death After Cardiac Operations. *Ann Thorac Surg*. 2016;101(4):1395-401.

[37] Meersch M, Schmidt C, Hoffmeier A, Van Aken H, Wempe C, Gerss J, et al. Prevention of cardiac surgery-associated AKI by implementing the KDIGO guidelines in high risk patients identified by biomarkers: the PrevAKI randomized controlled trial. *Intensive Care Med*. 2017;43(11):1551-61.

[38] Gocze I, Jauch D, Gotz M, Kennedy P, Jung B, Zeman F, et al. Biomarker-guided Intervention to Prevent Acute Kidney Injury After Major Surgery: The Prospective Randomized BigpAK Study. *Ann Surg*. 2018;267(6):1013-20.

In: Issues in Kidney Disease – Acute Kidney Injury
Editors: S. Z. Fadem and A. Arslan Yousuf Awan ISBN: 978-1-68507-002-1

Chapter 3

PRINCIPLES OF MANAGEMENT OF ACUTE KIDNEY INJURY

Michael W. Holliday, Jr.**, *MD, PhD
Selzman Institute for Kidney Health, Section of Nephrology,
Department of Medicine, Baylor College of Medicine, Houston, TX, USA
Michael E. DeBakey VA Medical Center, Houston, TX, USA

ABSTRACT

Acute kidney injury (AKI) is associated with increased morbidity, mortality, and health care utilization. Initial management of AKI through volume correction, discontinuation of nephrotoxins, and expedited workup, potentially including kidney biopsy, will ideally avoid the need for renal replacement therapy, resulting in stabilization and improvement in renal function and related patient outcomes.

Keywords: acute kidney injury, volume assessment, management

INTRODUCTION TO MANAGEMENT OF AKI

The goal of AKI treatment is to restore renal function and obviate the need for renal replacement therapy. Accurate diagnostic and prognostic assessments, as detailed in other chapters, are critical when formulating a personalized treatment plan for a patient with AKI. There are two key points to remember when beginning to assess the AKI patients:

One Size Does Not Fit All

Potential differential etiologies for AKI are as vast as the range of patient hemodynamic, volume, and metabolic parameters encountered in practice. Successful AKI treatment,

* Corresponding Author's E-mail: Michael.HollidayJr@bcm.edu.

therefore, epitomizes personalized medicine and requires a considered treatment plan customized to each patient.

Recognize Acuity and Anticipate Sequelae

For an anuric critically ill patient classified by AKI stage 3 with increasing serum potassium, the focus may be on renal replacement therapy, whereas for a patient with AKI stage 1 in setting of volume depletion, a course of replacement crystalloid fluid to restore intravascular volume and improve renal function is likely the most judicious course.

Formulating a Treatment Plan for AKI Begins WITH TARGETED HISTORY TAKING

Patient history and circumstances of presentation may frequently hint at etiology, therefore appropriate treatment for AKI through risk factor mitigation is implemented. It is essential to identify exposure to nephrotoxic agents, as well as recent changes to medications or other health issues that may be associated with AKI.

Table 1. Common factors associated with acute kidney injury [1]

Medications	Diagnostics/Procedures	OTC/Illicit Drugs	Other
Recent medication changes (also incorrect usage/non-compliance) ACEI/ARB Analgesics/NSAIDs Antibiotics Chemotherapies Diuretics Immunosuppressants Proton pump inhibitors	Bowel preparation Cardiac catherization Intravenous (IV) Iodinated contrast Surgery	Amphetamines Aristocholic acid (Chinese herbs) Cocaine/Levamisole Heroin Orlistat Synthetic marijuana	Burns GI illness Hx of urinary obstruction Inadequate PO intake Open wounds Recent infection Sepsis Syncope & orthostatic hypotension Thrombosis history Uncontrolled DM and glucosuria

For admitted patients, one should review the complete medication administration log and radiological studies to assess for nephrotoxic substance exposure. One should assess blood pressure and perioperative data for evidence of relative hypotension from patient's baseline blood pressure.

It is important to review intake and output balance during admission as well as weights over time. Recorded data are not always accurate. One should review the intake and output with patient, and observe the patient's room for presence of multiple drinks, outside food, etc.

> **Clinical pearls**
>
> Patients may frequently not be familiar with their medications. Consider reviewing the home medication list with the patient's family or caregiver. It is critical to accurately determine what the patient is actually taking.

Also, one should obtain an accurate list of the patient's home prescription and OTC medications and reconcile with the patient. Efficiency may be achieved through targeted medication review (Table 1). It is necessary to ask the patient and caregiver about GI symptoms including nausea, vomiting and diarrhea, as well nutritional and fluid intake over preceding days.

One should always ask the patient directly about prior issues: volume overload, heart and liver failure, prior acute kidney injury, obstructive uropathy (e.g., required foley catheter in the past, prior history of nephrolithiasis). Importantly, baseline serum creatinine levels are essential for accurate diagnosis and staging of AKI. Consider checking with prior institutions that have cared for patient to obtain baseline creatinine levels if none are available to you. If no baseline is available, trend creatinine during admission to assess for improvement with treatment.

Obstructive Uropathy

Patients with AKI should have an assessment for urinary tract blockage. Certain patient populations may be more likely to have blockage, such as those with known prostatic hypertrophy and concurrent UTI, those with neurogenic bladder, or those who have required foley catheter in the past. Nonetheless, even those patients without these complications may sustain complete or partial urinary obstruction, and such a diagnosis should be excluded.

> **Clinical pearls**
>
> UTI, pain medications, sedatives and anticholinergics all increase risk of urinary retention.
>
> Obstruction may lead to interstitial inflammation within the kidney, and tubular dysfunction may result in acidosis and hyperkalemia.

In high-risk individuals, rapid assessment for urinary retention could indicate the need for foley catheter. Bedside bladder scan augmented by point of care ultrasound may be employed in diagnosis of urinary retention. Relief of obstruction with foley catheter may precipitously improve the urine output. Subsequent measurement of urine output is necessary to address potential post-obstructive diuresis. Unilateral obstruction with resulting hydronephrosis may occur in setting of ureterolithiasis at the ureterovesical junction, or from local compression by an adjacent structure (metastatic cancer). Unilateral hydronephrosis on renal ultrasound indicates the obstruction, while the ureteral blockage may be better characterized on CT imaging. Bilateral obstruction may occur in setting of bladder outlet obstruction, such as prostatic hypertrophy, or in the form of bilateral ureteral pathology (stone, compression, or retroperitoneal fibrosis). Point-of-Care Ultrasound (POCUS) may be used to quickly assess for hydronephrosis, as well as for bladder distension. Hydronephrosis in setting of urosepsis may require urgent placement of percutaneous nephrostomy tube to relieve obstruction.

The Volume-Depleted Patient

The historical suggestion of volume depletion should be confirmed on physical examination and laboratory studies. When volume depletion is suspected in the context of acute kidney injury, it is useful to determine whether the patient has decreased effective intravascular volume or has a water deficit with hypernatremia and associated renal insufficiency (Table 2).

Table 2. Clues to diagnosing the volume-depleted state

Intravascular effective volume depletion or vasodilatory shock	Dehydration – water deficit
Collapsible IVC *Improvement in parameters with resuscitation* *Hyperdynamic LV* *Hypotension* *Lactic acidosis* *Low FENa (<1%) and FEUrea* *Meets criteria for sepsis* *Orthostatic hypotension* *Requiring pressors* *Tachycardia*	Renal vasoconstriction > AKI Dry mucous membranes and decreased skin turgor Hypernatremia Hyperosmolality Concentrated urine High thirst drive (unless neurologically impaired) *Suspect in patient relying on enteral feed and water supplementation; Dementia and failure to thrive.*

Patients with acute kidney injury in association with volume depletion with or without decreased systemic vascular resistance should be assessed for hemodynamic stability. The fulfillment of sepsis criteria in association with frank hypotension, lactic acidosis, or other signs of hypoperfusion typically indicate a likely benefit to supplementation with bolus crystalloid fluids (e.g., Ringer's lactate solution (LR), Plasmalyte, or Normal Saline). The goal of fluid resuscitation is to improve organ and renal perfusion and augment or sustain the mean arterial pressure without inducing sequelae of volume overload. Crystalloid fluids are generally preferred to colloidal preparations such as albumin. Starches are avoided. Bolus infusion at a rate of 0.5 to 1 L over an hour is more likely to augment the mean arterial pressure versus the use of a "maintenance" rate (100-200 cc per hour) [2, 3].

Certain patients may not be amenable to the typical aggressive early volume resuscitation. A history of advanced heart failure may indicate a patient may tolerate a lesser volume before needing transition to pressors to avoid worsening of pulmonary edema. Patients with intravascular low oncotic pressure such as those with liver failure or nephrotic syndrome may have rapid third-spacing of supplemented fluids. In scenarios where the patient may be fluid overloaded on presentation, or have such a history of fluid intolerance, stepwise administration of crystalloid fluid (such as in 500 cc volumes) with subsequent assessment of tolerance would be in order.

Consideration must be given to whether a patient has any concurrent increase in lung inflammation or pulmonary edema, or risk thereof, such as with developing acute respiratory distress syndrome; judicious bolus fluid administration should be considered in the context of a worsening alveolar-arterial oxygen gradient.

For hemodynamically stable patients with dehydration/hypernatremia and AKI, replacing free water would more likely resolve the hypernatremia in addition to augmenting overall volume status. Free water is typically replaced at a rate such that the sodium does not correct more than 10 milliequivalents per liter in 24 hours. For a hypernatremic patient with AKI and evidence of intravascular volume depletion, such as relative hypotension or in the setting of sepsis, isotonic crystalloids may be used initially to replace volume, with a subsequent transition to free water to further correct sodium [4]

Critical to accurate diagnosis of AKI etiology in the volume depleted patient is assessment of response to therapy. Correction of the intravascular volume deficit and stabilization of hemodynamic parameters may result in rapid improvement in renal function (serum creatinine level and urine output) due to restoration of renal perfusion. Failure of creatinine to stabilize or improve, or worsening oliguria, may indicate that the patient has sustained acute tubular injury. As described in accompanying chapters, urine microscopy to observe for muddy brown casts or increased renal tubular epithelial cells would be highly suggestive of acute tubular injury in the context of declining renal function/urine output despite restoration of adequate renal perfusion.

The Volume Overloaded Patient

Diagnosis and staging of AKI in the volume overloaded patient carries the caveat that the serum creatinine level may need adjustment based on fluid balance; in other words, in setting of volume overload, the serum creatinine level may underestimate stage of AKI [5].

Adjusted $S_{Cr} = S_{Cr}$ X correction factor

Correction factor = 1 + [cumulative fluid balance (L)/(admission body weight (kg) x 0.6)]

Commonly, patients with volume overload and AKI will have prior history of cardiac or liver dysfunction with associated hospital admissions. Prior records of cardiac function (echocardiography, cardiac catheterization) should be reviewed to assess for right- and left-sided heart failure, reduced ejection fraction, and valvular defects. If appropriate, current EKG and echocardiography should be reviewed for evidence of right heart strain/dysfunction that would result in preload dependent state (such as in setting of pulmonary embolism or hypertension) as well as changes to ejection fraction sustained from active cardiac disease (CAD, cardiomyopathy). For patients in which small changes in volume significantly affect cardiac output (i.e., patient has dilated left ventricle with reduced ejection fraction but no peripheral edema/obvious volume overload), B-type natriuretic peptide (BNP) measurement may be useful when compared to baseline measurement; however, BNP may be elevated in setting of AKI.

Patients with AKI associated with liver disease (e.g., cirrhosis, NAFLD) may have prior admissions for sequelae of liver failure such has GI bleeding, refractory ascites, infection, and altered mental status. Review prior GI evaluations for scoring of liver failure utilizing Model for End-Stage Liver Disease (MELD) and imaging for evidence of liver cirrhosis and fatty liver disease. Assess liver synthetic capacity with INR (international normalized ratio), serum albumin, and platelet count. Careful examination of blood, urine, and peritoneal fluid cultures in setting of decompensated liver disease commonly reveal infection.

New onset volume overload characterized by edema or anasarca with hypoalbuminemia and hyperlipidemia may indicate nephrotic syndrome (e.g., minimal change disease, primary FSGS) and need for kidney biopsy to characterize and treat the intrinsic renal disease.

Table 3. Clues to delineating the volume-overloaded state. *In setting of renal impairment, BNP may be elevated from baseline irrespective of volume status

Exacerbation of heart failure with AKI – cardiorenal syndrome type 1	AKI in setting of liver failure – hepatorenal syndrome type I	Nephrotic syndrome
No evidence of intrinsic renal disease Creatinine stable or improves with diuretics and reduction in patient weight/volume Elevated BNP from baseline* Hypokinetic/akinetic LV Hyponatremia Low cardiac index and systemic blood pressure Reduced EF Requirement for inotropic support Volume overload on exam (dependent interstitial tissue edema, increased jugular venous distension, pulmonary edema)	No evidence of intrinsic renal disease Abdominal compartment syndrome Esophageal varices Hyponatremia Hyperammonemia Hypoalbuminemia Increased renal venous pressure Inability to tolerate diuretics Refractory large volume ascites Portal hypertension Volume overload on exam (dependent pitting edema)	Abnormal urine analysis (hematuria) Foamy urine High urine protein: creatinine and urine albumin:creatinine Hypoalbuminemia Hypercoagulable state Hyperlipidemia Rapid-onset severe anasarca

Just as in the case of volume depletion or sepsis, those patients with volume overload presenting with AKI may sustain acute tubular injury. Tubular injury, with its related urine sediment characteristics, must be assessed before arriving at a physiologic explanation for AKI such as cardiorenal or hepatorenal syndrome. Cardiorenal syndrome type I results from acute decompensation in cardiac function or cardiogenic shock that results in decreased renal perfusion and function (AKI). Volume optimization with diuretics and inotropes are used to improve left ventricular function and cardiac output, with resultant improvement in diuretic responsiveness and serum creatinine levels [6]. Hepatorenal syndrome type I (HRS-1) occurs due to splanchnic vasodilation and renal vasoconstriction in context of decompensated liver cirrhosis with ascites. Intrinsic renal injury must be excluded, and cessation of diuretics and albumin supplementation (2 days of 1g/kg/d) are typically utilized to ensure absence of intravascular volume depletion. Once diagnosis is confirmed, albumin, octreotide, and midodrine or norepinephrine are utilized to reduce splanchnic vasodilation and improve mean arterial pressure [7].

The Euvolemic Patient

Exclusion of hypotensive insults or cardiac/liver issues in a patient with AKI and apparent euvolemia reinforces need for thorough assessment for intrinsic renal injury. Commonly, exposure to nephrotoxic substances may be revealed on history taking, and such substances should be discontinued. As an example, if patient has suspected AKI-related to toxicity of an antibiotic, switch to alternative agent with less renal toxicity. Beyond cessation of the offending substance in setting of AKI from drug related nephrotoxicity, care is typically supportive while additional evaluation is ongoing. Intravenous fluid supplementation may be used to support patient in setting of suspected volume depletion or inadequate intake to cover total daily losses. Typically, hemodialysis is not used for clearance of iodinated contrast dye. If patient has toxicity from an intoxicant with low protein-binding causing multi-organ dysfunction in the setting of inadequate renal clearance, dialysis may be considered.

Some commonly used medications such as non-steroidal anti-inflammatory drugs, antibiotics such as trimethoprim/sulfamethoxazole, and proton pump inhibitors have been associated with drug-induced acute interstitial nephritis. Patients commonly present with AKI and have active urine sediment with leukocyturia and may have rash and eosinophilia. A kidney biopsy is necessary for diagnosis of acute interstitial nephritis to facilitate appropriate steroid administration [8].

Renal imaging should also be assessed for evidence of arterial or venous obstruction to the kidneys that may result in oligo-anuria, such as, albeit rare, with thromboembolism or bilateral renal vein thrombosis.

When AKI is observed in concurrence with active urine sediment, inappropriate proteinuria, or evidence on serological workup of potential secondary cause (e.g., active hepatitis C, monoclonal gammopathy, low complement, etc.), kidney biopsy should be considered [9]. Potential risks versus benefits of kidney biopsy should always be considered and discussed with the patient. As an example, for a patient with longstanding history of progressive chronic kidney disease, and a new acute kidney injury with proteinuria and microscopic hematuria, the potential benefits of biopsy (less so given likely substantial interstitial fibrosis) should be weighed against the risk of holding aspirin e.g., given history of multiple prior cerebrovascular accidents.

Due to the variety of potential histological changes and associated therapies, kidney biopsy is preferred and necessary for appropriate diagnosis of glomerulonephritis and interstitial nephritis in adults. Certain circumstances exist in practice where the use of empiric therapy such as steroids might be considered.

1. Is the patient not a candidate for biopsy? Would there be a likely benefit to empiric therapy if patient has had long course of chronic, progressive, and advanced disease?
2. What is the pre-test probability of the diagnosis? Consider a known FSGS patient with recurrence of proteinuria on steroid withdrawal, where the diagnosis is comfortably assumed, versus an adult patient with new nephrotic syndrome, where multiple diagnoses are still considered, and treatment may vary greatly.
3. Will empiric drug exposure interfere with interpretation of kidney biopsy, such as in acute interstitial nephritis?

ROLE FOR DIALYSIS IN AKI

Patients with acute kidney injury may, despite volume correction, have progression of intrinsic renal injury, whether from acute tubular injury or nephritis. Such progression may result in decline, or complete cessation of urine output and stall of metabolic clearance. Hemodialysis may be employed for optimization of volume status in this scenario should diuretics fail, as well as for clearance of uremia associated substances. Urgent or emergent hemodialysis may be required for treatment of intoxications (e.g., ethylene glycol or other renally-cleared toxicants), hyperkalemia, severe hypercalcemia, uremia with altered mental status, severe metabolic acidosis, and for volume optimization in setting of pulmonary edema and inadequate response to high-dose diuretics.

For patients that are hemodynamically stable or that require rapid clearance of intoxicants, standard hemodialysis may be employed. For critically ill patients requiring vasopressors to maintain mean arterial pressure, either prolonged intermittent renal replacement therapy (e.g., 12 hours) or continuous renal replacement therapy are employed. The latter modalities utilize less clearance per unit time versus standard hemodialysis, however, may be more well-tolerated with regard to effects on blood pressure [10].

MEDICATION DOSING IN AKI

An important component of AKI management is ensuring that medications are adequately dosed based on renal function. Small changes in creatinine (when the baseline level is within normal range) indicate a large percentage drop from normal. As an example, an increase in creatinine from 1.0 mg/dL to 1.5 mg/dL represents a 25% decline in glomerular filtration rate. Commonly used outpatient medications such as gabapentin and metformin should be adjusted or discontinued depending on the slope of estimated glomerular filtration rate (eGFR) decline and urine output.

Antibiotics are generally administered initially at the usual dose in setting of sepsis or infection, irrespective of kidney function - this is to ensure adequate peak levels to facilitate pathogen clearance. Subsequent maintenance doses may be adjusted based on renal function and/or subsequent trough levels [11].

The following chapters in this book will describe in detail the diagnosis and management of renal disorders briefly introduced above.

REFERENCES

[1] Perazella MA. Pharmacology behind Common Drug Nephrotoxicities. *Clin J Am Soc Nephrol*. 2018;13(12):1897–908.

[2] Howell MD, Davis AM. Management of Sepsis and Septic Shock. *JAMA*. 2017;317(8):847.

[3] Khwaja A. KDIGO Clinical Practice Guidelines for Acute Kidney Injury. *Nephron Clin Pract*. 2012;120(4):c179–84.

[4] Sterns RH. Evidence for Managing Hypernatremia: Is It Just Hyponatremia in Reverse? *Clin J Am Soc Nephrol*. 2019;14(5):645-647.

[5] Thongprayoon C, Hansrivijit P, Kovvuru K, Kanduri SR, Torres-Ortiz A, Acharya P, et al. Diagnostics, Risk Factors, Treatment and Outcomes of Acute Kidney Injury in a New Paradigm. *J Clin Med*. 2020;9(4):1104.

[6] Rangaswami J, Bhalla V, Blair JE, Chang TI, Costa S, Lentine KL, et al. Cardiorenal Syndrome: Classification, Pathophysiology, Diagnosis, and Treatment Strategies: A Scientific Statement From the American Heart Association. *Circulation*. 2019;139(16):e840–78.

[7] Runyon BA. AASLD. Introduction to the revised American Association for the Study of Liver Diseases Practice Guideline management of adult patients with ascites due to cirrhosis 2012. *Hepatology*. 2013;57(4):1651–3.

[8] Moledina DG, Perazella MA. Drug-Induced Acute Interstitial Nephritis. *Clin J Am Soc Nephrol*. 2017;12(12):2046–9.

[9] Summary of Recommendation Statements. *Kidney Int Suppl*. 2012;2(2):143–53.

[10] Gaudry S, Hajage D, Benichou N, Chaïbi K, Barbar S, Zarbock A, et al. Delayed versus early initiation of renal replacement therapy for severe acute kidney injury: a systematic review and individual patient data meta-analysis of randomised clinical trials. *Lancet*. 2020;395(10235):1506–15.

[11] Crass RL, Rodvold KA, Mueller BA, Pai MP. Renal Dosing of Antibiotics: Are We Jumping the Gun? *Clin Infect Dis*. 2018;68(9):1596–602.

In: Issues in Kidney Disease – Acute Kidney Injury
Editors: S. Z. Fadem and A. Arslan Yousuf Awan

ISBN: 978-1-68507-002-1

Chapter 4

DIAGNOSIS OF ACUTE KIDNEY INJURY – BIOMARKERS AND OTHER NOVEL TESTS

Ingrid Hougen, MD, Edward Clark, MD and Swapnil Hiremath*, MD, MPH, FASN

Division of Nephrology, Department of Medicine, University of Ottawa, Ottawa, Canada

ABSTRACT

Acute kidney injury (AKI) is classically defined on the basis of a change in creatinine and/or urine output. However, creatinine has several limitations, including a lack of discrimination of causal etiology, apart from the well-known issues with inability to diagnose AKI early. Biomarkers can step into this niche, allowing for not just superior diagnostics, but possibly with predictive and prognostic capabilities. The term 'biomarker' is a portmanteau of 'biological marker' and broadly refers to an objective measurement of a clinical state which can be reproduced accurately. Biomarkers in AKI can enhance clinical aspects of care, including early diagnosis, precise pinpointing of the etiology of AKI, and the ability to tailor care based on the predictive abilities. They may allow for diagnosis of etiology, such as acute interstitial nephritis, without a kidney biopsy. In certain settings, the lack of a rise in biomarkers discordant with a rise in creatinine may allow us to safely continue therapy. Conceptually, biomarkers could be added to AKI staging, as being positive or negative in the presence of a rise in creatinine or a fall in urine output. Similarly, in clinical research, the embedding of biomarkers can make for more efficient clinical trials. Several biomarkers have shown such abilities, and a few are already approved, however further validation is needed before their widespread use. In addition to classical biomarkers, there are other tests and technological features that can inform early diagnosis and prognosis, such as renal functional reserve, the furosemide stress test, and the use of artificial technology in the form of neural networks.

* Corresponding Author's E-mail: shiremath@toh.ca.

Keywords: acute kidney injury, biomarkers, AKI, diagnosis, nephrocheck, hypercreatininemia, creatinine; renal functional reserve, acute kidney disease, furosemide stress test

INTRODUCTION

Acute renal failure was historically defined as a sudden and abrupt decline in kidney function. What was missing in this classic definition, was details about the magnitude of this decline, as well as the time course over which this decline occurred, apart from subjective criteria of the suddenness. Over the last two decades, initially with Risk, Injury, Failure, Loss, End Stage Renal Disease (RIFLE), then Acute Kidney Injury Network (AKIN), and then Kidney Disease Improving Global Outcomes (KDIGO), the definition has evolved into a more objective version with clear guidance about the magnitude and the speed of this decline in kidney function [1] [2] [3]. Earlier chapters in this volume already described these criteria, and in this section, we will explain what is possibly the next frontier for diagnosis of acute kidney injury (AKI), namely the use of biomarkers. AKI has always been defined, not just by urine output, but mostly by change in creatinine. Creatinine is a filtration marker, with a minor secretory component, and really is not a marker of tubular injury, the most common pathway to AKI. It also does not tell anything about the etiology of AKI. Thus, there are several limitations to creatinine, and the only reason it has survived so far, is because of the convenient laboratory testing, tradition, and ease of daily monitoring. We do need something better than creatinine, and the research in the last 2 decades has thrown up several promising biomarkers which will, hopefully, revolutionize the practice of medicine in the coming years. Biomarkers in AKI are often markers of tubular injury, but also have diverse roles in pathophysiological processes in AKI, including inflammation, repair, and fibrosis. In this chapter, we will discuss what biomarkers are, the specific need for biomarkers in AKI, specific AKI biomarkers, and the current evidence and the way forward.

ACUTE KIDNEY DISEASE AND WORSENING KIDNEY FUNCTION

Before we discuss biomarkers, a few concepts based on creatinine are worth considering in a little bit more detail. Though the AKI criteria are well known, less attention has been paid to the acute kidney disease, or AKD, which was part of the KDIGO criteria (see Table 1). AKD refers to kidney damage that has happened in the last 90 days, with much broader criteria. In a cohort study of 1.1 million Canadian residents, James and colleagues demonstrated that these AKD criteria were useful, and identified patients who did not meet existing criteria for CKD or AKI [4]. These patients did have an increased risk of incident as well as progressive CKD (hazard ratio, HR 3.17, 95% confidence interval [CI], 3.10-03.23) end-stage kidney disease (ESKD, HR 8.56, 95 CI 7.32 - 10.01), and death (HR 1.42, 95% CI 1.39 - 1.45). Worsening renal function (WRF) is another such definition, and is defined as an increase of ≥0.3 mg/dL in the serum creatinine level compared with the value on admission, and is commonly used in the setting of decompensated acute heart failure [5] [6]. The prognostic implication of this has been questioned, and will be discussed briefly in the next section on permissive hypercreatininemia.

Table 1. Classical definitions of acute kidney injury and disease, and worsening renal function

	Acute Kidney Injury (AKI)	**Acute Kidney Disease (AKD)**	**Worsening Renal Function (WRF)**
Duration	< 7 days	≤ 3 months	During hospitalization, usually in setting of acute heart failure
Urine output criteria	Oliguria ≥ 6 hours	Not defined	Not defined
Creatinine or GFR criteria	Increase by > 0.3 mg/dl in 48 hours, OR Increase by >50% in 7 days	AKI, or GFR <60 ml/min/1.73m2, or Decrease in GFR by >35%, or Increase in creatinine >50%	Increase by > 0.3 mg/dl from baseline at admission
Structural alteration	Not defined	Marker of kidney damage (albuminuria)	Not defined

GFR: glomerular filtration rate

Table 2. Pitfalls of Creatinine for kidney function in acute kidney injury

Characteristic	**Explanation**	**Comments**	**Role for biomarkers**
Early diagnosis	By the time creatinine increases, kidney injury has already set in and may be established	Early detection clinically may allow examination of interventions in clinical trials	Multiple biomarkers approved and undergoing evaluation
Inaccurate Low creatinine despite AKI	In certain conditions, the serum creatinine may remain in normal range despite kidney injury, e.g., hepatorenal syndrome	Low muscle mass and liver synthetic failure may result in lower serum creatinine	
Inaccurate Inhibited tubular secretion	Drugs that inhibit creatinine secretion may show a larger creatinine rise than true kidney injury	Egg drugs such as cimetidine, trimethoprim, fenofibrate; possibly also sometimes with vancomycin	
Inaccurate Hemodynamic changes	In certain conditions, a rise in creatinine may reflect clinical improvement, e.g., with decongestion in acute decompensated heart failure	Understand 'permissive hypercreatininemia', with use of diuretics, renin-angiotensin system blockade, or sodium-glucose cotransporter-2 inhibitors	Markers of injury may be normal, helping to differentiate hemodynamic changes from true injury
Accurate GFR estimation	Creatinine cannot be used to calculate accurate GFR when not in steady state	Matters especially for drugs with narrow therapeutic window; may use alternate formulae such as kinetic GFR based on creatinine kinetics	Not yet available in AKI; cystatin C may be useful in chronic kidney disease

GFR: glomerular filtration rate; AKI: acute kidney injury

The Need for Biomarkers

The term biomarker is a portmanteau of 'biological marker' and broadly refers to an objective measurement of a clinical state which can be reproduced accurately. The National Institutes of Health Biomarkers Definitions Working Group in 1998 defined a biomarker as a characteristic that is objectively measured and evaluated as an indicator of normal biological processes, pathogenic processes, or pharmacologic responses to a therapeutic intervention [7]. Another workgroup from the World Health Organization defined a biomarker as any substance, structure, or process that can be measured in the body or its products and influence or predict the incidence of outcome or disease [8]. Thus, even urea and creatinine are basically biomarkers. However, creatinine has several limitations (see Table 2 for a concise list).

In addition, biomarkers can be thought of to be diagnostic, prognostic, predictive, safety, and pharmacodynamic or response biomarkers. In AKI, biomarkers could play a role in each of these areas, so it is important to understand the differences briefly [9, 10]. A diagnostic biomarker detects or confirms the presence of a disease or condition of interest, or identifies an individual with a subtype of the disease. A prognostic biomarker is used to identify the likelihood of a clinical event, disease recurrence, or disease progression in patients with a disease or medical condition of interest. A predictive biomarker is defined by the finding that the presence or change in the biomarker predicts an individual or group of individuals more likely to experience a favorable or unfavorable effect from the exposure to a medical product or environmental agent. A safety biomarker is measured before or after an exposure to a medical intervention or environmental agent to indicate the likelihood, presence, or extent of a toxicity as an adverse event. Lastly, when the level of a biomarker changes in response to exposure to a medical product or an environmental agent, it can be called a pharmacodynamic/response biomarker. As one contemplates these, it is clear that any particular biomarker cannot be easily pigeonholed into these categories, and may have overlapping roles in any specific clinical setting, and the same applies to AKI.

Biomarkers in AKI: Clinical Role

Though biomarkers in AKI are often thought to be useful for early diagnosis, there are many other possible roles and uses, using the biomarker framework described above. Indeed, biomarkers may detect AKI earlier than the rise in creatinine and/or fall in urine output, as is described below with artificial intelligence (AI) [11, 12]. In other specific conditions, where creatinine is not helpful for diagnosis (e.g., hepatorenal syndrome, discussed below), novel biomarkers can allow for a correct diagnosis as well. Some biomarkers (e.g., interleukin-9) show promise in identifying specific etiology of AKI, in this case acute interstitial nephritis. Much more research and development has focused on being able to differentiate prerenal and reversible AKI from irreversible acute tubular necrosis, which would have diagnostic, predictive and prognostic aspects to it. Several biomarkers, in particular the furosemide stress test (FST, discussed below), Neutrophil gelatinase-associated lipocalin (NGAL) and urinary insulin-like growth factor-binding protein (IGFBP-7) and tissue inhibitor of metalloproteinase (TIMP-2, both combined as "Nephrocheck"), have shown varying levels of utility in this area. These biomarkers are particularly useful in focusing on appropriate management (e.g., either more intravenous fluids, or early nephrology involvement and planning for renal replacement therapy). In the kidney transplantation arena, use of biomarkers of tubular injury may help reduce discard of organs being considered for transplant. Lastly, biomarkers may allow for prognostication, in identification of patients with recovery of kidney function. Apart from NGAL, proenkephalin-A, urinary dickkopf-3 and albuminuria have shown to be useful in individual studies. Overall, biomarkers may eventually allow better phenotyping of AKI in almost all aspects [13].

Table 3. Summary of biomarkers in AKI

	Characteristic	Applicability
NGAL	Present in neutrophil granules; released with tissue injury and freely filtered. Urine NGAL represents intrarenal production	Approved in Europe (Conformité Europέene [CE]), Australia (Therapeutics Goods Administration), South Africa (South African National Accreditation System), and Canada (Health Canada)
Kidney injury molecule	Transmembrane glycoprotein induces on proximal tubular apical membrane with injury	Mixed results; few supporting data in heart failure
Nephrocheck (insulin-like growth-factor binding protein 7 and tissue inhibitor of metalloproteinases)	Cell cycle arrest proteins expressed with cellular stress or injury	Several validity studies done; approved in United States and Europe
Interleukin 18	Proinflammatory cytokines, expresses in proximal tubules with injury	Promising data in kidney transplantation population; mixed results in the setting of heart failure
Liver-type fatty acid-binding protein	Part of lipid-binding protein superfamily, binds with fatty acids and elevated with ischemia reperfusion injury	Predictor of AKI after cardiac surgery; approved in Japan
N-acetyl-β-D-glucosaminidase	Lysosomal enzyme, found in proximal tubular cells and presence in urine reflects tubular injury	Promising data in chronic kidney disease; mixed results in the setting of heart failure
Procalcitonin	116-amino acid peptide, upregulated in many tissues during infections compared with chronic inflammatory states	High levels seen in infectious conditions and heart failure (with or without AKI)
Copeptin	The C-terminal segment of the arginine vasopressin prohormone, with high ex vivo stability that is easy to measure	Theoretically would be useful as an indirect measure of vasopressin activation in decompensated heart failure

AKI, acute kidney injury; NGAL, neutrophil gelatinase-associated lipocalin. Schematic depicting that the implications of acute elevations in serum creatinine are context dependent. AKI, acute kidney injury; RAAS, renin angiotensin system; SGLT2i, sodium glucose transporter inhibitors. From Sriperumbuduri et al. [6], used with permission

Clinical Pearls

- A rise in creatinine and recognition of AKI may reflect well established AKI, and prophylactic strategies in this setting may often be too late
- A rise in creatinine may also reflect favorable hemodynamic and volume changes, e.g., with intensive blood pressure lowering and decongestion, and not true tubular injury
- Use of formulae based on creatinine kinetics, such as kinetic GFR, may be used for dosing drugs with narrow therapeutic window in the setting of creatinine not in steady state
- Biomarkers can be not just diagnostic, but prognostic, predictive, pharmacodynamic, and safety biomarkers
- Biomarkers also require analytic and clinical validation in different settings before widespread use
- Nephrocheck (combination of insulin-like growth-factor binding protein 7 and tissue inhibitor of metalloproteinases) have been approved for clinical use, however, have been only validated in critically ill patients, and may have lower validity in other settings.
- Biomarkers in AKI may be able to make clinical research more efficient by smarter patient choice, and faster outcome detection

Permissive Hypercreatininemia

Though the management of worsening renal function is beyond the scope of this particular chapter, increasing creatinine in the setting of heart failure often leads to reactive changes in medications, often including stopping renin-angiotensin system blockers, diuretics, or other useful drugs. These medications are often useful for decongestion as well as the overall prognosis. Stopping these medications may often improve the creatinine number, without improving clinical outcomes. This concept has been called 'permissive hypercreatininemia' [14]. In the setting of acute decompensated heart failure, inducing AKI, with an increase in the creatinine number, does not mean there is acute kidney injury per se. This should be differentiated from spontaneous AKI, for example that which occurs with sepsis or hypotension. This requires clinical judgment and careful assessment of the patient including the volume status and overall course. However, and understanding of this concept, will allow proper management, including continuation of useful therapeutic agents. This is conceptually explained in Figure 1. Biomarkers are different in this respect, since they often do represent actual kidney injury, rather than hemodynamic changes, which an increase in creatinine represents in this scenario. Indeed, biomarkers may allow for a greater confidence in the permissive nature of allowing continuation of perceived 'nephrotoxic' drugs.

Biomarkers in AKI: Research Aspects

Clinical research is necessary to validate most of these biomarkers in the setting of AKI. In addition to that, there are several different ways that biomarkers might prove useful for conducting better and faster studies [15]. Clinical research in AKI relies on identifying eligible patients on the basis of creatinine or urine output. Adding validated biomarkers of injury could allow enrichment of the patient population to select those that are at highest risk of requiring, e.g., renal replacement therapy. This would allow recruitment of a smaller patient population, accrue endpoints faster, and make clinical research faster and cheaper, and ultimately more efficient. Another way of making trials more efficient is by recruiting a more homogenous population. The syndromic diagnosis of AKI often includes different etiologies, making for a heterogenous population. Hence interventions designed to work in a certain pathophysiologic pathway may not work in another population. Use of diagnostic biomarkers which could identify specific causes of AKI can allow research focused on a particular etiological mechanism of AKI. Similarly, if predictive biomarkers can identify those with a lower chance of kidney recovery, these patients could either be included, or excluded, depending on the intervention being studied. Lastly, pharmacodynamic biomarkers could serve as surrogate endpoints to identify changes early on, and focus on promising interventions.

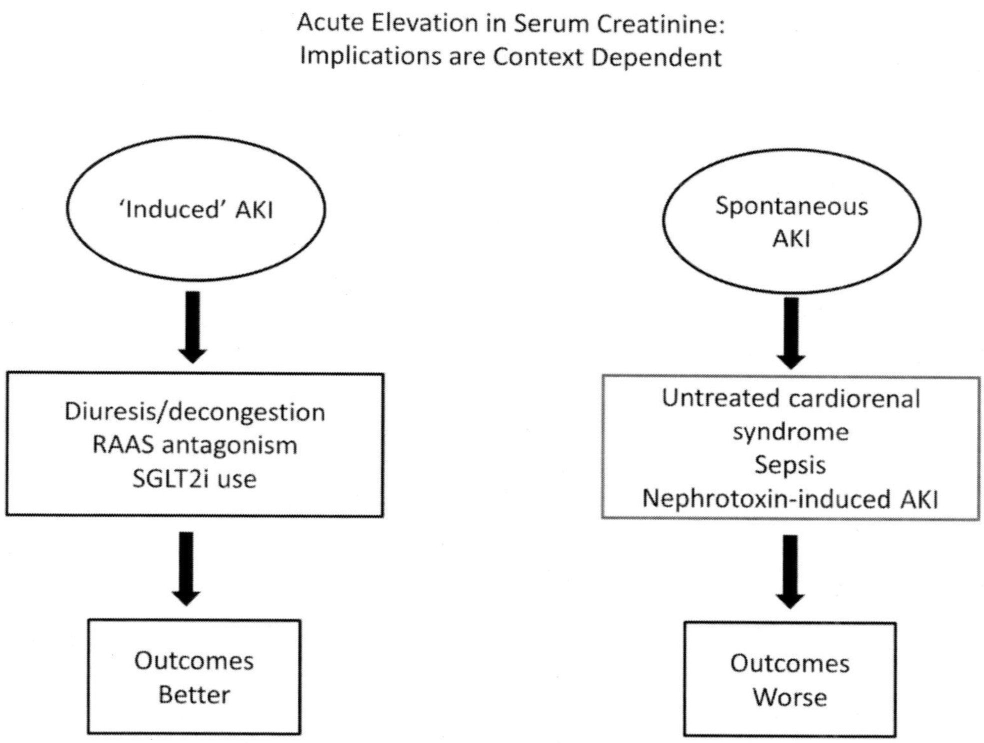

Figure 1. Schematic depicting that the implications of acute elevations in serum creatinine are context-dependent. AKI, acute kidney injury; RAAS, renin angiotensin system; SGLT2i, sodium glucose transporter inhibitors. From Sriperumbuduri et al. [6], used with permission.

INDIVIDUAL AKI BIOMARKERS

Neutrophil Gelatinase-Associated Lipocalin

Neutrophil gelatinase-associated lipocalin (NGAL) is a 25 kDa protein belonging to the lipocalin superfamily. It was initially found in activated neutrophils, however, many other cells, like kidney tubular cells, may produce NGAL in response to various insults. Both serum and urinary NGAL have been studied as markers of early tubular injury. Indeed, NGAL is probably the most researched biomarker in AKI [16].

Nephrocheck

Insulin-like growth factor-binding protein-7 (IGFBP-7) and tissue inhibitor of metalloprotease-2 (TIMP-2) have been implicated during the early stage of cellular stress in G1 cell-cycle arrest via blocking the effect of cyclin-dependent protein kinase complexes. Performed together, they have been marketed as 'Nephrocheck' (Astute Medical Inc.) and is the only test approved by the United States Federal Drug Administration [17].

Kidney Injury Molecule-1

Kidney injury molecule-1 (KIM-1) is a transmembrane glycoprotein expressed by proximal tubular cells in response to kidney injury and functions in the clearance of apoptotic cells.

Albuminuria

Albuminuria has been well recognized in chronic kidney disease, but even in AKI, it associates with occurrence of AKI, severity of AKI, and subsequent non-recovery of AKI and dialysis dependence [18].

Interleukin-18

Interleukin-18 (IL-18) is an 18 kDa molecule that is released into the urine following tubular damage. In particular, it has been reported to be elevated after acute interstitial nephritis [19].

Liver-Type Fatty Acid-Binding Protein

Liver-type fatty acid-binding protein (L-FABP) is a 14 kDa molecule, found in hepatocytes and proximal tubular cells and is freely filtered and absorbed, but is found in the urine in the setting of tubular injury.

Dickkopf-3

This is a 38 kDa glycoprotein, stress-induced and released from kidney tubular epithelium, and secreted into the urine under conditions of tubular stress.

Uromodulin

Uromodulin (UMOD), also known as Tamm–Horsfall protein, is expressed by renal tubular epithelial cells localized in the thick ascending limb of the loop of Henle and is the most abundant protein in the urine of healthy individuals.

Proenkephalin A

This is an endogenous polypeptide hormone in adrenal medulla, nervous system, immune system and the renal tissue, and elevated levels in the plasma are associated with AKI, severity and recovery [20].

Osteopontin

Osteopontin (OPN) is a glycoprotein expressed in tubular cells and interstitial infiltrating cells in areas of tubulointerstitial damage.

Others

Several other biomarkers have been described in single studies such as retinol binding protein, tumor necrosis factor, epithelial growth factor (EGF), netrin-1, chitinase-3-like protein 1 (YKL-40), alkaline phosphatase, hepcidin, and this field is expected to grow and expand.

Thus, biomarkers in AKI can be classified in many different ways. For tubular injury markers, based on the site in the tubule, they could be from the proximal tubule (e.g., KIM-1, L-FABP, NGAL), loop of Henle (UMOD, OPN), or the distal tubule (NGAL, OPN). Apart from markers of tubular injury, there are biomarkers of inflammation (OPN, IL-18), biomarkers of fibrosis (TGF-beta), and biomarkers of repair (YKL-40).

Furosemide Stress Test

In addition to biomarkers, researchers are looking at functional measures to diagnose and predict acute kidney injury. One such measure is termed the furosemide stress test (FST), as described by Chawla et al. [21]. They looked at critically ill patients with early AKI (AKIN I or II) and whether response to furosemide at a dose of 1.0 or 1.5mg/kg could predict progression to more severe stage AKI. In a retrospective cohort of 23 patients, and a multicenter prospective cohort of 54 patients, they found that those who progressed to AKIN stage-III had significantly lower urine output each hour for the first 6 hours following FST compared to those whose AKI did not progress to that stage ($p<0.001$). In the first 2 hours following FST, a urine volume of less than 200ml had a sensitivity of 87.1% and specificity of 84.1% of predicting AKI progression. They did not include patients with evidence of volume depletion, and the study protocol included replacement of hourly urine output with Ringer's lactate or Normal Saline for 6 hours to minimize hypovolemia.

Other studies looking at the FST have since followed. A recent meta-analysis identified 11 trials, totaling 1366 participants, which looked at the FST with outcomes of risk of AKI progression, renal replacement therapy or mortality [22]. For risk of AKI progression, they calculated a pooled sensitivity and specificity of 0.81 (95% CI 0.74-0.87) and 0.88 (95% CI 0.82-0.92), with a positive LR 5.45 (95% CI 3.96-7.50) and negative LR 0.26 (95% CI 0.19-0.36), area under the receiver operator curve (AUROC) 0.88, with low to moderate heterogeneity between studies. For predicting renal replacement therapy, they calculated sensitivity 0.84 (95% CI 0.72-0.91), specificity 0.77 (95% CI 0.64-0.87), positive LR 3.16 (95% CI 2.06-4.86) and negative LR 0.25 (95% CI 0.14-0.44), with high heterogeneity between studies, and AUROC 0.86. Subgroup analysis showed better diagnostic performance in the early AKI population.

Renal Functional Reserve Testing

Another functional measure is the renal functional reserve (RFR). This refers to the capacity of the intact nephron mass to increase GFR from baseline, in response to a physiologic stress. Comparing patients with the same GFR, a lower RFR may signal a greater risk of AKI than a patient with higher RFR. It is defined as the difference between baseline GFR and the maximal GFR that can be attained in response to a renal functional demand. In studies it is measured by administering an oral protein or amino acid load followed by measuring creatinine clearance [23].

The RFR has been studied in perioperative cardiac surgery patients [24]. In 110 patients with GFR >60ml/min/1.73m^2, pre-operative RFR was lower in those who experienced post-op AKI ($p < 0.001$) and predicted AKI with an area under the receiver operating curve 0.83 (95% CI 0.70-0.96). They used an oral protein load of 1.2g/kg red meat protein delivered after an 8 hour fast with hydration. Both resting GFR and stress GFR were calculated using endogenous creatinine clearance. The difference between stress GFR and resting GFR was defined as the RFR, and a normal RFR was considered greater or equal or 30ml/min/1.73m^2. They estimated a pre-operative RFR of 15ml/min/1.73m^2 had 67% sensitivity and 94% specificity for predicting AKI. Further studies are warranted to assess the use of RFR in identifying patients at risk of AKI.

Artificial Intelligence and AKI

Advanced technology is also being investigated as a tool for earlier prediction of AKI. The DeepMind team is creating models that use artificial intelligence to predict AKI [12]. They used a deep learning technique called a recurrent neural network. It processes data from individual electronic health records to build an internal memory of relevant information up to that point. At a given time point the model will predict the probability of AKI within the next 48 hours. The model was trained using data from a multicenter retrospective dataset of over 700,000 patients at the US Department of Veterans Affairs. They report 55.8% of inpatient AKI events were predicted with their model up to 48 hours in advance. They had a high false positive ratio of 2 false predictions for every true prediction. The model was better at predicting severe AKI requiring dialysis, correctly predicting 84.3% of AKI requiring dialysis within 30 days, and 90.2% of AKI requiring dialysis within 90 days. Further prospective studies are needed to validate this model.

Evidence for Biomarkers and AKI Prediction

Biomarkers have not only been studied as markers of kidney injury but are also being investigated as predictors of developing AKI, or progression to requiring renal replacement therapy. As discussed above, the biomarker that has been shown to have superior predictive value for developing AKI is the product of urine insulin-like growth factor-binding protein 7 (IGFBP7) and tissue inhibitor of metalloproteinases-2 (TIMP-2) [25]. These are both inducers of G1 cell cycle arrest, which is a key mechanism implicated in AKI. In the Sapphire study with 744 critically ill patients without AKI at enrollment, urine IGFBP7 and TIMP-2 together had an AUC of 0.80 for predicting KDIGO stage 2 or 3 AKI within 12 hours, which was superior to previously described markers of AKI they evaluated such as NGAL, plasma cystatin-C, KIM-1, IL-18, pi-GST and L-FABP ($p < 0.002$). The product of urine IGFBP7 and TIMP2 as a biomarker has since been FDA approved and is commercially available in the United States as an adjunct to clinical evaluation for critically ill patients.

A recent meta-analysis looked at trials evaluating biomarkers for prediction of requiring renal replacement therapy in AKI [26]. They included 41 studies, with 13 different biomarkers. NGAL had the largest body of evidence, with a pooled AUC for urine NGAL of 0.720 (95% CI 0.638-0.803) and blood NGAL 0.755 (0.706-0.803). Serum creatinine and cystatin C had pooled AUCs of 0.764 (0.732-0.796) and 0.768 (0.729-0.807). Urine interleukin-18, cystatin C and the product of IGFBP7 and TIMP2 had pooled AUCs of 0.668 (0.606-0.729), 0.722 (0.575-0.868) and 0.857 (0.789-0.925) respectively. They found that several of these biomarkers showed reasonable prediction for renal replacement therapy in this population. However, further studies to strengthen the findings are warranted before implementation in routine practice.

Biomarkers in Contrast Associated AKI

AKI of course encompasses a variety of different etiologies and mechanisms of kidney injury. Studies have looked more closely at biomarkers for particular AKI mechanisms, such as contrast-associated AKI, post-operative AKI and hepatorenal syndrome.

Several studies have looked specifically at the association between NGAL and contrast-associated AKI. A meta-analysis of 14 studies and 1520 patients found NGAL had a pooled AUC for predicting contrast-associated AKI of 0.93, with a diagnostic odds ratio 42.52, sensitivity 83.98%, specificity 89.03% using a mean cut-off NGAL value of 52.4mg/ml [27].

A sub study of the Prevention of Serious Adverse Events Following Angiography (PRESERVE) trial looked at pre-angiography biomarkers of injury and repair as predictors of contrast-associated AKI, including KIM-1, NGAL, IL-18, MCP-1, UMOD and YKL-40 [28].

They measured serum biomarkers in 916 patients and urine biomarkers in 797 patients. They found several markers were associated with major adverse kidney events and death (MAKE-D), but with only modest discriminatory capacity. Plasma KIM-1 was the only biomarker significantly associated with contrast associated AKI. This study and a subsequent study front he same group indeed suggests that the pathophysiology of contrast associated AKI, which is often transient in nature and recovers, may not be tubular injury and may require clinical adjudication rather than biomarkers [29, 30].

A recent prospective study of 490 patients undergoing coronary angiography looked at urine NGAL, KIM-1 and calprotectin <24 hours before angiography as predictors of contrast - associated AKI [27, 31]. They found that the 30 patients who developed AKI had 3.1-fold higher baseline urinary NGAL/creatinine ratios than those who did not develop AKI. Urine NGAL/creatinine ratio had an AUC of 0.68 (95% CI 0.60-0.81) and negative predictive value of 96.5% for NGAL/creatinine ratio <56.4ug/mg. There was no significant difference in KIM-1 or calprotectin. Although there are some conflicting results between studies, it seems NGAL may be a useful biomarker in contrast-associated AKI, particularly for its negative predictive value.

Biomarkers in Postoperative AKI

Several studies have also looked at the use of biomarkers to predict post-operative AKI. In a 2015 meta-analysis of 28 studies reporting intraoperative or early postoperative biomarkers for patients undergoing cardiac surgery, they found modest predictive ability of serum and urine biomarkers, with AUROC values <0.7 or <0.75, including urine NGAL, KIM-1, NAG, cystatin C, liver-type fatty acid binding protein, and IL-18 [27, 31, 32]. In the Translational Research Investigating Biomarker Endpoints in Acute Kidney Injury (TRIBE-AKI) prospective cohort of 1199 patients undergoing cardiac surgery, post-operative urinary biomarkers IL-18, NGAL, KIM-1, L-FABP and albumin were also examined as predictors of duration of AKI [33]. They found 34% of the population developed at least stage 1 AKI. Higher concentrations of all biomarkers were associated with greater odds of a longer duration of AKI. Similar studies have been conducted in the post-operative liver transplant population. A recent systematic review identified 11 studies with 563 patients where urine and plasma NGAL was studied to predict post-operative AKI after liver transplant [34]. They found AUROC values ranging from 0.5-0.83 for urine and 0.54-0.86 for plasma NGAL. These studies show while there is an association between biomarkers and post-operative AKI, the results thus far are modest and variable between studies, both in study design and findings. Further prospective studies are warranted.

Biomarkers in Hepatorenal AKI

In patients with cirrhosis, urinary biomarkers have also been shown to be associated with AKI progression and death. In a multicenter, prospective study of 188 patients with cirrhosis and AKI (defined by AKIN stage 1 criteria), they found NGAL, IL-18, KIM-1, L-FABP and albuminuria were independently associated with a combined outcome of AKI progression and death [35]. No biomarker was associated with progression of AKI alone. FeNa was also not associated with AKI progression. Other studies in this population have focused on the use of biomarkers to differentiate between causes of AKI.

BIOMARKERS USED TO DIFFERENTIATE TUBULAR INJURY FROM HYPERCREATININEMIA

Biomarkers have not only been studied for prediction of AKI, but also in differentiating the cause of AKI. In patients with cirrhosis for example, NGAL has been studied as a biomarker to differentiate between acute tubular necrosis vs. functional injury such as pre-renal AKI or hepato-renal syndrome, with the expectation that biomarkers would be higher in cases of tubular injury. NGAL had an AUC of 0.79 in differentiating ATN from HRS [35]. Urine NGAL and IL-18 also were shown to have good discrimination between ATN and other types of AKI in a systematic review of patients with cirrhosis, with AUCs of 0.89 and 0.88 respectively [35, 36].

Another study looked at patients presenting to the emergency room who had AKI based on AKIN serum creatinine criteria [37]. They measured urinary NGAL using a dipstick and ELISA method, and correlated this with whether patients had transient, sustained or undetectable changes in serum creatinine during admission. They found NGAL had high specificity 0.91 and negative predictive value 0.97 for identifying tubular injury. They propose this as a rapid bedside assay which may help identify kidney injury in real time without waiting for creatinine accumulation, identify cases of tubular injury where serum creatinine is not elevated due to renal reserve, and those with more severe tubular injury versus hemodynamically reversible changes in creatinine.

ROLE OF BIOMARKERS IN RESEARCH

While further study is needed before routine implementation of biomarkers in clinical practice, there may also be a promising role for the use of biomarkers in clinical trials. In particular, biomarkers associated with increased risk of kidney injury may help in selecting study populations which are more likely to experience outcomes and complications. This in turn can reduce sample size requirements, and study costs. In the PRESERVE trial substudy which looked at biomarkers associated with contrast associated AKI and major adverse kidney events and death, authors calculated that if they had screened patients using the 50th percentile of pre-angiography plasma KIM-1 or YKL-40, this would have reduced the sample size requirement by 30%, or about 2000 participants [28, 37].

Another trial used both KDIGO staging and plasma NGAL>150ng/ml as enrollment criteria in their trial comparing early versus delayed initiation of renal replacement therapy for patients with severe acute AKI [38]. They chose to include NGAL as inclusion criteria to select a population that was at greater risk for requiring renal replacement therapy (RRT). Among 231 participants, all patients in the early RRT group received RRT, and nearly all patients (108 out of 119) in the delayed group received RRT. Few patients however were actually excluded on the basis of having NGAL<150ng/dl (3 participants) after first screening for KDIGO stage 2 or greater and other initial exclusion criteria.

Similarly, Srisawat et al. used plasma NGAL at enrollment of ICU patients with RIFLE criteria AKI to separate patients into high pNGAL (> or equal to 400ng/ml), or low pNGAL (<400 ng/ml), and then randomized those in the high pNGAL group to early or standard RRT initiation [38, 39]. Amongst 40 patients in the high pNGAL group, they had more severity of illness and worse clinical outcome, but those randomized to early RRT did not have a difference in 28-day mortality compared to the standard group. In their study, all patients randomized to early RRT received RRT, 40% in the standard RRT group with high NGAL required RRT, while none in the low NGAL group required RRT. Thus, the utility of biomarkers in trial participant selection likely depends on the study population as well as cutoff values of biomarkers utilized. The optimal role for biomarkers in trials requires further study.

Acute Dialysis Quality Initiative Consensus Statement

A recent consensus document from the Acute Dialysis Quality Initiative (ADQI) covers this topic, and provides guidance for clinical aspects, as well as research in this area [11]. The workgroup has come up with 11 different consensus statements, and the entire document makes for useful reading for the reader interested in this subject. The actual consensus statements follow:

1. The decision to perform a Kidney Health Assessment (KHA) to gauge AKI susceptibility should integrate patient factors, including demographic characteristics, comorbidities, and previous AKI episodes with the expected intensity of a planned exposure that carries AKI risk. (Grade B, strong)
2. The types of functional and/or damage biomarker evaluation to be performed should be driven by the results of the KHA for AKI susceptibility. (Grade B, strong)
3. Biomarkers of acute damage are not interpretable prior to a kidney insult and should not be used for AKI risk assessment. (Grade A, strong)
4. Use validated biomarkers to identify patient populations for whom preventive interventions have been shown to improve outcomes. (Grade A, strong)
5. Combine clinical assessment and validated biomarkers to triage patients and optimize the timing and type of interventions designed to improve processes of care and patient outcomes. (Grade C, strong)
6. A combination of damage and functional biomarkers, along with clinical information, should be used to improve the diagnostic accuracy of AKI, to recognize the different pathophysiological processes, to discriminate AKI etiology, and to assess AKI severity. (Grade B, conditional)
7. A combination of biomarkers may assist the planning of therapy and management of AKI. (Grade C, conditional)
8. Inclusion of biomarker data with clinical assessments can be used to identify patients who will need KRT and facilitate optimal timing of KRT initiation. (Grade C, conditional)
9. Novel biomarkers can be used for prediction of duration and recovery of AKI. (Grade C, weak)

10. There is insufficient evidence to recommend the routine use of novel biomarkers to refine acute kidney disease staging. (Grade C, strong)
11. Biomarkers predictive of CKD staging and progression should be incorporated into a comprehensive post-AKI care bundle and KHA. (Grade C, strong)

Conceptually, biomarkers could be added to AKI staging, as being positive or negative in the presence of a rise in creatinine or a fall in urine output. This could allow a substage of AKI staging into A (biomarker negative) and B (biomarker positive). In addition, the workgroup conceptualized a 1S stage, with no AKI based on traditional criteria, but with a positive biomarker [11]. Needless to say, these stages provide a theoretical framework to think about and perform clinical research.

Conclusion

Creatinine has been the marker of kidney function, in both chronic as well as acute kidney injury. It has several weaknesses, which are especially glaring in the field of acute kidney injury. Specifically, creatinine does not give an early enough warning about AKI, nor does it help discriminate among causes of AKI. In the last 2 decades, several biomarkers have been described, most with diagnostic properties, but also some with predictive and prognostic associations stronger than creatinine. Some biomarkers (NGAL, Nephrocheck) are now even commercially available. Biomarkers can also be extremely useful in the setting of clinical research, allowing for more efficient clinical trials. The recent ADQI consensus statement provides a clear path forward for the further development and implementation of biomarkers in AKI.

References

[1] Bellomo R, Ronco C, Kellum JA, Mehta RL, Palevsky P; Acute Dialysis Quality Initiative workgroup. Acute renal failure - definition, outcome measures, animal models, fluid therapy and information technology needs: the Second International Consensus Conference of the Acute Dialysis Quality Initiative (ADQI) Group. *Crit Care.* 2004;8(4):R204–12.

[2] Mehta RL, Kellum JA, Shah SV, Molitoris BA, Ronco C, Warnock DG, et al.; Acute Kidney Injury Network. Acute Kidney Injury Network: report of an initiative to improve outcomes in acute kidney injury. *Crit Care.* 2007;11(2):R31.

[3] Kellum JA, Lameire N; KDIGO AKI Guideline Work Group. Diagnosis, evaluation, and management of acute kidney injury: a KDIGO summary (Part 1). *Crit Care.* 2013;17(1):204.

[4] James MT, Levey AS, Tonelli M, Tan Z, Barry R, Pannu N, et al. Incidence and Prognosis of Acute Kidney Diseases and Disorders Using an Integrated Approach to Laboratory Measurements in a Universal Health Care System. *JAMA Netw Open.* 2019;2(4):e191795–191795.

[5] Mullens W, Abrahams Z, Francis GS, Sokos G, Taylor DO, Starling RC, et al. Importance of venous congestion for worsening of renal function in advanced decompensated heart failure. *J Am Coll Cardiol*. 2009;53(7):589–96.

[6] Sriperumbuduri S, Clark E, Hiremath S. New Insights Into Mechanisms of Acute Kidney Injury in Heart Disease. *Can J Cardiol*. 2019;35(9):1158–69.

[7] Biomarkers Definitions Working Group. Biomarkers and surrogate endpoints: preferred definitions and conceptual framework. *Clin Pharmacol Ther*. 2001;69(3):89–95.

[8] Biomarkers IR. *Validity and Validation*. [cited 26 Feb 2021]. Available: http://www.inchem.org/documents/ehc/ehc/ehc222.htm

[9] *FDA-NIH Biomarker Working Group. BEST (Biomarkers, EndpointS, and other Tools) Resource*. 2016 [cited 27 Feb 2021]. Available: https://www.ncbi.nlm.nih.gov/books/NBK326791/

[10] Califf RM. Biomarker definitions and their applications. *Exp Biol Med* (Maywood). 2018;;243(3):213–21.

[11] Ostermann M, Zarbock A, Goldstein S, Kashani K, Macedo E, Murugan R, et al. Recommendations on Acute Kidney Injury Biomarkers From the Acute Disease Quality Initiative Consensus Conference: A Consensus Statement. *JAMA Netw Open*. 2020;3(10):e2019209–2019209.

[12] Tomašev N, Glorot X, Rae JW, Zielinski M, Askham H, Saraiva A, et al. A clinically applicable approach to continuous prediction of future acute kidney injury. *Nature*. 2019;572(7767):116–9.

[13] Moledina DG, Parikh CR. Phenotyping of Acute Kidney Injury: Beyond Serum Creatinine. *Semin Nephrol*. 2018 Jan;38(1):3–11.

[14] Coca SG. Ptolemy and Copernicus Revisited: The Complex Interplay between the Kidneys and Heart Failure. *Clin J Am Soc Nephrol*. 2018;13(6):825–8.

[15] Parikh CR, Moledina DG, Coca SG, Thiessen-Philbrook HR, Garg AX. Application of new acute kidney injury biomarkers in human randomized controlled trials. *Kidney Int*. 2016;89(6):1372–9.

[16] Haase-Fielitz A, Haase M, Devarajan P. Neutrophil gelatinase-associated lipocalin as a biomarker of acute kidney injury: a critical evaluation of current status. *Ann Clin Biochem*. 2014;51(Pt 3):335–51.

[17] *Product Information*. [cited 27 Feb 2021]. Available: https://www.nephrocheck.com/global/product-information/

[18] Hiremath S, Clark EG. Albuminuria as a risk factor for acute kidney injury: what is the evidence? *Nephrol Dial Transplant*. 2020;35(12):2026–9.

[19] Coca SG, Yalavarthy R, Concato J, Parikh CR. Biomarkers for the diagnosis and risk stratification of acute kidney injury: a systematic review. *Kidney Int*. 2008;73(9):1008–16.

[20] Legrand M, Hollinger A, Vieillard-Baron A, Dépret F, Cariou A, Deye N, et al.; French and euRopean Outcome reGistry in ICUs (FROG-ICU) Investigators. One-Year Prognosis of Kidney Injury at Discharge From the ICU: A Multicenter Observational Study. *Crit Care Med*. 2019;47(12):e953–61.

[21] Chawla LS, Davison DL, Brasha-Mitchell E, Koyner JL, Arthur JM, Shaw AD, et al. Development and standardization of a furosemide stress test to predict the severity of acute kidney injury. *Crit Care*. 2013;17(5):R207.

[22] Chen JJ, Chang CH, Huang YT, Kuo G. Furosemide stress test as a predictive marker of acute kidney injury progression or renal replacement therapy: a systemic review and meta-analysis. *Crit Care*. 2020;24(1):202.

[23] Jufar AH, Lankadeva YR, May CN, Cochrane AD, Bellomo R, Evans RG. Renal functional reserve: from physiological phenomenon to clinical biomarker and beyond. *Am J Physiol Regul Integr Comp Physiol*. 2020;319(6):R690–702.

[24] Husain-Syed F, Ferrari F, Sharma A, Danesi TH, Bezerra P, Lopez-Giacoman S, et al. Preoperative Renal Functional Reserve Predicts Risk of Acute Kidney Injury After Cardiac Operation. *Ann Thorac Surg*. 2018;105(4):1094–101.

[25] Kashani K, Al-Khafaji A, Ardiles T, Artigas A, Bagshaw SM, Bell M, et al. Discovery and validation of cell cycle arrest biomarkers in human acute kidney injury. *Crit Care*. 2013;17(1):R25.

[26] Klein SJ, Brandtner AK, Lehner GF, Ulmer H, Bagshaw SM, Wiedermann CJ, et al. Biomarkers for prediction of renal replacement therapy in acute kidney injury: a systematic review and meta-analysis. *Intensive Care Med*. 2018;44(3):323–36.

[27] Wang K, Duan CY, Wu J, Liu Y, Bei WJ, Chen JY, et al. Predictive Value of Neutrophil Gelatinase-Associated Lipocalin for Contrast-Induced Acute Kidney Injury After Cardiac Catheterization: A Meta-analysis. *Can J Cardiol*. 2016;32(8):1033.e19–29.

[28] Parikh CR, Liu C, Mor MK, Palevsky PM, Kaufman JS, Thiessen Philbrook H, et al. Kidney Biomarkers of Injury and Repair as Predictors of Contrast-Associated AKI: A Substudy of the PRESERVE Trial. *Am J Kidney Dis*. 2020;75(2):187–94.

[29] Liu C, Mor MK, Palevsky PM, Kaufman JS, Thiessen Philbrook H, Weisbord SD, et al. Postangiography Increases in Serum Creatinine and Biomarkers of Injury and Repair. *Clin J Am Soc Nephrol*. 2020;15(9):1240–50.

[30] Hiremath S, Velez JC. Preventing a nonexistent entity: the curious case of contrast and acute kidney injury. *Curr Opin Nephrol Hypertens*. 2020;29(1):152–60.

[31] Seibert FS, Heringhaus A, Pagonas N, Rudolf H, Rohn B, Bauer F, et al. Biomarkers in the prediction of contrast media induced nephropathy - the BITCOIN study. *PLoS One*. 2020;15(7):e0234921.

[32] Ho J, Tangri N, Komenda P, Kaushal A, Sood M, Brar R, et al. Urinary, Plasma, and Serum Biomarkers' Utility for Predicting Acute Kidney Injury Associated With Cardiac Surgery in Adults: A Meta-analysis. *Am J Kidney Dis*. 2015;66(6):993–1005.

[33] Coca SG, Nadkarni GN, Garg AX, Koyner J, Thiessen-Philbrook H, McArthur E, et al.; TRIBE-AKI Consortium. First Post-Operative Urinary Kidney Injury Biomarkers and Association with the Duration of AKI in the TRIBE-AKI Cohort. *PLoS One*. 2016;11(8):e0161098.

[34] Yeung AC, Morozov A, Robertson FP, Fuller BJ, Davidson BR. Neutrophil Gelatinase-Associated Lipocalin (NGAL) in predicting acute kidney injury following orthotopic liver transplantation: A systematic review. *Int J Surg*. 2018;59:48–54.

[35] Belcher JM, Sanyal AJ, Peixoto AJ, Perazella MA, Lim J, Thiessen-Philbrook H, et al.; TRIBE-AKI Consortium. Kidney biomarkers and differential diagnosis of patients with cirrhosis and acute kidney injury. *Hepatology*. 2014;60(2):622–32.

[36] Puthumana J, Ariza X, Belcher JM, Graupera I, Ginès P, Parikh CR. Urine Interleukin 18 and Lipocalin 2 Are Biomarkers of Acute Tubular Necrosis in Patients With Cirrhosis: A Systematic Review and Meta-analysis. *Clin Gastroenterol Hepatol*. 2017;15(7):1003–1013.e3.

[37] Stevens JS, Xu K, Corker A, Gopal TS, Sayan OR, Geraghty EP, et al. Rule Out Acute Kidney Injury in the Emergency Department With a Urinary Dipstick. *Kidney Int Rep*. 2020;5(11):1982–92.

[38] Zarbock A, Kellum JA, Schmidt C, Van Aken H, Wempe C, Pavenstädt H, et al. Effect of Early vs Delayed Initiation of Renal Replacement Therapy on Mortality in Critically Ill Patients With Acute Kidney Injury: The ELAIN Randomized Clinical Trial. *JAMA*. 2016;315(20):2190–9.

[39] Srisawat N, Laoveeravat P, Limphunudom P, Lumlertgul N, Peerapornratana S, Tiranathanagul K, et al. The effect of early renal replacement therapy guided by plasma neutrophil gelatinase associated lipocalin on outcome of acute kidney injury: A feasibility study. *J Crit Care*. 2018;43:36–41.

In: Issues in Kidney Disease – Acute Kidney Injury
Editors: S. Z. Fadem and A. Arslan Yousuf Awan
ISBN: 978-1-68507-002-1

Chapter 5

NON-INVASIVE IMAGING IN ACUTE KIDNEY INJURY

Forrest F. Lindsay-McGinn[1], MD, Ira H. Blau[2], MD, Devin M. McKelvey[2], DO and Nathaniel C. Reisinger[2,*], MD

[1]Department of Emergency Medicine, Penn Medicine, Philadelphia, PA, USA
[2]Division of Renal, Electrolyte and Hypertension, Penn Medicine. Philadelphia, PA, USA

ABSTRACT

The incidence and recognition of acute kidney injury (AKI) has been steadily rising for decades. AKI is associated with poor outcomes and increased need for kidney replacement therapy. Performing timely imaging is critical in AKI to establish the correct diagnosis. Ultrasound is the modality of choice for the initial imaging in AKI due to its low cost, wide availability, and lack of ionizing radiation. Ultrasound readily identifies AKI due to obstruction and can add data for differentiating AKI versus chronic kidney disease (CKD) in patients with decreased kidney function of unknown duration. Point-of-care ultrasound (POCUS) employs ultrasound devices at the bedside to rapidly exclude obstruction and add data on the patient's volume status to guide fluid, diuretic, and ultrafiltration therapies. Computed tomography (CT), magnetic resonance imaging (MRI), and nuclear medicine studies complement ultrasound, adding additional information specific to the presenting complaint.

Keywords: acute kidney injury, ultrasound, point-of-care ultrasound, computed tomography, magnetic, resonance imaging, nuclear scintigraphy, contrast-enhanced ultrasound

INTRODUCTION

The incidence and recognition of acute kidney injury (AKI) has been steadily rising for decades. AKI is associated with poor outcomes and increased need for kidney replacement

---

* Corresponding Author's E-mail: ncreisinger@gmail.com.

therapy. Anatomic data on the kidney are key to excluding obstruction while parenchymal characteristics such as size, cortical thickness, echogenicity, and presence of hydronephrosis can lend clues to the etiology of AKI. However, the retroperitoneal position of the kidneys and free-floating relation to surrounding structures make physical examination unreliable and history alone does not reliably exclude obstructive nephropathy. Ultrasound is the modality of choice for initial imaging of the kidney given its safety with no ionizing radiation, wide availability, and low cost. Point-of-care ultrasound (POCUS) is imaging at the bedside performed by the provider and allows for more rapid medical decision making and assessment of change over time evaluating response to therapeutic maneuvers. Other imaging modalities such as computed tomography (CT), magnetic resonance imaging (MRI), and nuclear medicine imaging add additional information specific to the presenting complaint [1]. This textbook chapter serves as a guide for non-invasive imaging for AKI for the practicing nephrologist.

ULTRASOUND

Introduction

Ultrasound is the modality of choice for the initial non-invasive kidney imaging given its safety, ease of use, and wide availability. B-mode ultrasound imaging provides reliable data on chronicity of kidney disease such as kidney size, echogenicity, and cortical thickness as well as detecting most pathologic features including cysts, calculi, masses, and hydronephrosis. Doppler imaging adds functional assessment of kidney arterial and venous anatomy.

History

Properties of acoustics—the science of sound—date back as far as the 6th century BCE when Pythagoras described the mathematical principles of stringed instruments. Ultrasound was not known until 1794 when the Italian priest Lazzaro Spallanzani first described echolocation in bats. The development of technology employing ultrasound was made possible by the discovery of the piezoelectric effect by the brothers Pierre and Jacques Curie in 1880. Subsequent developments in ultrasound technologies accelerated with the advent of sonar for nautical applications in the 1910s following the Titanic disaster and submarine warfare of the first world war. Ultimately these principles were used for medical applications beginning with the neurologist Karl Dussik in the 1940s and developed into modern diagnostic ultrasonography by Howry and Holmes (a nephrologist) in the 1960s [2].

Basics of Ultrasound Physics

Ultrasound, like other medical imaging modalities, is a form of tomography or imaging by sections using a penetrating wave. Ultrasound employs sound waves with frequency of 2-10 MHz (megahertz) well above the range of human hearing which is around 20 kHz (kilohertz). Sounds are generated by a specialized crystal called a piezoelectric. Piezoelectrics generate an electric field when mechanical strain is applied—termed the direct piezoelectric effect—and generate mechanical strain when and electric field is applied—termed the reverse piezoelectric effect. When used in medical imaging, piezoelectrics, principally lead zirconate titanate, are aligned in the ultrasound transducer which produce pulses of sound waves as rapidly alternating voltages deform the crystals. The sound waves emanate into the desired structure and those that are scattered or refracted are lost while those that are reflected to the piezoelectric generate an electric current in response to the mechanical strain. This is termed the pulse-echo principle. These electric currents are analyzed by the computer which creates a greyscale image. Table 1 provides additional key terminology in ultrasound [3].

Table 1. Key Terminology in Medical Ultrasound

Term	Description
Depth	The distance of a structure from the ultrasound transducer.
Gain	Overall brightness setting of a B-mode image.
Echogenicity	Relative brightness of a given structure.
Hypoechoic	A structure that appears darker relative to a reference structure.
Hyperechoic	A structure that appears brighter relative to a reference structure.
Isoechoic	A structure that appears the same brightness as a reference structure.
Anechoic	A structure that appears completely lacking in all echoes. Fluids and fluid-filled structures such as cysts tend to be anechoic.
Acoustic Shadow	Anechoic stripe deep to a highly reflective structure such as a stone or bone due to poor penetration of sound waves.
Posterior acoustic enhancement	Hyperechoic stripe deep to a fluid-filled structure such as the bladder or a kidney cyst due to exuberant sound wave penetration.

Transducer Selection

Depending on the application of ultrasound, different ultrasound transducers are selected. Generally speaking, the higher the frequency of the ultrasound used, the higher the spatial resolution and the lower the depth of beam penetration. Conversely, using an ultrasound with lower frequency provides a greater depth of beam penetration at the expense of less spatial resolution. Linear transducers are high frequency transducers with a narrow, flat interface intended for superficial applications such as the assessment of skin or the evaluation of hemodialysis access. Lower frequency transducers are ideal for imaging deeper structures and their shapes are optimized to application. Cardiac transducers have a small footprint fitting to narrow windows in the intercostal spaces while abdominal transducers have a wide and curved footprint ideal for fitting abdominal viscera into the same ultrasound image [3].

Ultrasound Modes

B-mode (brightness mode) is the default mode of most ultrasound devices and is the most commonly used mode in ultrasound. B-mode is a two-dimensional mode with depth determined by the time to the echo return and brightness determined based on the intensity of reflected signal, also termed greyscale. The extent of reflection of the sound wave back to the transducer determines how bright the signal appears, termed echogenicity. B-mode generates a map of structures with relative positions and brightness.

M-mode (motion mode) tracks motion over time along a single axis in a B-mode image tracking the anatomic relationships between structures as they change over time. This is particularly useful in cardiac ultrasonography to capture relative positions of the chambers and valves through the cardiac cycle.

Doppler mode is imaging of the relative motion and velocity of tissues and fluids in the body with respect to the ultrasound transducer. This mode uses the Doppler effect to determine the relative motions by measuring the frequency shift of ultrasound echoes emanating from objects in motion such as red blood cells. Blood flow can be visually assessed as either moving away from or towards the transducer probe by calculating the frequency shift of a sample of blood. By default, flow away from the transducer is colored blue and flow toward the transducer is colored red. A handy mnemonic for this directionality is "Blue Away, Red Towards" (BART).

Basic Technique

To image the kidneys, the patient is placed in the supine position. The curvilinear transducer is selected, though a cardiac transducer can be used to obtain views through an intercostal space. As kidneys are estimated to move by as much as 4-5 cm with respiration, the patient is asked to hold a breath at maximal inspiration. The transducer is placed in the posterior axillary line rotated 15-30 degrees posteriorly to align the transducer with the long axis of the kidney. The ultrasonographer sweeps the beam from end to end visualizing the entire kidney in the long axis. The operator then rotates 90 degrees counterclockwise to image the kidney in the short axis, sweeping from superior pole to inferior pole. On the right, the liver is used as an acoustic window. On the left, the spleen is used as an acoustic window. Owing to the more superior and posterior position of the left kidney, the transducer is positioned more posteriorly. The patient can be shifted to the right lateral decubitus position to further aide in imaging. Transplanted kidneys are visualized in their heterotopic location most typically in the right lower quadrant of the abdomen. Ultrasonographers should be aware of congenitally ectopic kidneys such as horseshoe kidneys (occurring in 1 in 500) and pelvic kidneys (occurring in fewer than 1 in 2200) as well as unilateral renal agenesis (occurring in 1 in 1000)[4].[4]

Kidney Appearance

The kidneys appear as ellipsoids with a hyperechoic inner layer comprising the fat-filled medullary sinus and hypoechoic outer layer consisting of cortex and medulla. The medullary pyramids appear hypoechoic compared to the remainder of the parenchyma. Normal kidney cortical echogenicity is isoechoic or hypoechoic compared with the liver on the right and spleen on the left. A thin fibrous capsule surrounds the kidneys. At the hilum, renal artery and vein as well as the ureter enter the sinus. Typical kidney size is 9-13 cm in length, 3-7 cm wide, and 3-6 cm thick with the left kidney slightly larger than the right. Typical parenchymal thickness is 1.1-2.5 cm [3].

Advantages of Ultrasound

Ultrasound is the preferred initial imaging modality for AKI. Low cost makes ultrasound ubiquitous, even in resource limited locations. Portability allows use even in clinically unstable patients in critical care units. The use of harmless sound waves as opposed to ionizing radiation of x-ray computed tomography makes ultrasound ideal even for pre-natal imaging and imaging in children. Caution should be used with more advanced Doppler techniques due to thermal risk and cavitation from excessive scanning.

Echogenicity

Kidney ultrasound provides critical information on the presence or absence of pathology in AKI. Findings of increased cortical echogenicity provide supporting evidence of pathology. Increased echogenicity is observed with interstitial inflammation or fibrosis. However, kidneys can appear echogenic in the context of AKI, as with acute tubular necrosis or glomerulonephritis, as well as in CKD. Increased cortical echogenicity, thus, does not differentiate AKI from CKD. Further, echogenicity is judged on a relative scale by comparing kidney cortical echogenicity to the neighboring liver or spleen. The presence of pathology in these organs can be a confounding factor in assessing kidney echogenicity such as with increased liver echogenicity in fatty liver disease.

Size and Cortical Thickness

Findings of decreased kidney size less than 9 cm and decreased cortical thickness less than 1 cm support a diagnosis of CKD. The combination of both small size and increased cortical echogenicity is strongly associated with non-recovery of kidney function. However, these are relatively late findings in the course of CKD with numerous exceptions with size being preserved in diabetic kidney disease, HIV-associated nephropathy, and infiltrative diseases such as amyloidosis. Further, the kidneys are obliquely oriented in the body with the superior pole relatively posteromedial and the inferior pole relatively anterolateral. Thus, when scanning, the ultrasound transducer must be oriented in the same plane or the kidney is imaged off axis leading to underestimation of kidney size. Small size is relatively specific for the presence of CKD, but insensitive [5].

Hydronephrosis

Obstruction may occur at any point along the urinary tract, most commonly at the ureteropelvic junction, ureterovesical junction, and the urethra. Ultrasound of the kidneys and bladder is sufficient for the detection of hydronephrosis in most patients, though often fails to localize the level of obstruction owing to changes in acoustic impedance as sound waves pass through bowel gas. Hydronephrosis is the sonographic hallmark of obstructive nephropathy. Hydronephrosis is visualized as anechoic space representing the dilated collecting system interdigitating withing the hyperechoic renal sinus. Hydronephrosis can be distinguished from prominent renal vasculature with color flow Doppler. Sonographic severity of hydronephrosis correlates with duration of obstruction. Hydronephrosis is graded as mild, moderate, or severe based on extent of the calyceal dilatation. In mild hydronephrosis, enlarged calyces are visible, but renal parenchymal architecture including both papillae and pyramids is preserved.

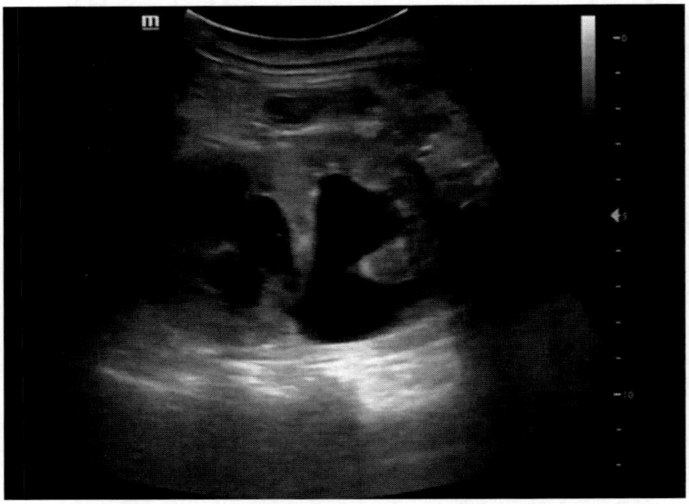

Figure 1. Long axis ultrasound of the right kidney demonstrating severe hydronephrosis in a patient presenting with ureteral obstruction due to obstructing urothelial malignancy.

With moderate hydronephrosis, major and minor calyces are dilated, and papillae and pyramids appear blunted. In severe hydronephrosis, medullary structures are completely obliterated, and cortical effacement is present. Care should be taken in clinical correlation of hydronephrosis, particularly with mild hydronephrosis which may be present in high flow states such as post-ATN diuresis and diabetes insipidus as well as in pregnancy [6]. Figure 1 demonstrates severe hydronephrosis.

Renal Calculi

The most common cause of post-renal obstruction, renal calculi appear as discrete, well-circumscribed hyperechoic structures that cast an acoustic shadow, an anechoic stripe deep to the structure resulting from absence of passage of sound waves. Ultrasound has relatively low sensitivity in detecting stones as obstructing ureteral stones are often obscured by bowel gas overlying the course of the ureter. Non-contrast CT is generally considered the modality of choice for the detection of stones disease. However, a randomized controlled trial of 2759 patients presenting to the emergency department with suspected nephrolithiasis showed no difference in high-risk diagnosis with complications, serious adverse events, or repeat acute care utilization among those with initial imaging modality of ultrasound, point-of-care ultrasound performed by emergency physicians, or abdominal computed tomography. Patients initially imaged with ultrasound had lower cumulative radiation exposure [7].

Other Findings

When ultrasound is undertaken to evaluate AKI, it is common to encounter a variety of other benign findings as well as pathologic processes unrelated to the etiology of AKI. Developmental variants are common and of no clinical significance but can be inaccurately interpreted as pathology or cause distress to the patient when appearing on a radiologist's report. Fusion defects ranging from a simple junctional parenchymal defect or hypertrophied column of Bertin to completely duplicated collecting systems may occur. The presence of persistent fetal lobulation or a Dromedary hump owing to the impression of the spleen on the left kidney can be misconstrued as potentially neoplastic. The presence of an extrarenal pelvis is easily mistaken for hydronephrosis but lacks the characteristic calyceal dilatation [8].

Renal cysts are very common with simple cysts appearing anechoic with smooth, thin walls and exhibit posterior acoustic enhancement which appears as a hyperechoic stripe deep to the cyst owing to more exuberant passage of sound waves through the fluid-filled structure than surrounding parenchyma. The presence of septations, poorly defined walls, internal echoes, and mixed solid-cystic components should raise suspicions for complex cysts or renal masses such as renal cell carcinoma and angiomyolipoma. The presence of multiple simple cysts raises the prospect of polycystic kidney disease [9].

Kidney Transplant Allograft

Owing to the more superficial location of the typical kidney transplant allograft in the iliac fossa, ultrasound is the imaging modality of choice. Technique is similar to native kidneys with images taken in both long and short axes taking care to align the transducer with the long axis of the kidney noting that orientation is highly variable. Hydronephrosis is easily visualized in the transplant allograft, though it is common to have mild hydronephrosis owing to reflux from the uretero-vesical anastomosis. Relative echogenicity is difficult to evaluate without a neighboring solid organ for comparison. Fluid collections including lymphocele, hematoma, and urinoma are frequent complications in the immediate post-transplant period. All appear initially as anechoic fluid adjacent to the kidney, though more echogenic layering occurs with hematoma as blood clots [10].

Contrast-Enhanced Ultrasound

Visualization of microcirculation of the kidneys as well as advanced assessment of renal masses is limited. Contrast-enhanced ultrasound (CEUS) using intravenously administered gas-filled microbubbles is an emerging technology for assessing vascular abnormalities and for better delineation of renal masses. Sulfur hexafluoride lipid type A microspheres and perflutren lipid microspheres are novel ultrasound contrast agents comprising a microparticle 1-6 micrometers in diameter, consisting of an outer phospholipid coat and inner fluorine-based gas. The first of these agents was approved by the FDA in 2016 and they are used clinically in echocardiography to better delineate the endocardial border. In contrast to CT and MRI, these intravenous agents can be administered safely in patients with AKI. For renal imaging, the lipid microspheres are administered intravenously and transit to the arterial side within 1-2 minutes where they enhance echogenicity of vasculature allowing better characterization of microcirculation and provide enhancement for complex masses. Following disruption of the lipid layer, the inert gas travels to the lung where it is exhaled. Data regarding efficacy are limited, but early studies have shown good sensitivity for detection of renal malignant lesions [11].

POINT-OF-CARE ULTRASOUND

Introduction

Clinician performed ultrasound at the bedside, also known as point-of-care ultrasound (POCUS), is an increasingly accessible and powerful imaging modality due to advances in technology and reductions in cost and size of devices. Many providers find POCUS preferable to referral radiology studies in specific situations because they can answer clinical questions quickly and providers can directly correlate their findings with their knowledge of the patient at that moment in time. POCUS provides several major advantages for assessing AKI. The first advantage is that the physician can immediately identify urinary tract obstruction. The second advantage is to provide the clinician with objective data pertaining to the intravascular volume status of the patient which is essential for management of AKI. Third, POCUS can aid in the rapid differentiation of shock and assessment of cardiac function, which frequently are the underlying cause for AKI. POCUS has several strengths for assessing volume status in the setting of AKI because it is noninvasive, provides instantaneous data for decision making, and can be repeated as many times as necessary to monitor progress. The most common studies for volume assessment include cardiac, IVC, and lung ultrasound [12].

Kidney Ultrasound

Rapid identification of obstructive uropathy as the cause of AKI is essential because it requires a fundamentally different treatment approach from other causes of AKI and often requires consultation with urology or interventional radiology to mechanically resolve the cause of obstruction. The assessment for obstructive uropathy consists of the evaluation of both kidneys for hydronephrosis, ureteral jets, and a post void residual volume of the bladder. POCUS is not the gold standard for hydronephrosis but has moderate sensitivity and specificity. Emergency physicians using POCUS to evaluate patients with suspected kidney stones for hydronephrosis were found to be able to identify hydronephrosis with a sensitivity of 81% and specificity of 59% when compared to a CT reference standard interpreted by radiologists. Specificity increases with severity of hydronephrosis [13]. False positive diagnosis of hydronephrosis can be caused by parapelvic cysts, hypoechoic renal pyramids, or a full urinary bladder where no attempt to void has been made prior to imaging [14].

Bladder Ultrasound

Bladder ultrasound can aid in assessing true bladder volumes compared to bladder scanners and to visualize ureteral jets. The bladder is one of the simplest organs to evaluate with ultrasound given that a fluid filled structure is most conducive to the passage of ultrasound waves. Transverse and sagittal views of the bladder are obtained preferably with an abdominal transducer, though a cardiac transducer can be used. With the patient supine, the transducer is placed on the abdominal wall just superior the symphysis pubis with the indicator facing the patient's right. The sonographer sweeps the transducer through the full length of the bladder superiorly to inferiorly to obtain transverse axis images, then rotates the transducer 90 degrees with indicator facing superiorly to obtain sagittal views, again sweeping through the length of the bladder. The image is frozen on the largest dimensions which are measured. Bladder volume is calculated as:

$$volume = 0.52 \cdot length \cdot width \cdot height.$$

This method is superior to a simple bladder scan. Bladder scanners are unreliable when a patient has progressively worsening kidney injury because estimations of bladder volume can be confounded by abdominal ascites, bladder diverticulum, midline abdominal masses, and user error [15]. Figure 2 demonstrates a markedly distended bladder due to urethral obstruction in patient presenting with AKI and fluid overload.

The expression of urine from the ureteral orifice into the bladder is termed ureteral jet. Ureteral jets are visualized with ultrasound using color Doppler. Their frequency and duration can be assessed in the setting of suspected ureteral obstruction to shed light on the grade of obstruction. Frequent ureteral jets every 15-20 seconds, lasting less than a second is useful for ruling out high grade obstruction. However, merely visualizing a single ureteral jet cannot reliably rule out high grade obstruction.

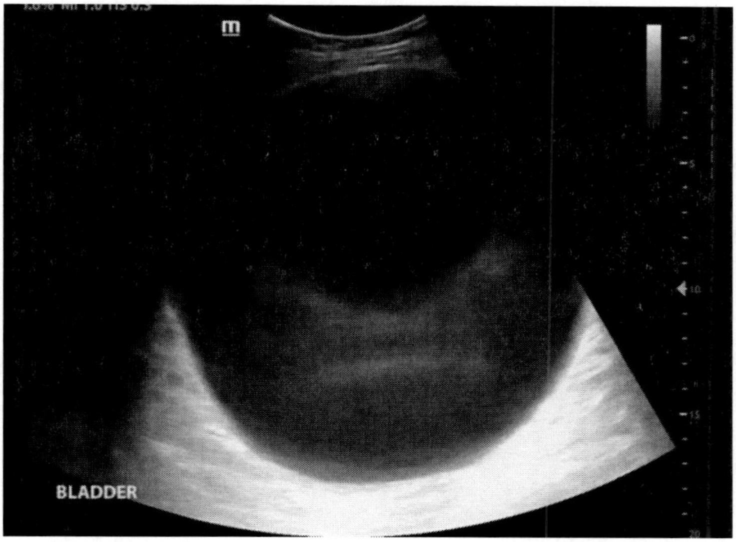

Figure 2. Transverse plane ultrasound of a markedly distended bladder due to urethral obstruction in patient presenting with AKI and fluid overload.

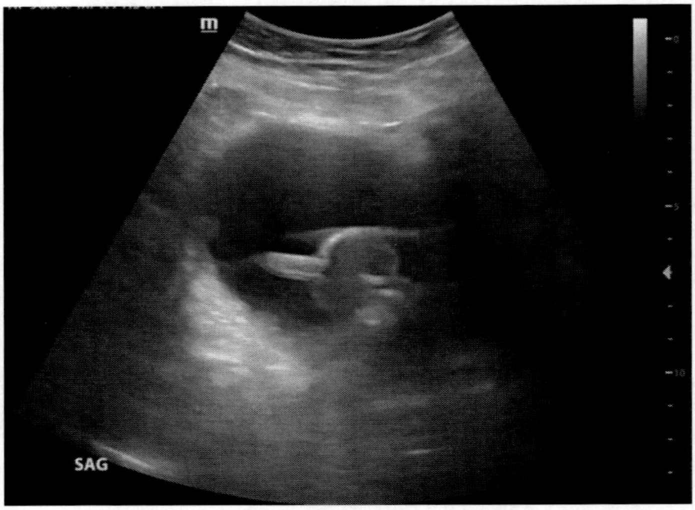

Figure 3. Sagittal ultrasound showing an obstructed urinary catheter with filled balloon seen in bladder.

Bladder ultrasound can also give helpful information in the situation of a urinary catheter that is not functioning. In patients with an appropriately positioned urinary catheter that is obstructed, the catheter balloon will be visualized within a full bladder. In the case of hematuria, blood clots within the bladder are easily visualized. If the urinary catheter is not in the bladder it can often be visualized in the vagina or prostatic urethra or even in the distal ureter. If a patient with abdominal ascites is thought to have an obstructed urinary catheter due to decreased urine output, POCUS is superior to bladder scanners because the provider can differentiate the abdominal ascites from the bladder. Figure 3 demonstrates an obstructed urinary catheter with balloon seen in bladder. Figure 4 shows a urinary catheter balloon seen within the bladder with thickened wall and blood clots. Figure 5 illustrates the sagittal view of bladder at right with adjacent abdominal ascites at left.

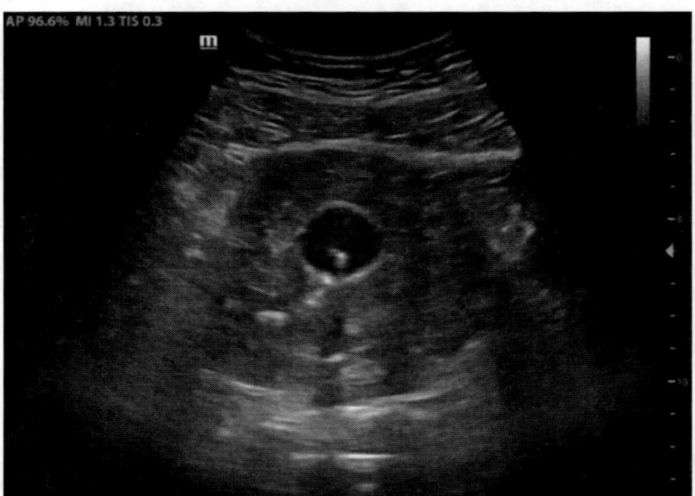

Figure 4. Sagittal ultrasound with urinary catheter balloon seen within bladder with thickened wall and blood clots.

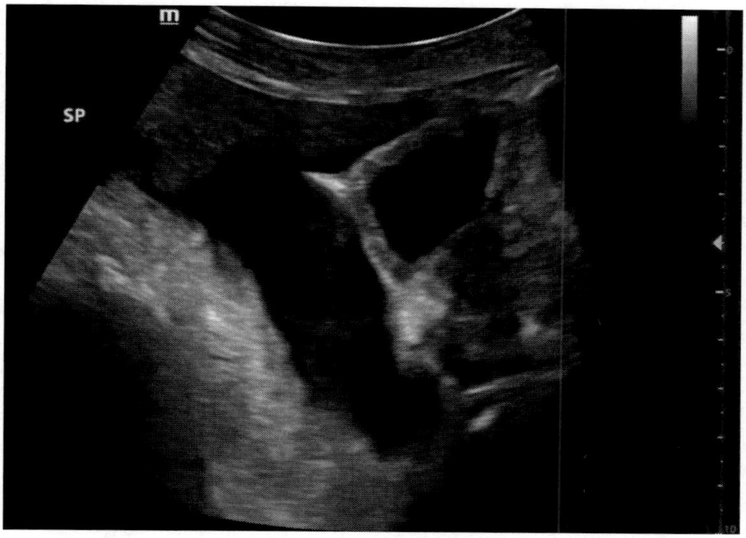

Figure 5. Sagittal ultrasound of bladder at right with adjacent abdominal ascites at left.

Ultrasonographic Assessment of Intravascular Volume: IVC and JVP

Accurately determining the volume status of a patient with AKI is crucial for their successful treatment [16]. Assessment of the inferior vena cava (IVC) with POCUS has been described by nephrologists for assessing volume status in dialysis patients. IVC assessment has proven more useful than physical exam alone for assessing volume status in hemodialysis patients [17]. Interpretation of IVC measurements includes the maximum diameter and the degree of variation over the respiratory cycle, sometimes called collapsibility index. These measurements are most useful for clinical decision making at the extremes. In the presence of a flat IVC, AKI is more likely to be the result of intravascular depletion. Conversely, patients with dilated IVCs with minimal respiratory variation should raise the suspicion for cardiorenal syndrome type 1 due to renal venous congestion. However, it is critical to be aware of conditions that cause large IVC diameter without intravascular overload, including tricuspid regurgitation, cardiac tamponade, positive pressure ventilation, pulmonary hypertension, or right heart failure. Unrelated conditions causing a flat IVC include increased intraabdominal pressure as with intraabdominal hypertension or abdominal compartment syndrome. Abdominal masses, usually hepatic, can also cause a flat IVC in an otherwise fluid overloaded patient. Figure 6 represents a distended IVC seen in long axis view using a cardiac transducer in the subxiphoid window.

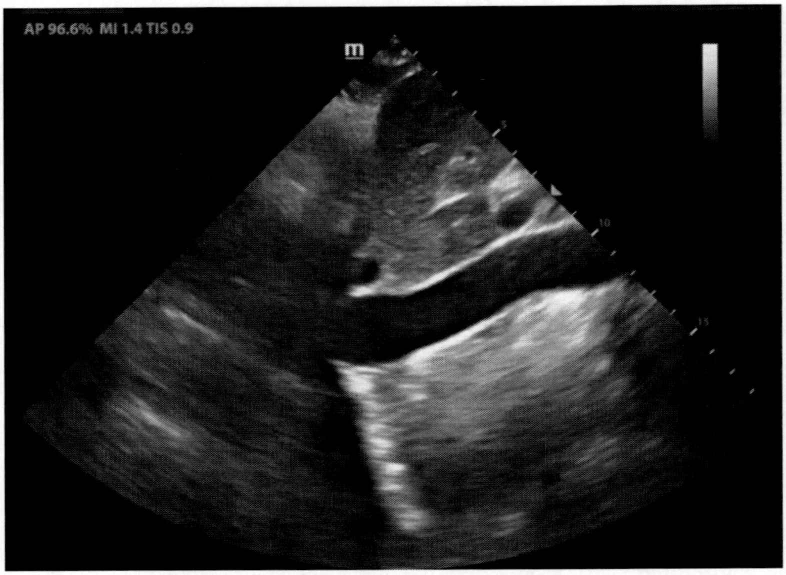

Figure 6. Distended IVC seen in long axis view using a cardiac ultrasound transducer in the subxiphoid window.

POCUS has also been used to estimate jugular venous pressure by visualizing the height of pulsatility in the vein and calculating in the same manner as visual estimation. It has been found to correlate with transduced pressures from the right atrium. It may be most useful in assessing patients with large neck circumference where visual estimation becomes unreliable [18].

Lung Ultrasound

It should first be noted that lung ultrasound is not routinely performed by radiology departments and was developed primarily as a POCUS technique. Lung ultrasound can diagnose pulmonary edema, pneumonia, pleural effusions, and pneumothorax. The most useful ultrasonographic signs suggestive of fluid overload are ultrasonographic B-lines and pleural effusions. It should be noted that B-lines can also be present in interstitial pneumonia, interstitial lung disease, ARDS, and pulmonary carcinomatosis [19]. However, in the context of acute dyspnea it is specific for pulmonary edema.

Ultrasonographic B-lines are caused by a reverberation artifact owing to increased interstitial fluid in the lungs. B-lines appear as hyperechoic vertical lines originating at the pleural line, obliterating the normal horizontal A-line pattern, and extending to the bottom of the screen. The presence of B-lines has been shown to be highly sensitive (94%) and specific (92%) for acute cardiogenic pulmonary edema in patients presenting to the emergency department with dyspnea [20]. Physical exam consisting of lung auscultation and assessment of peripheral edema is both insensitive and non-specific for the detection of increased extravascular lung water compared with lung ultrasound [21]. Lung ultrasound is consistently superior to chest x-ray which tends to only identify moderate and severe pulmonary edema [22]. Ultrasonographic B-lines also correlate with NT-proBNP in terms of its ability to differentiate between cardiogenic and noncardiogenic dyspnea [23]. NT-proBNP is less specific in the setting of AKI.

B-lines have also been shown to correlate in real time with intravascular volume. Patients scanned before and after ultrafiltration during dialysis have been shown to have a consistent decrease in B-lines [24]. Additionally, patients who are diuresed on presentation to the emergency department for acute decompensated heart failure have been shown to have decreased total B-lines at 3 and 24 hours [25]. Figure 7 illustrates ultrasonographic B-lines due to pulmonary edema in setting of suspected fluid overload.

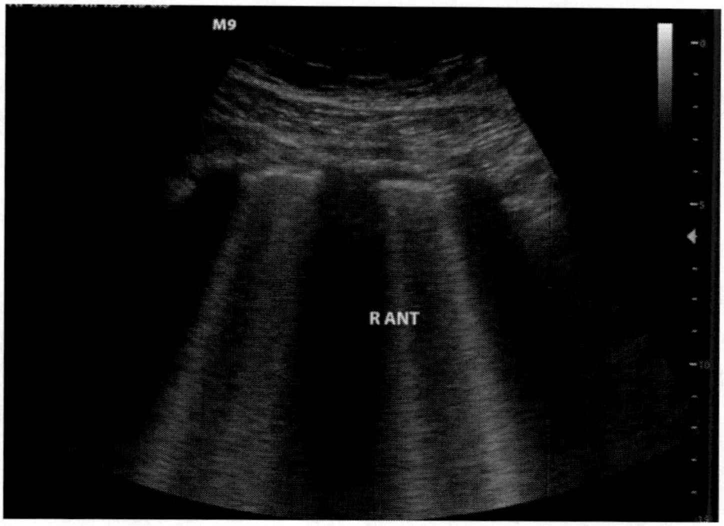

Figure 7. Thoracic ultrasound with numerous ultrasonographic B-lines due to pulmonary edema in setting of suspected fluid overload.

Pleural effusions are also easily visualized with ultrasound and ultrasound is more sensitive for pleural effusions than chest x-ray [26]. Pleural effusions appear as anechoic fluid collections above the diaphragm surrounding lung tissue. Septations and debris can also be visualized and are suggestive of an exudative etiology. A systematic review and meta-analysis of 12 retrospective and prospective studies including 1554 patients showed pooled sensitivity of 94% and specificity of 98% for the diagnosis of pleural effusion with POCUS compared with gold standard [27].

Cardiac Ultrasound

One of the major advantages of POCUS is that the bedside provider can rapidly assess cardiac function during their examination if their history and physical exam is suspicious for concomitant heart failure. In a study of emergency department patients with acute dyspnea the combined findings of decreased left ventricular ejection fraction, full IVC, and increased B-lines was found to be 100% specific for a final diagnosis of acute decompensated heart failure [28]. Ultrasound can also be used to identify diastolic heart failure, which is frequently unreported in patients' medical records. In cases where there are not clear signs of systolic heart failure, one can compare the mitral valve diastolic inflow velocity with the mitral annulus velocity as a ratio of E/E'. In patient presenting with acute dyspnea and preserved left ventricular ejection fraction, a cut-off value of 13-15 was found to be 76%–82% sensitive and 88%–91% specific for a diagnosis of heart failure which was similar to the test characteristics of BNP for a cutoff value of 100-150 pg/mL [29, 30]. This can be a great aid in diagnosing cardiorenal syndrome in a patient who does not previously carry a diagnosis of heart failure. Additionally, ultrasound can be used to support a diagnosis of right heart failure at the bedside. The parasternal short axis view may show a loss of crescent shape morphology of the right ventricle, interventricular septal flattening, or paradoxical septal wall motion. The apical four chamber view can show right ventricular dilation relative to the left ventricle. In patients being treated for pulmonary embolism in the intensive care unit, critical care fellows were found to be able to identify right ventricular dysfunction with a sensitivity and specificity of 83% and 88% when compared to echocardiograms performed by sonographers and interpreted by cardiologists [31]. Figure 8 is demonstrative of systolic heart failure with enlarged left-ventricular end diastolic volume seen in the parasternal long axis.

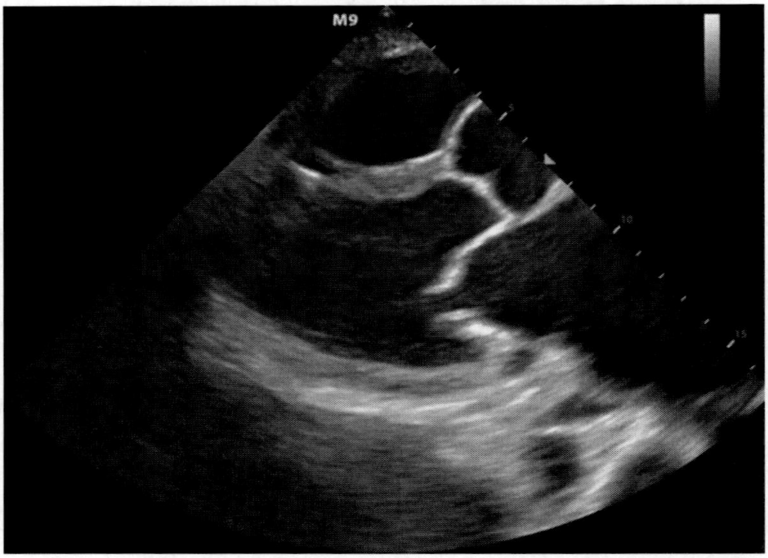

Figure 8. Transthoracic ultrasound of the heart in parasternal long axis demonstrating systolic heart failure with enlarged left-ventricular end diastolic volume.

CT Imaging

Computed tomography (CT) uses ionizing radiation (x-rays) to create cross sectional images of the body and can be performed with or without intravenous contrast agents. CT is often considered the gold standard to identify hydronephrosis and nephrolithiasis, except in pregnant patients. The role of CT in the evaluation of AKI is not well-studied but many of the same principles apply to the use of ultrasound, primarily to rule out obstructive nephropathy in the acute presentation. CT is superior for evaluating structural abnormalities of the genitourinary tract, especially between the UPJ and UVJ where ultrasound is limited by the presence of bowel gas. CT is also superior for the evaluation polycystic kidney disease, retroperitoneal bleeding, mass effect from tumor, or abdominal aortic aneurysm when compared to ultrasound. CT is preferred by many emergency providers for the evaluation of suspected renal colic in elderly patients where the differential diagnosis includes other life-threatening causes of pain. However, it should be noted that abdominal aortic dissection, which can cause AKI and mimic renal colic, will not be detected without intravenous contrast.

Due to the concern for contrast-associated nephropathy related to intravenous administration of iodinated intravenous contrast, the use of contrast in patients with AKI or CKD has been widely discouraged by guidelines and hospital policies. However, recent evidence suggests that this risk has been overstated but still recommends limitation of IV contrast in patients with CKD and GFR less than 30 mL/min/1.73m^2 and those with recent AKI [32-34]. Although not widely recommended, contrast enhanced CT offers several potential benefits in the evaluation of AKI. CT angiography has long been used as a gold standard for many vascular studies, especially due to advancements in 3D reconstruction, which aid with visualization of malformations. It is an excellent modality for identifying renal artery stenosis or aortic dissection into the renal arteries. Due to the rapid acquisition of modern 64 sensor spiral CT, one contrast bolus can be used to image parenchyma and the collecting system. During the nephrographic phase of contrast enhanced CT imaging, which comes 30-40 seconds after contrast bolus, one can visualize the parenchyma and cortex of the kidneys, at which point infarcted tissue, septic emboli, renal tumors, and parenchymal disease can be seen. During the excretory phase a CT urogram can be obtained which provides detailed information about the grade and cause of ureteral obstruction. Additionally, functional CT with intravenous contrast can be used to calculate GFR normalized to renal volume because some contrast agents have very similar properties to inulin [35]. Figure 9 shows a characteristic beaded-string appearance in patient with renal artery stenosis due to fibromuscular dysplasia. Figure 10 illustrates right-sided hydronephrosis due to an obstructing stone at the ureteropelvic junction. Figure 11 shows an obstructing stone in the left mid-ureter.

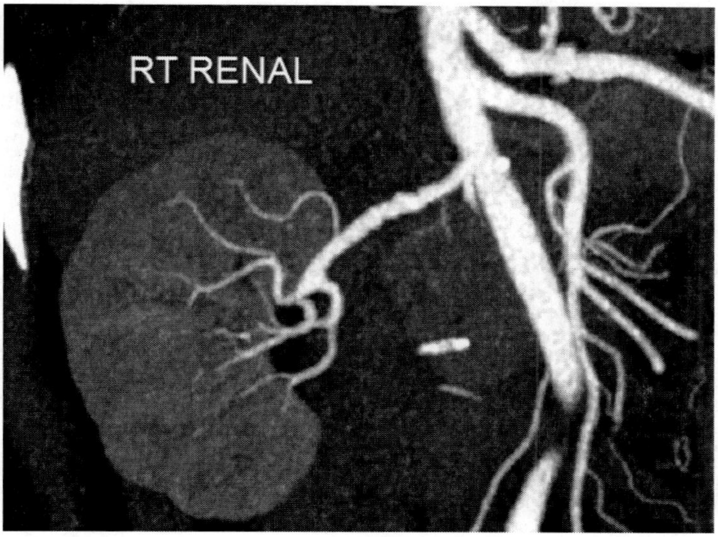

Figure 9. CT digital reconstruction of the right kidney demonstrating characteristic beaded-string appearance in patient with renal artery stenosis due to fibromuscular dysplasia.

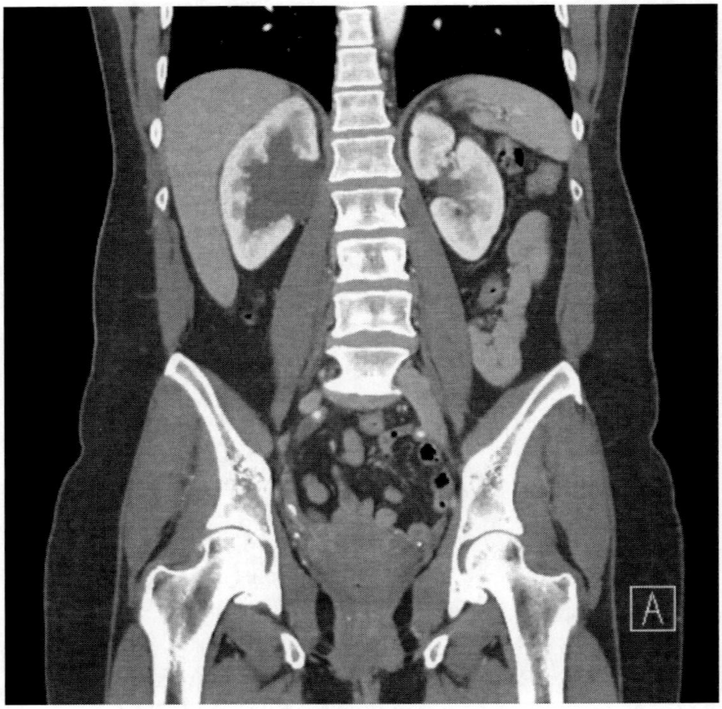

Figure 10. Coronal CT imaging of the abdomen illustrating right sided hydronephrosis due to an obstructing stone at the ureteropelvic junction.

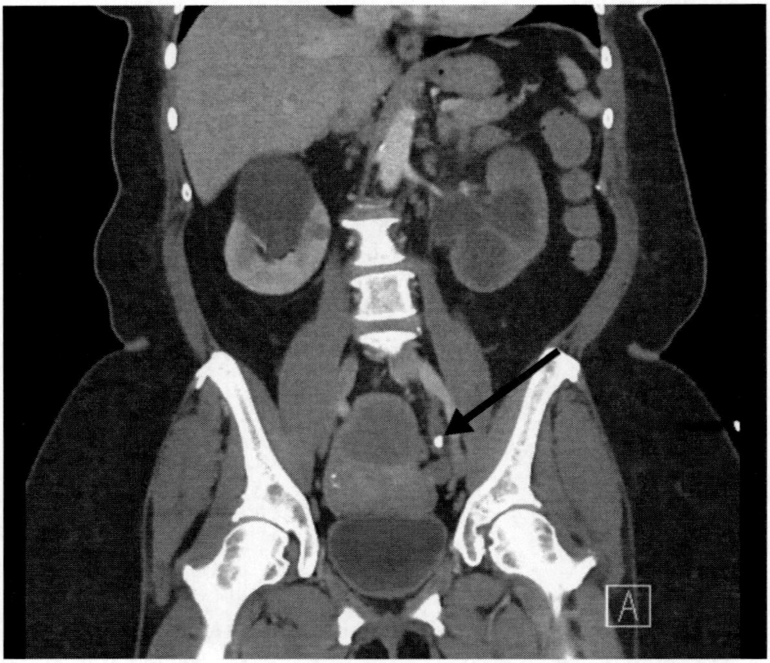

Figure 11. Coronal CT image showing an obstructing stone in the left mid-ureter (arrow).

MRI IMAGING IN AKI

The use of magnetic resonance imaging (MRI) has led to major breakthroughs in understanding structure and function within the body and is highly valued for its ability to generate high quality, high contrast imaging of anatomic structures. In 1988 the development of gadolinium-based contrast agents then made functional MR imaging possible. Particularly within the kidneys where gadolinium (Gd), a highly paramagnetic element (due to 7 unpaired electrons in its outermost orbital) with size smaller than 1 kD, is freely filtered by the glomeruli and neither absorbed nor secreted by the tubules, Gd played a crucial role in understanding renal physiology and was able to demonstrate glomerular filtration and concentrating ability within the kidneys [36].

MRI works through non-ionizing radio waves. Rather than exposing patients to x-ray radiation and nephrotoxic contrast agents as in CT imaging, MRI utilizes an alternating external magnetic field to induce a spin polarization in the nuclei of hydrogen atoms in the water molecules and fat stored within soft tissue using radio frequency energy. This spin polarization is then able to generate a radio frequency signal that is picked up by antennas within the MRI machine. By varying the pulse sequence, different contrasts may be generated to distinguish between tissue types based on the relaxation properties of the hydrogen atoms within these tissues. As there is no ionizing radiation, MRI imaging is optimal for pediatric or pregnant patients where the use of radiation could be harmful.

The use of MRI imaging in AKI has the potential for future clinical applications. By enhancing nuclear relaxation rates, the use of contrast agents such as gadolinium can increase utility of MRI imaging by improving characterization of blood vessels, detecting inflammation, and enhancing contrast within tissues. However, given the risk of nephrogenic systemic fibrosis (NSF) in AKI, where the true GFR is unknown, there is currently no role for MRI in the guidelines for work up and management in AKI [37]. While there is variability in the incidence of NSF among different gadolinium-based agents, the risk of this rare but highly morbid condition often outpaces the benefits of the study.

One promising alternative to gadolinium-based contrast agents is ultrasmall superparamagnetic iron oxides (USPIOs) such as ferumoxytol and ferumoxtran-10 which may change how we utilize MRI imaging in AKI in the future [38]. Similar to gadolinium, USPIOs enhance T1 and T2 relaxation time and are small enough to have a similar biodistribution to gadolinium, though at 20-40 nm they are still too large to be freely filtered across the glomeruli which is generally limited to molecules < 7 nm. However, USPIOs have excellent safety profiles in patients with low GFR, including ESRD patients on hemodialysis [39].

One unique property of USPIOs as iron particles is that of being almost entirely phagocytized by macrophages and will therefore localize to areas of inflammation. This process has been used to show kidney inflammation in acute ischemia in rat models and could provide a way to clarify these ischemic and inflammatory disease processes in the future. Additional future directions in MRI imaging will utilize functional MRI and will include modalities such as blood oxygen-level-dependent (BOLD) MRI, arterial spin labeling (ASL), and diffusion weight imaging (DWI) [40]. BOLD MR has already demonstrated that it is able to assess intrarenal oxygenation changes by using the paramagnetic properties of deoxyhemoglobin as an endogenous contrast agent, as deoxyhemoglobin changes the spin properties of nearby water molecules, accelerating spin dephasing [41]. This spin dephasing rate has been termed R2*, where R2* is equal to the inverse of spin-spin relaxation T2 images on MRI. In other words, the higher the medullary and cortical R2* values, the higher the concentration of deoxyhemoglobin and the lower the oxygenation within the tissue. Previous studies have demonstrated a negative correlation between cortical R2* and eGFR as well as an increased risk of AKI in CKD patients with higher cortical R2* values [42, 34]. BOLD MRI in the future may have diagnostic benefit in assessing ischemic ATN in patients where the diagnosis is unclear.

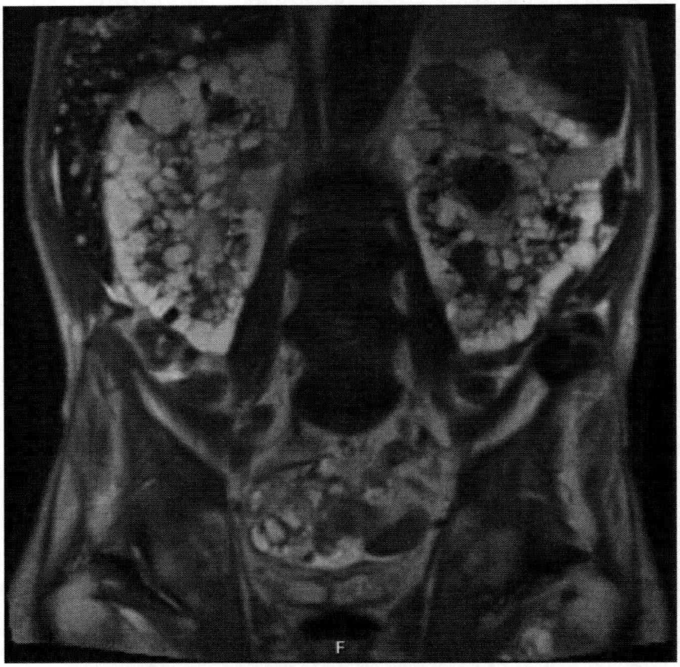

Figure 12. Magnetic resonance urogram of the abdomen in the coronal plane demonstrating multiple cystic lesions to the kidneys bilaterally.

Whereas BOLD MRI offers quantitative information into tissue oxygenation, ASL and DWI offer information on the perfusion and diffusion in the kidney, respectively. Arterial spin labeling magnetically tags protons in water within the blood and utilizes these signals as an endogenous contrast agent. When the water enters the kidneys and is exchanged for non-labeled water a difference in magnetization is observed and quantified, providing an imaging of perfusion within the kidney. Previous studies have shown a significant quantitative difference in renal perfusion in patients with AKI versus patients with healthy kidneys [44]. Another study has shown in mouse models that the use of ASL may provide follow up benefit in patients recovering from AKI, where an increase in renal perfusion indicating likelihood and progression of recovery. DWI on the other hand utilizes the motion of water molecules within the renal microvasculature to quantify an apparent diffusion coefficient (ADC) [45]. ADC has been previously shown to be severely decreased in AKI [46]. How and when these modalities should be incorporated into clinical decision making in patients with AKI has yet to be defined.

MRI imaging does have unique drawbacks when compared to other imaging modalities. The time required to obtain images is considerably longer than CT. This means that patients have to remain stationary within the tube, and very sick patients in extremis or pain may not be capable of remaining this way for long. MRI also require patients to be able to lay flat for this duration. It is also enclosed which may generate severe anxiety in claustrophobic patients, and while open MRIs attempt to solve this problem, they are compromised by lower contrast and quality images due to lower power magnets that they utilize. Figure 12 illustrates a magnetic resonance urogram of the abdomen in the coronal plane demonstrating multiple cystic lesions to the kidneys bilaterally.

Nuclear Imaging In AKI

Compared to the other types of imaging discussed here which can provide some degree of functional imaging but are primarily structural and anatomic modalities, nuclear medicine is entirely based on functional outcomes and provides little anatomic visualization when used alone.

Nuclear medicine takes advantage of the decay of radioactive isotopes, termed radiopharmaceuticals, to assess the uptake of tracers within an organ to assess organ function. This radiation is the picked up by a gamma camera detector and is then converted into an image for analysis. When assessing kidney function using nuclear medicine the radiopharmaceutical used is a technetium isotope, 99m Technetium (Tc), bound to ligands of either dimethylenetriaminepentaacetic acid (DTPA) or mercaptoacetyltriglycine (MAG3). DTPA and MAG3 have both been used to assess GFR and renal blood flow (RBF), respectively, in the past and attempts have been made to establish their utility in AKI [47]. In the case of MAG3 this would look like a delay in uptake in the radioactive tracer in ischemic injury or decreased RBF, whereas the uptake would be negligible in obstructive nephropathy, possibly shedding light on the etiology of the injury. However, this imaging modality is not routinely utilized to date.

Current use of the MAG3 in the clinical setting is centered on assessing differential function between left and right kidneys, such as in the case of unilateral obstruction due to nephrolithiasis. This test allows the isolation of the blockage and provides comparative function between the kidneys. Figure 13 demonstrates Tc-99m MAG3 imaging of the kidneys in the coronal plane with differential function of 67% by the left kidney and 33% by the right.

Positron emission tomography (PET) offers another avenue in nuclear imaging that may provide useful information in kidney imaging in the future. Whereas other nuclear studies such as the MAG3 scan assess pooling of the radioactive tracer, PET imaging measures the uptake and utilization of the tracers at the cellular level in order to assess the overall metabolic activity of the cells being imaged and elucidating particular physiologic and biochemical properties of the organs being visualized.

PET scans have already seen widespread use in oncology and cardiology to assess metabolism and to infer perfusion and overall function. To accomplish this very different radioisotope tracers are used than the nuclear studies mentioned above. Renal blood flow studies can be performed with O-15-labeled water, N-13-labeled ammonia, and other agents. With these tracers, RBF can be quantified using a modified microsphere kinetic model. Glomerular filtration can be imaged and quantified with gallium-68 EDTA or cobalt-55 EDTA. Measurements of RBF with PET have potential applications in renovascular disease, in transplant rejection or acute tubular necrosis, in drug-induced nephropathies, ureteral obstruction, before and after revascularization, and before and after the placement of ureteral stents [48].

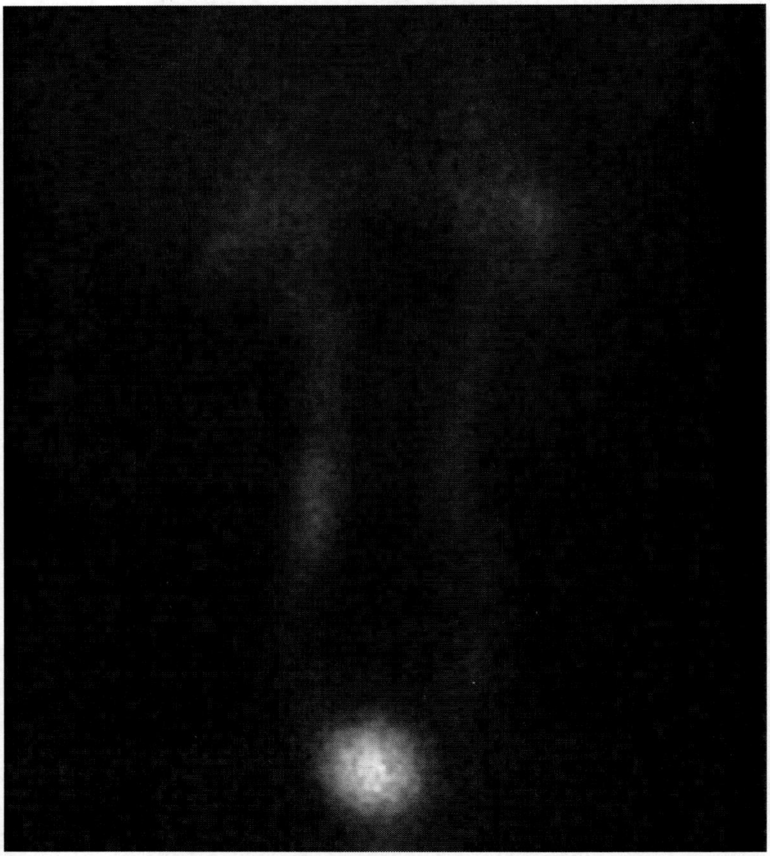

Figure 13. Tc-99m MAG3 imaging of the kidneys in the coronal plane demonstrating differential function of 67% by the left kidney and 33% by the right.

Future applications of PET would employ more advanced, disease specific molecular probes and could see broad application in renovascular disease, obstructive nephropathy, and monitoring of acute nephrotoxicity in the setting of chemotherapeutics which are proving to be a growing cause of AKI. Such markers would include probes for reactive oxygen species in AKI, as well as evidence of recovery and cellular survival mechanisms after AKI such as with peptic nucleic acid tracers [49]. Sub-acute loss of GFR that is secondary to diabetic nephropathy could be elucidated through the use of VEGF probes, helping to distinguish this entity from other causes of AKI in a patient who may already have nephrotic range proteinuria without the use of biopsy [50].

Clinical Pearls

- Ultrasound is the imaging modality of choice for the initial evaluation of the patient with AKI.
- Hydronephrosis is the sonographic hallmark of obstructive nephropathy and is easily established with ultrasound.
- Small size and decreased cortical thickness support a diagnosis of CKD but are relatively insensitive being present only late in the course of the disease.
- Point-of-Care Ultrasound quickly establishes presence or absence of obstructive nephropathy and adds information on clinical volume status.
- CT is the imaging modality of choice in patients with suspected nephrolithiasis.
- MRI is an emerging modality in the evaluation of AKI and iron-based contrast agents are a potential alternative to gadolinium.
- Nuclear medicine studies add functional data and are useful in lateralizing obstruction.

CONCLUSION

Knowledge of the roles of various non-invasive imaging is critical to the practicing nephrologist for the diagnosis and treatment of AKI. Ultrasound is the imaging modality of choice as it can rapidly rule in or rule out obstructive AKI by demonstrating a distended bladder or hydronephrosis. Ultrasound is widely available, easy to use, and free of potentially harmful ionizing radiation and adds information helpful to determine the duration of kidney dysfunction of unknown duration by evaluating kidney length, echogenicity, and cortical thickness. Ultrasound can be used at the point-of-care to more rapidly exclude obstruction, determine cardiac function, and assess volume status. CT is the imaging modality of choice for the assessment of suspected nephrolithiasis as most obstructing stones are present in the ureters which are often obscured by bowel gas making them inaccessible to ultrasound. MRI remains an investigational tool and gadolinium-containing contrast should be used with caution in AKI owing to the risk of NSF. Nuclear imaging plays a limited role in determining relative function of the kidneys and lateralizing obstruction.

REFERENCES

[1] Fried JG, Morgan MA. Renal Imaging: Core Curriculum 2019. *Am J Kidney Dis.* 2019;73(4):552-565.

[2] Freimanis K, Wild J, Bliss WR, *Joseph I. of Diagnostic Ultrasound: The Role of American Radiologists with engineers.* 1993:189-194.

[3] Soni NJ. *Point of Care Ultrasound.* 2nd edition. Elsevier; 2019.

[4] Baston CM. *Pocket Guide to POCUS Point-of-Care Tips for Point-of-Care Ultrasound.*; 2019.

[5] O'Neill WC. *Atlas of Renal Ultrasonography.* Saunders; 2001.

[6] O'Neill WC. Renal relevant radiology: Use of ultrasound in kidney disease and nephrology procedures. *Clin J Am Soc Nephrol.* 2014;9(2):373-381.

[7] Smith-Bindman R, Aubin C, Bailitz J, et al. Ultrasonography versus Computed Tomography for Suspected Nephrolithiasis. *N Engl J Med.* 2014;371(12):1100-1110.

[8] Faubel S, Patel NU, Lockhart ME, Cadnapaphornchai MA. Renal relevant radiology: Use of ultrasonography in patients with AKI. *Clin J Am Soc Nephrol*. 2014;9(2):382-394.

[9] Reisinger N, Koratala A, Goral S. Use of Point-of-Care Ultrasound to Assess CKD. *Am J Kidney Dis*. 2021.

[10] 10. Sharfuddin A. Renal relevant radiology: Imaging in kidney transplantation. *Clin J Am Soc Nephrol*. 2014;9(2):416-429.

[11] Chang EH, Chong WK, Kasoji SK, et al. Diagnostic accuracy of contrast-enhanced ultrasound for characterization of kidney lesions in patients with and without chronic kidney disease. *BMC Nephrol*. 2017;18(1):1-13.

[12] Koratala A, Bhattacharya D, Kazory A. Point of care renal ultrasonography for the busy nephrologist: A pictorial review. *World J Nephrol*. 2019.

[13] Pathan SA, Mitra B, Mirza S, et al. Emergency Physician Interpretation of Point-of-care Ultrasound for Identifying and Grading of Hydronephrosis in Renal Colic Compared With Consensus Interpretation by Emergency Radiologists. *Acad Emerg Med*. 2018;25(10):1129-1137.

[14] Alnaif B, Drutz HP. The accuracy of portable abdominal ultrasound equipment in measuring postvoid residual volume. *Int Urogynecol J*. 1999;10(4):215-218.

[15] Brouwer TA, van den Boogaard C, van Roon EN, Kalkman CJ, Veeger N. Non-invasive bladder volume measurement for the prevention of postoperative urinary retention: validation of two ultrasound devices in a clinical setting. *J Clin Monit Comput*. 2018;32(6):1117-1126.

[16] Velez JCQ, Petkovich B, Karakala N, Huggins JT. Point-of-Care Echocardiography Unveils Misclassification of Acute Kidney Injury as Hepatorenal Syndrome. *Am J Nephrol*. 2019;50(3):204-211.

[17] Brennan JM, Ronan A, Goonewardena S, et al. Handcarried ultrasound measurement of the inferior vena cava for assessment of intravascular volume status in the outpatient hemodialysis clinic. *Clin J Am Soc Nephrol*. 2006;1(4):749-753.

[18] Newman J, Pillarella J, Laubham M, Raichlin E LM. Bedside ultrasound improves the accuracy of jugular venous pressure assessment. *J Card Fail*. 2018;24(8):S51-S52.

[19] Reisinger N, Koratala A. Lung ultrasound: a valuable tool for the assessment of dialysis patients with COVID-19. *Clin Exp Nephrol*. 2020.

[20] Al Deeb M, Barbic S, Featherstone R, Dankoff J, Barbic D. Point-of-care ultrasonography for the diagnosis of acute cardiogenic pulmonary edema in patients presenting with acute dyspnea: A systematic review and meta-analysis. *Acad Emerg Med*. 2014;21(8):843-852.

[21] Torino C, Gargani L, Sicari R, et al. The agreement between auscultation and lung ultrasound in hemodialysis patients: The LUST study. *Clin J Am Soc Nephrol*. 2016;11(11):2005-2011.

[22] Maw AM, Hassanin A, Ho PM, et al. Diagnostic Accuracy of Point-of-Care Lung Ultrasonography and Chest Radiography in Adults With Symptoms Suggestive of Acute Decompensated Heart Failure: A Systematic Review and Meta-analysis. *JAMA Netw open*. 2019.

[23] Gargani L, Frassi F, Soldati G, Tesorio P, Gheorghiade M, Picano E. Ultrasound lung comets for the differential diagnosis of acute cardiogenic dyspnoea: A comparison with natriuretic peptides. *Eur J Heart Fail*. 2008;10(1):70-77.

[24] Noble VE, Murray AF, Capp R, Sylvia-Reardon MH, Steele DJR, Liteplo A. Ultrasound assessment for extravascular lung water in patients undergoing hemodialysis: Time course for resolution. *Chest*. 2009;135(6):1433-1439.

[25] Cortellaro F, Ceriani E, Spinelli M, et al. Lung ultrasound for monitoring cardiogenic pulmonary edema. *Intern Emerg Med*. 2017.

[26] Eibenberger KL, Dock WI, Ammann ME, Dorffner R, Hörmann MF GF. Quantification of pleural effusions: sonography versus radiography. *Radiology*. 1994;191(3):681-684.

[27] Yousefifard M, Baikpour M, Ghelichkhani P, et al. Screening Performance Characteristic of Ultrasonography and Radiography in Detection of Pleural Effusion; a Meta-Analysis. *Emerg (Tehran, Iran)*. 2016;4(1):1-10.

[28] Anderson KL, Jenq KY, Fields JM, Panebianco NL, Dean AJ. Diagnosing heart failure among acutely dyspneic patients with cardiac, inferior vena cava, and lung ultrasonography. *Am J Emerg Med*. 2013;31(8):1208-1214.

[29] Arques S, Roux E, Sbragia P, et al. Accuracy of tissue Doppler echocardiography in the diagnosis of new-onset congestive heart failure in patients with levels of B-type natriuretic peptide in the midrange and normal left ventricular ejection fraction. *Echocardiography*. 2006;23(8):627-634.

[30] Dokainish H, Zoghbi WA, Lakkis NM, Quinones MA, Nagueh SF. Comparative accuracy of B-type natriuretic peptide and tissue Doppler echocardiography in the diagnosis of congestive heart failure. *Am J Cardiol*. 2004;93(9):1130-1135.

[31] Filopei J, Acquah SO, Bondarsky EE, et al. Diagnostic accuracy of point-of-care ultrasound performed by pulmonary critical care physicians for right ventricle assessment in patients with acute pulmonary embolism. *Crit Care Med*. 2017;45(12):2040-2045.

[32] Aycock RD, Westafer LM, Boxen JL, Majlesi N, Schoenfeld EM, Bannuru RR. Acute Kidney Injury After Computed Tomography: A Meta-analysis. *Ann Emerg Med*. 2018;71(1):44-53.e4.

[33] Davenport MS, Perazella MA, Yee J, et al. Use of Intravenous Iodinated Contrast Media in Patients With Kidney Disease: Consensus Statements from the American College of Radiology and the National Kidney Foundation. *Kidney Med*. 2020;2(1):85-93.

[34] Hinson JS, Ehmann MR, Fine DM, et al. Risk of Acute Kidney Injury After Intravenous Contrast Media Administration. *Ann Emerg Med*. 2017;69(5):577-586.e4.

[35] Tsushima Y, Blomley MJK, Kusano S, Endo K. Use of contrast-enhanced computed tomography to measure clearance per unit renal volume: A novel measurement of renal function and fractional vascular volume. *Am J Kidney Dis*. 1999;33(4):754-760.

[36] Choyke PL, Austin HA, Frank JA, et al. Hydrated clearance of gadolinium-DTPA as a measurement of glomerular filtration rate. *Kidney Int*. 1992;41(6):1595-1598.

[37] Grobner T, Prischl FC. Gadolinium and nephrogenic systemic fibrosis. *Kidney Int*. 2007;72(3):260-264.

[38] Jo SK, Hu X, Kobayashi H, et al. Detection of inflammation following renal ischemia by magnetic resonance imaging. *Kidney Int*. 2003;64(1):43-51.

[39] Provenzano R, Schiller B, Rao M, Coyne D, Brenner L, Pereira BJG. Ferumoxytol as an intravenous iron replacement therapy in hemodialysis patients. *Clin J Am Soc Nephrol*. 2009;4(2):386-393.

[40] Zhou HY, Chen TW, Zhang XM. Functional Magnetic Resonance Imaging in Acute Kidney Injury: Present Status. *Biomed Res Int*. 2016;2016(Ivim).

[41] Prasad P V., Edelman RR, Epstein FH. Noninvasive evaluation of intrarenal oxygenation with BOLD MRI. *Circulation*. 1996;94(12):3271-3275.

[42] Srivastava A, Cai X, Lee J, et al. Kidney functional magnetic resonance imaging and change in eGFR in individuals with CKD. *Clin J Am Soc Nephrol*. 2020;15(6):776-783.

[43] Prasad P V., Thacker J, Li LP, et al. Multi-parametric evaluation of chronic kidney disease by MRI: A preliminary cross-sectional study. *PLoS One*. 2015;10(10).

[44] Dong J, Yang L, Su T, et al. Quantitative assessment of acute kidney injury by noninvasive arterial spin labeling perfusion MRI: A pilot study. *Sci China Life Sci*. 2013;56(8):745-750.

[45] Hueper K, Gutberlet M, Rong S, et al. Acute Kidney Injury: Arterial Spin Labeling to Monitor Renal Perfusion Impairment in Mice—Comparison with Histopathologic Results and Renal Function. *Radiology*. 2013;270(1):130367.

[46] Hueper K, Rong S, Gutberlet M, et al. T2 relaxation time and apparent diffusion coefficient for noninvasive assessment of renal pathology after acute kidney injury in mice: Comparison with histopathology. *Invest Radiol*. 2013;48(12):834-842.

[47] Kalantarinia K. Novel imaging techniques in acute kidney injury. *Curr Drug Targets*. 2009;10(12):1184-1189.

[48] Szabo Z, Xia J, Mathews WB, Brown PR. *Future Direction of Renal PET*. 2007;36(1):36-50.

[49] Szabo Z, Xia J, Mathews WB. Radiopharmaceuticals for Renal Positron Emission Tomography Imaging. *Semin Nucl Med*. 2008;38(1):20-31.

[50] Cooper ME, Vranes D, Youssef S, et al. Increased renal expression of vascular endothelial growth factor (VEGF) and its receptor VEGFR-2 in experimental diabetes. *Diabetes*. 1999;48(11):2229-2239.

In: Issues in Kidney Disease – Acute Kidney Injury
Editors: S. Z. Fadem and A. Arslan Yousuf Awan

ISBN: 978-1-68507-002-1

Chapter 6

OBSTRUCTIVE UROPATHY

Jacob L. Kraus[1,2], James Anaissie[1,2], MD, Utsav K. Bansal[1,2], MD, Richard E. Link[1,2], MD, PhD and Wesley A. Mayer[1,2,*], MD

[1]Baylor College of Medicine, Houston, TX, USA
[2]The Scott Department of Urology at the Baylor College of Medicine, Houston, TX, USA

ABSTRACT

Obstructive uropathy is a urinary tract pathology caused by the acute or chronic obstruction of urinary flow, accounting for nearly 10% of renal failure cases [1]. Obstructive uropathy encompasses a diverse collection of etiologies originating in both the upper and lower urinary tract, each with specific diagnostic and treatment considerations. Prompt diagnosis and effective management are vital to limit permanent kidney injury with significant morbidity and mortality. This chapter reviews the epidemiology, physiology, etiology, diagnosis, and management of obstructive uropathy. The pathologic changes that occur in both unilateral and bilateral obstruction, as well as factors affecting the recovery of renal function, are explored. Finally, the physiology, risk factors, and management of post obstructive diuresis is reviewed. A disease-specific approach can help avoid common pitfalls and ensure that the best care is provided to patients.

Keywords: hydronephrosis, ureteral obstruction, urethral obstruction, urinary bladder neck obstruction, urinary retention

* Corresponding Author's E-mail: Wesley.Mayer@bcm.edu.

INTRODUCTION

Obstructive uropathy (OU) is a disorder of the urinary tract characterized by the partial or complete obstruction of urinary flow and can occur at any point along the urinary tract, including the kidneys, ureters, bladder, and urethra. Obstruction can affect one (unilateral) or both (bilateral) kidneys, and accounts for approximately 10% of all cases of renal failure [1]. OU may result from a variety of etiologies and can affect both genders in all age groups. Hydronephrosis, or dilation of the renal collecting system, which may signal OU, occurs in approximately 0.5-1.0% of all neonates [2].

PATHOPHYSIOLOGY

Unilateral Renal Obstruction

In the setting of unilateral ureteral obstruction (UUO), the kidney experiences a triphasic pattern of hemodynamic changes [3, 4]. The first phase of UUO lasts 1 to 2 hours. As the flow of urine becomes obstructed, hydrostatic pressure increases within the renal tubules, causing a concurrent decrease in glomerular filtration rate (GFR). The renal vasculature initially counteracts this through the production of vasodilatory molecules such as nitric oxide (NO) and prostaglandin E2 (PGE_2) to increase renal blood flow (RBF) [5,6]. In the second phase, RBF begins to decline as ureteral pressure continues to rise and the renal vasculature can no longer compensate [3]. This phase lasts for 3 to 4 hours. In the final phase, which starts about 5 hours after obstruction, both RBF and ureteral pressure begin to decrease as afferent arteriolar constriction occurs due to a lack of NO production after prolonged obstruction. A concurrent decrease in renal function and GFR follows [7]. In response to UUO, a normal contralateral kidney is usually able to maintain fluid balance through the release of NO, thus increasing RBF and subsequently GFR [8].

Bilateral Renal Obstruction

Bilateral Ureteral Obstruction (BUO) results in a biphasic pattern of hemodynamic changes. During the first 90 minutes, GFR decreases bilaterally due to increasing hydrostatic pressure in the renal tubules. The renal vasculature attempts to compensate through the production of vasodilatory molecules, increasing RBF [4]. This is followed by a second phase marked by decreased RBF bilaterally due to persistently elevated ureteral pressures. A concomitant decrease in GFR results for reasons similar to those described above. However, because of a lack of contralateral functioning renal unit, a subsequent increase in intravascular volume occurs. Atrial natriuretic peptide is released as a response to the excess intravascular volume, causing dilation of the afferent arterioles, constriction of the efferent arterioles, and inhibition of the renin-angiotensin-aldosterone system (RAAS) [9]. This combination of changes increases glomerular capillary pressure as an attempt to compensate for the loss of GFR at the cost of reduced RBF due to prolonged efferent arteriolar vasoconstriction.

In both UUO and BUO, the resultant increase in hydrostatic pressure causes dilation of the urinary system. Progressive distention of the collecting system increases intratubular pressure leading to an eventual reduction in RBF with a concurrent decrease in GFR. Parenchymal ischemia ensues and is further perpetuated by the activation of RAAS. Ultimately, renal fibrosis results from the combination of ischemic changes and hydrostatic stress, resulting in permanent functional loss [7].

Post-Obstructive Diuresis

Following relief of obstruction, patients may experience an excessive loss of both water and electrolytes through urinary excretion known as post-obstructive diuresis (POD). A urine output of greater than 200 ml/hr for two consecutive hours or greater than three liters in 24 hours following relief of obstruction qualifies as POD [10]. The pathophysiology is theorized to involve several mechanisms including an osmotic diuresis of retained solutes, reduced collecting duct sensitivity to antidiuretic hormone (ADH), loss of the corticomedullary concentration gradient, and an increased production of diuretic hormones in response to fluid overload [9, 11, 12]. Most patients who are lucid and able to self-regulate oral fluid consumption can generally compensate for POD. However, POD can be life-threatening for patients unable to self-regulate fluid intake and requires careful monitoring and possibly parenteral fluid replacement.

Management of Post-Obstructive Diuresis

POD can be either physiologic or pathologic. Physiologic POD is usually self-limited, resolving within 24 hours. Several risk factors, as demonstrated in Table 1, can lead to pathologic POD, and if lasts greater than 48 hours and may cause severe electrolyte derangements [10]. Specific gravity, a surrogate for osmolality, can be used to differentiate between physiologic and pathologic POD. A urine specific gravity of 1.010 is equivalent to that of serum, suggesting a physiological diuresis. A urine specific gravity of less than 1.010 is consistent with the inability of the kidneys to concentrate urine properly, indicating pathologic POD [13].

Table 1: Risk factors for pathologic POD

Risk factors
• Bilateral obstruction
• Obstruction of a solitary kidney
• Congestive heart failure
• Chronic kidney disease

Patients at high risk for progressing to pathologic POD should be admitted for observation. Strict inputs and outputs should be assessed every 2 hours and daily weights should be recorded [13]. Serum electrolytes should be monitored periodically and corrected accordingly. Intravenous hydration should be limited to patients who are unable to self-regulate and restricted to 50% of the preceding hour's urine output in an effort to achieve a negative fluid balance [14].

Clinical Pearls
• Patients at high risk for progressing to pathologic POD should be admitted for observation. In cases where the patient is unable to adequately self-regulate fluid intake, careful repletion of urine output with parenteral fluids is appropriate.

RECOVERY OF FUNCTION

Recovery of renal function is affected by several factors including the age of onset, duration, baseline function of the ipsilateral kidney, and condition of the contralateral kidney [15-17]. The immature kidney is more susceptible to the effects of OU due to the impairment of nephrogenesis, which can lead to progressive renal atrophy and fibrosis. In a systematic review of infants treated endoscopically for posterior urethral valves (PUV), a pediatric cause of BOU, 22% of patients progressed to chronic kidney disease (CKD) following treatment and 11% progressed to end-stage renal disease (ESRD) [18]. Regarding the mature kidney, younger patients have shown improved recovery compared to older patients. In a retrospective review of 138 patients undergoing pyeloplasty for ureteropelvic junction obstruction, patients under 35 years of age were more likely to recover renal function when compared to older patients [19].

Baseline function of the ipsilateral kidney predicts recovery of renal function. In a study of 4,400 patients receiving treatment for obstructing urinary calculi, Kukreja et al. found that increased baseline preoperative serum creatinine was significantly associated with further decline in renal function following definitive surgical treatment [17]. Mishra et al. found that a decreased GFR 5 days following initial decompression of bilateral obstructive urolithiasis with percutaneous nephrostomy (PCN) predicted progression of CKD in patients with pre-existing renal insufficiency [20]. There may be less resilience to prolonged obstruction of kidneys with baseline CKD from medical causes like hypertension and diabetes. In a prospective review of 160 patients undergoing percutaneous nephrostomy placement for urinary tract obstruction, Sharma et al. found that decreased cortical thickness, corticomedullary differentiation, and parenchymal echogenicity negatively predicted the recovery of renal function [16]. On the other hand, normal functioning contralateral kidney positively predicted recovery of renal function.

The longer a kidney has been obstructed, the less likely that full recovery of baseline renal function will occur. Leahy et al. induced partial UUO in three groups of canines for 14, 28, and 60 days respectively [21]. The entire 14-day group recovered normal function after relief, while only 8% of the 60-day group recovered normal function. These results have been used to justify the approach of giving patients with obstructing stones and manageable symptoms 4 – 6 week "trials of stone passage" without significant concern for long-term renal functional compromise. However, there are limitations to the conclusions we can draw from studies on normal canine kidneys performed > 30 years ago.

Chronic obstruction at the level of the bladder outlet can also lead to upper urinary tract dysfunction. Over time, outlet obstruction can cause bladder hypertrophy, progressive denervation, increased collagen deposition, reduction in compliance, and decreased contractility [22]. These changes then lead to exacerbation of the lower urinary tract OU and cause upper tract deterioration over time [23]. Leng et al. treated 9 men with non-neurogenic BOO with either transurethral incision, resection of the prostate, or transurethral balloon dilation of urethral stricture [24]. Bladder compliance improved from 3.06 to 13.53 cm/H2O following treatment of obstruction.

Clinical Pearls

- Recovery of renal function depends on several factors, including patient age at onset, duration, and baseline ipsilateral and contralateral kidney function.

PRESENTATION AND DIAGNOSIS

Clinical Presentation

The clinical presentation of OU varies depending on the location, duration, and etiology of the obstruction. It is important to begin with a detailed patient history, including onset, location, duration, and characterization of pain, as well as any aggravating or relieving factors [4, 25]. Classic signs and symptoms of upper urinary tract obstruction include flank pain with or without radiation to the groin, nausea, and vomiting [4, 26]. Obstruction of the distal ureter, lower urinary tract, or bladder outlet may cause urgency, frequency, nocturia, or dysuria. These patients may also present with the inability to void, or a weak, slow, or staccato stream. Hematuria can also be associated with several causes of OU such as urolithiasis, malignancies, or benign prostatic hyperplasia (BPH). Fever can indicate an accompanying infection, which often requires emergent drainage in the setting of obstruction.

Following the patient history, a thorough physical exam with special focus on the abdominal and genitourinary (GU) components should be performed. For example, palpation of the bladder may help assess for urinary retention. Percussion and palpation of the flank may help determine laterality of pathology. A digital rectal exam may identify a prostatic, gastrointestinal, or pelvic floor etiology [25].

Laboratory Tests

The laboratory evaluation of patients may vary depending on etiology. A basic metabolic panel to assess renal function is essential [25]. OU can result in post-renal azotemia due to inadequate renal filtration, particularly with bilateral obstruction. Findings would generally demonstrate fractional excretion of sodium (FENa) of greater than 2 with a blood urea nitrogen:creatinine ratio (BUN:Cr) ratio of less than 20:1 [27]. A routine urinalysis should be performed if the patient is making urine and urine culture sent if pyuria and/or bacteria is present or if a urologic intervention is being planned [28]. If surgical intervention is indicated to relieve obstruction, a pre-operative complete blood count (CBC) is generally indicated. Note that a mildly elevated WBC count is common in patients experiencing painful renal colic due to the effect of stress hormones on WBC trafficking from bone marrow and may not indicate active infection. In the event a PCN is required, coagulation studies should be obtained [29].

POD requires specific laboratory monitoring. Following decompression of an obstructed solitary kidney or BUO, serum electrolytes and urine output should be carefully monitored. This is particularly critical for patients with cognitive impairment who cannot self-regulate fluid intake or in patients with medical issues such as CKD or congestive heart failure that may limit their tolerance for POD.

The laboratory assessment of UO continues to evolve as our understanding of the molecular mechanisms advances. In a series of studies in rats, the expression of aquaporin 1, aquaporin 2-3, and caveolin 1 was significantly higher in the setting of BOO [30-31]. When looking at bladder urothelium in patients with BOO, Araki et al. found significantly higher expression of epithelial sodium channels than in controls without BOO [32]. Another study found significantly increased Creatinine:Cystatin C ratio in 15 patients with obstructive acute kidney injury (AKI) compared to 46 patients with azotemia from a non-obstructive etiology (6.9 vs. 4.4, p-value = 0.007) [33]. Hung et al. studied 854 with lower urinary tract symptoms (LUTS) secondary to BPH and found that elevated levels of C reactive protein (CRP) and higher prostate specific antigen (PSA) levels were significantly associated with increased lower urinary tract symptoms [34]. Older age and elevated International Prostate Symptom Score (IPSS) were also found to be significant predictors of an elevated CRP.

Imaging Modalities

Ultrasound

Due to its accessibility, cost-effectiveness, and lack of ionizing radiation, renal bladder ultrasound (RBUS) can be a useful initial imaging study when screening patients for OU, providing anatomic information for both the kidneys and bladder. Ultrasound kidney anatomy can be divided into the renal parenchyma (outer cortex, inner medullary pyramids) and the renal sinus (fat, vasculature and the collecting system). Normal renal parenchyma is slightly hypoechoic when compared to adjacent organs (liver on the right and spleen on the left). The renal sinus should appear hyperechoic due to the presence of blood vessels and fat. The nondilated collecting system can be difficult to visualize in most non-obstructed kidneys [35].

In obstructed kidneys, hydronephrosis appears as dilation of the collecting system with anechoic fluid. Often, the renal pelvis can be clearly discerned from the calyces. Depending on the level of obstruction, the proximal ureter may also appear dilated [35]. The degree of hydronephrosis can be classified into 4 grades [36]. Isolated dilation of the renal pelvis without associated caliceal dilation is termed pelviectasis and may not always reflect obstruction.

Duplex doppler imaging allows for the calculation of the resistive index (RI), which is proportional to vascular resistance and compliance. As hydronephrosis increases, both resistance to blood flow through the renal artery and RI increase as well. An RI of 0.70 or greater may indicate possible obstruction [37]. Color doppler has also shown efficacy in assessing "ureteral jets" in the bladder, the absence of which can suggest ureteral obstruction. Jandahgi et al. suggested that a ureteral jet frequency of 1.5 jets/min or less, a decreased peak ureteral jet velocity, and decreased duration of ureteral jets can be diagnostic of ureteral obstruction in patients with urolithiasis [38].

Ultrasound plays a particularly important role when ionizing radiation is relatively contraindicated, such as in pregnancy or in pediatric patients. RBUS in expert hands can provide valuable information to suggest an etiology for obstruction. However, RBUS is relatively insensitive for identifying ureteral pathology such as ureteral stones, particularly in more obese patients. A RBUS showing hydronephrosis without a clear etiology may require either CT or magnetic resonance imaging (MRI) to establish an etiology.

Computed Tomography

Computed tomography (CT) of the abdomen and pelvis is often the test of choice for radiographic assessment of obstruction, particularly in the setting of acute flank pain. Non-contrast CT (NCCT) is the gold standard for imaging suspected urolithiasis with a sensitivity of near 95% and a specificity of 98% [39]. NCCT may be useful in determining stone composition through the measurement of Hounsfield units [39].

CT with intravenous (IV) contrast plays an important role in the diagnosis of GU malignancy. Triphasic CT urography, also referred to as the CT Urogram (CTU), consists of non-contrast, nephrogenic, and pyelographic/delayed phases, the latter of which can be useful for the assessment of upper urinary tract obstruction. CTU can identify filling defects that could represent tumors, blood clots, or stones among many other things. The combination of positron emission tomography (PET) with CT can occasionally aid in detecting malignancy as a cause of OU [40], although this is generally not a modality available in the acute setting. CT is also helpful for diagnosing retroperitoneal fibrosis (RPF) or anatomic variants (such as a retrocaval ureter) associated with OU [41, 42]. CT scans require exposing the patient to ionizing radiation, which is a particular concern if multiple serial imaging tests are anticipated. In the case of pregnant women requiring CT, the fetus is most sensitive to the negative effects of ionizing radiation during the first trimester [43, 44]. In select cases later in pregnancy, such as when identification of an obstructing ureteral stone might dramatically change therapeutic intervention, low dose CT protocols exist that may limit fetal exposure risk. Additionally, a GFR of <30 mL/min is considered a relative contraindication for contrast administration during CT scans due to the risk of contrast-induced acute kidney injury. If a contrast-enhanced CT is necessary in these patients, one should consider peri-procedural IV hydration, although the data in this domain is conflicting [45].

Clinical Pearls

- Indications for CT should be carefully considered in pediatric patients and pregnant women who are at higher risk for the deleterious effects of ionizing radiation. However, in some specific circumstances the benefits of a low dose CT may outweigh the risks in these patients.

Nuclear Scintigraphy

Nuclear scintigraphy, which provides overall renal functional information as well as differential renal function between kidneys, can also be used to differentiate between obstructive and non-obstructive hydronephrosis. After radionuclide administration, a diuretic such as furosemide may be given to increase urine production and radionuclide washout from the kidney is calculated and compared to reference standards. There are a variety of radionuclides used in nuclear renography, each with their own advantages and disadvantages. Radiotracers are often divided into several categories including those eliminated through tubular secretion, those eliminated through glomerular filtration, and those retained in the renal tubules after endocytosis from the glomerular filtrate.

Radiotracers that are eliminated through tubular secretion, such as MAG-3, are more commonly used than those eliminated through glomerular filtration, such as Dimercaptosuccinic acid (DMSA), due the relative ease with which the kidney can extract them from plasma [46, 47]. This allows for more effective measurement of radiotracer washout when assessing for urinary tract obstruction. Traditionally, the T1/2, or the time from furosemide administration to when 50% of peak radionuclide activity remains in the collecting system, has been used to determine obstruction. A T1/2 of less than 10 minutes suggests that no physiologically significant obstruction exists. A T1/2 of greater than 20 minutes suggests possible physiologically significant obstruction [47]. However, recent studies have challenged the notion that T1/2 is the most important parameter for assessing obstruction. Bao et al. created a predictive model for assessing the probability of normal drainage using MAG-3 diuretic scan [48]. They found that time to maximum cortical activity, 20-minute activity to maximum activity ratio, and postvoid to maximum activity ratio were the most significant in predicting normal renal drainage. In a retrospective review of 37 patients with ureteropelvic junction obstruction (UPJO) following pyeloplasty, von Rundstedt et al. suggested the percent of maximal tracer still present 40 minutes after administration increased the sensitivity of renal scintigraphy for obstruction from 49% to 73% compared to T1/2 alone [49].

DMSA is another commonly used radiopharmaceutical that allows for the evaluation of renal scarring and differential renal function in the pediatric population following episodes of acute pyelonephritis [50]. Diethylenetriamine pentaacetate is excreted through glomerular filtration and allows for accurate measurement of GFR as well as the visualization of urinary flow from the renal calyces through to the bladder.

Pyelography

Pyelography involves using X-ray imaging of the urinary tract (plain films or fluoroscopy) with the aid of intraluminal contrast administered through a retrograde, antegrade, or parenteral fashion [51]. Retrograde pyelography via a retrograde pyelogram (RPG) involves cystoscopic access and catheterization of the ureter, usually under anesthesia. It can be utilized in the evaluation of OU for patients in which IV contrast is contraindicated, such as poor renal function or contrast allergy. Anterograde pyelography is usually performed by passing contrast through a PCN tube directly into the kidney, and observing it travel through the urinary system. These techniques can delineate the level and extent of ureteral obstruction, assess for ureteral injury and urine leak, perform cancer surveillance, and evaluate causes of hematuria. Pyelography is also important during endoscopic procedures such as ureteroscopy, ureteral stent placement, and attaining percutaneous renal access. Intravenous pyelography, during which contrast is administered parenterally and excreted into the collecting system, was historically the preferred modality for assessing urothelial tumors, stones, and GU tuberculosis but has been largely marginalized due to the superiority of CTU in modern imaging protocols [40, 52].

Whitaker Test

The Whitaker test is a flow test used to differentiate obstructive versus non-obstructive dilation of the urinary tract by measuring the difference in pressure between renal pelvis and the bladder. The test is most often performed via a nephrostomy tube with a simultaneous bladder catheter in place. The upper urinary tract is then perfused at a constant rate of 10 mL/min with either diluted contrast or saline [54]. The relative pressure is calculated by subtracting the bladder pressure from the absolute pressure of the renal pelvis [55]. These pressures may then be used to differentiate between obstructive and non-obstructive urinary tract dilation. Because of its invasiveness and a general lack of experience with the technique in both urology and radiology hands, the Whitaker test is not commonly performed. It is generally reserved for cases of suspected upper urinary tract obstruction where initial testing is equivocal or in clinical dilemmas where surgical intervention is contemplated [54].

Etiology, Diagnosis, and Treatment of Obstructive Uropathy

Intrinsic Causes

Calculi

Background

Urolithiasis is a common cause of OU. The lifetime incidence of nephrolithiasis in the United States is approximately 1 in 11 [56]. Men are affected at a rate 1.3 times greater than women and patients with a history of a previous stones have a 42.7% chance of recurrence within ten years [57, 58]. The most common cause of nephrolithiasis is low urine volume due to insufficient hydration. Other factors that contribute to stone formation include diets high in sodium and/or animal protein, anatomic abnormalities that cause urinary stasis, medications, genetic diseases such as cystinuria, and urinary tract infections (UTI) with urea splitting organisms [59]. Bladder stones are another source of urinary calculi. They tend to form in the bladder and do not often represent stones of kidney origin. Their causes include BOO, intravesical foreign bodies, or anatomic abnormalities that prevent complete emptying (such as urethral strictures or large bladder diverticulae). Up to 10% of men with BPH will develop bladder stones and they represent an indication for surgical management [60].

Diagnosis

Urolithiasis may present asymptomatically on imaging or with acute or chronic symptoms such as flank pain that may radiate towards the groin. The pain may be associated with nausea and/or vomiting due to ureteral spasm [62]. A recent meta-analysis of 49 studies found that 84% percent of patients with proven urolithiasis and 77% of those experiencing acute renal colic also have concurrent microhematuria [63]. Patients should have a metabolic panel with a creatinine and BUN as well as a urinalysis [64]. Signs of infection in the setting of obstruction include fever, chills, hypotension, and tachycardia. If infection is suspected or surgical intervention planned, a urine culture as well as CBC is also warranted [28]. The initial imaging of a patient with suspected urolithiasis consists of a NCCT of the abdomen and pelvis or a RBUS and/or plain x-ray of the kidneys, ureter, and bladder [39, 64]. Although contrast CT scans are appropriate for circumstances in which other abdominal pathology (appendicitis, diverticulitis, perforated viscus, trauma) is likely to be responsible for pain, contrast in the collecting system can obscure urinary tract calculi and may exacerbate an acute kidney injury.

In pregnant women and children, ultrasound is preferred to avoid ionizing radiation [39]. If a diagnosis cannot be made on ultrasound and further characterization with CT is needed, a low dose radiation protocol can be used [63].

Treatment

Treatment of obstructing urolithiasis depends on the level of the obstruction. Management begins with IV fluids, pain management, and antiemetics [60]. Urgent upper tract urinary drainage may be indicated in certain clinical scenarios, as demonstrated in Table 2.

Table 2: Indications for urgent urinary drainage in obstructive uropathy

• Inability to tolerate oral intake
• Uncontrollable pain
• Bilateral ureteral obstruction or obstruction of a solitary kidney • Signs of infection
• Acute kidney injury

Urgent decompression can be achieved with either a ureteral stent or PCN tube, depending on specific clinical circumstances [28]. This is usually a temporizing measure, and definitive treatment of the obstructive etiology should be delayed until any infection has been treated. In patients with acute sepsis of urinary tract origin, there is retrospective evidence favoring PCN over ureteral stents to avoid the risks associated with general anesthesia [66] and provide the most reliable drainage. However, in a clinical trial comparing PCN versus ureteral stent drainage of obstructing ureteral calculi in 42 patients with suspected infections, Pearle et al. found no significant difference in the effectiveness of drainage or subsequent recovery between the two methods [67].

If indications for immediate drainage are not met, treatment depends on several factors. Observation can be offered to patients with uncomplicated ureteral stones, although spontaneous passage rates for stones 6 mm or greater in size drop below 60% [68]. Medical expulsive therapy (MET) consisting of an alpha-receptor blocker such as tamsulosin or a calcium channel blocker has been described as facilitating stone passage and, as a result, is a described treatment option in the 2016 American Urological Association (AUA) guideline on the management of stone disease [28, 69-72] However, more recent data has called the effectiveness of MET into question. Meltzer et al. studied 512 patients randomized to placebo or tamsulosin treatment groups for stones less than 9 mm in size found that there was no significant difference in stone passage rates after 28 days of treatment with tamsulosin compared to placebo [73]. Similarly, the Spontaneous Urinary Stone Passage Enabled by Drugs (SUSPEND) trial found no benefit of MET with either tamsulosin or nifedipine compared to placebo for passage of stones less than 5 mm in size [74].

Patients who fail a trial of passage symptomatically or prefer intervention can be offered surgical treatment [28]. Symptomatic renal stone treatment depends on the location, amount of the total stone burden, stone density, anatomic considerations, and patient habitus. Treatment options include extracorporeal shock wave lithotripsy (ESWL), ureteroscopy (URS) with or without laser lithotripsy, or percutaneous nephrostolithotomy (PCNL). Common stone burden variables and recommended treatments can be seen in Table 3 below.

In terms of the lower urinary tract, bladder stones can be treated through a variety of methods including transurethral (most common), laparoscopic, open surgical, and percutaneous approaches [60].

Table 3: Treatment algorithm for surgical management of nephrolithiasis

Location		**Stone burden**	**First line treatment**
Renal	Non-Lower Pole	≤ 20 mm	URS or ESWL
		> 20 mm	PCNL (ESWL also acceptable in pediatric patients)
	Lower Pole	≤ 10 mm	URS or ESWL
		> 10 mm	URS or PCNL
Ureteral	Proximal	≤ 10 mm	URS
		> 10 mm	URS or ESWL
	Distal	≤ 10 mm	URS
		> 10 mm	URS or ESWL
Legend	URS: Ureteroscopy, ESWL: Extracorporeal Shockwave Lithotripsy, PCNL: Percutaneous Nephrolithotomy		

Genitourinary Malignancy

Background

OU secondary to GU malignancy can occur at any level of the urinary tract. GU malignancy can cause intrinsic or extrinsic obstruction through local extension, invasion, and compression of urinary tract structures [75]. For example, up to 10% of patients with prostate cancer will experience upper tract obstruction and up to 57.9% of patients with muscle invasive bladder cancer will have preoperative hydronephrosis due to invasion of the ureteral orifices [76, 77]. Lymphadenopathy from GU malignancies can result in extrinsic compression of the ureter resulting in obstruction. Blood clots from upper tract cancers such as renal cell carcinoma can also cause ureteral obstruction.

Diagnosis

Presenting symptoms can include hematuria, flank pain, anorexia, nausea, vomiting, and urinary retention. Advanced GU malignancy may result in constitutional symptoms such as weight loss or fever [25]. CT and MRI play critical roles in the diagnoses and staging of GU malignancies. Renal cell carcinoma is primarily diagnosed and staged through either multiphasic CT or MRI [4]. Urinary tract cancers can be seen as contrast "filling defects" in the urinary system during a RPG or CTU. Further evaluation is guided by the particular cancer diagnosed.

Treatment

Initial treatment depends on the location and type of cancer causing the obstruction in conjunction with patient comorbidities. Renal or ureteral obstruction can be relieved with either retrograde ureteral stent placement or PCN. PCN may be necessary in complex patients with significant ureteral tumor involvement, if the ureteral orifices are obscured due to pathology at the bladder level, or with abnormal or difficult to navigate anatomy due to prior treatment, such as with urinary diversions [75, 76]. For bladder outlet or urethral obstruction, urethral catheterization or suprapubic cystostomy may be utilized. Suprapubic cystostomy should be avoided in cases of bladder cancer due to the risk of tumor seeding [75]. Palliative urinary drainage for advanced cancers should be carefully discussed with patients. Regular exchange of these tubes is essential to minimize the risk of encrustation, dysfunction, and infection; and these frequent exchanges can be burdensome and costly. While obstructive symptoms may be relieved, symptoms due to the growth and metastasis of the tumor are unlikely to resolve with decompression alone and drainage tubes increase the risk for UTI [75].

Clinical Pearls

- PCN for upper tract drainage is preferred over ureteral stenting for patients with significant ureteral tumor involvement, obscured ureteral orifice, or complex anatomy such as urinary diversions that limit retrograde access.
- Regular PCN and ureteral stent exchanges are needed for chronic indwelling tubes to minimize the risk of encrustation, dysfunction, and infection.

Strictures

Background

GU strictures can occur anywhere in the urinary tract. A urethral stricture is a narrowing of the urethra caused by fibrosis of the surrounding corpus spongiosum [78]. Men older than 65 years of age are most affected, but urethral strictures can present at any age, resulting from a variety of etiologies with iatrogenic and idiopathic causes being the most common [79]. Additional causes include infection, trauma, radiation, lichen sclerosis and complications of circumcision [78]. The most common location for a urethral structure in a male is the bulbar urethra, followed by the penile urethra.

A ureteral stricture is a narrowing of the ureter that may cause obstruction of urinary flow. Strictures have a variety of causes including iatrogenic injury, stone impaction, trauma, GU malignancy, and radiation. Fam et al. studied 77 patients undergoing treatment for impacted ureteral calculi and found a stricture rate of 7.8% following rigid ureteroscopy [80].

Diagnosis

Urethral strictures present with obstructive voiding symptoms, dysuria, urinary retention, and in some cases frequency, urgency, or recurrent UTIs. Spongiofibrosis may be detectable upon palpation of the penis [78]. Definitive diagnosis focuses on determining the location and length of the stricture, often by performing a retrograde urethrogram (RUG). Ultrasound, particularly using intraluminal probes, can be used in conjunction with RUG to help further characterize stricture length and the extent of spongiofibrosis [81]. While strictures may be diagnosed by cystoscopy, stricture length is less accurately ascertained via endoscopy and should be used to complement a RUG [78]. Antegrade urethrograms can also be considered in patients with suprapubic tubes particularly in cases of severe stricturing of the bulbar urethra [82]. VCUG is suggested in cases were bladder outlet or posterior urethral involvement is suspected [79].

Ureteral strictures may present with ipsilateral flank pain, calculi, hematuria, nausea and/or vomiting, renal dysfunction, and recurrent UTIs or pyelonephritis. They can be diagnosed via CTU, RPG, antegrade nephrostogram, diuretic renal scintigraphy, ureteroscopy, or a combination of these [83].

Treatment

Initial treatment of urethral strictures depends on the location and size, as seen in Table 4. Acute retention should be managed with suprapubic cystotomy if urethral catheterization is not feasible [84]. Both endoscopic management and urethroplasty may be considered for definitive treatment [79, 81]. Endoscopic management can include either dilation and/or direct visual internal urethrotomy [84, 86]. For strictures 2 cm or less in size, endoscopic management achieves patency in up to 60% of cases [85]. Urethroplasty is preferred for strictures greater than 2 cm as well as multi-focal, bulbar, and penile strictures. Tissue transfer techniques (such as buccal mucosal grafting) can be highly effective at repairing urethral strictures. Urethroplasty is also preferred in pediatric patients due to the high rate of recurrence with endoscopic treatment [86]. If urethroplasty is contraindicated, a combination of endoscopic management and maintenance clean intermittent catheterization can be used [84].

Table 4: Indications for endoscopy vs. Urethroplasty in surgical management of urethral strictures

Endoscopy	Urethroplasty
• ≤ 2 cm in length	• 2 cm in length
• Single stricture	• Penile or bulbar location
• Poor surgical candidates	• Multi-focal
• Treatment-naïve	• Pediatric patients
	• Failed previous endoscopic attempt

Management of ureteral strictures depends on the etiology, location, and length. For short strictures (< 2 cm) with benign etiologies, endoscopic balloon dilation has shown variable efficacy (33-100%) [83]. Endoureterotomy has shown success rates ranging from 60% to 86% across all techniques in well-selected patients with short strictures. Ureteral strictures may also be managed with chronic indwelling stent or PCN, particularly in cases where patients are poor surgical candidates. This carries the risk of encrustation and infection as well as the burden of frequent exchanges. In cases of extrinsic ureteral compression, particularly malignant ureteral obstruction, PCNs have been shown to be more effective due to stent failure rates as high as 58% [83, 87]. Metallic stents are also an option and offer promising, albeit more expensive alternative to traditional stents. Kim et al. compared the efficacy of metallic stents versus ureteral stents in 19 patients with MUO [88]. Patency rates were significantly higher in the metallic stent group at both 3 and 6 months (90% and 57%) post placement compared to the ureteral stent group (35% and 21%). Chung et al., in a comparative study, found that 65.3% of ureters with MUO managed with metallic stents remained patent after 24 months compared to only 37.8% of those managed with double J-stents [89].

If initial endoscopic management fails or is not advisable, reconstructive surgery should be considered. Surgical options depend on stricture location/extent and include ureteral reimplantation with or without a psoas hitch, Boari flap creation, ureteroureterostomy, transureteroureterostomy, pyeloplasty, ileal ureter, and autotransplantation [90]. More recently, buccal mucosal graft augmented ureteroplasty has been described as a promising technique with success rates of 71% to 83% [91]. These reconstructions may be performed using minimally invasive laparoscopic and robotic techniques in many cases. In a retrospective series reviewing the outcomes of 250 patients who underwent robotic upper urinary tract reconstruction, there was a 97% symptomatic success rate at a mean follow up of 17.1 months [92].

Ureteroenteric strictures (strictures at the junction of ureteral anastomoses to bowel segments in urinary diversion) have shown high rates of recurrence with endoscopic treatment and often necessitate reconstructive surgery [93]. In a retrospective series of 161 patients comparing endoscopic treatment to open reconstruction, patients who received open surgical reconstruction maintained a patency rate of 69% at 60 months versus only 27% in patients who received endoscopic treatment [94].

Radiation can lead to OU through progressive fibrosis and stricture formation in the urinary tract. Radiation induces direct DNA damage and free radical formation causing cell death. Rapidly dividing cells, such as those in cancer, are preferentially affected, but surrounding tissues and vascular basement membranes may also be harmed. Thrombosis and occlusion of vasculature follows, leading to tissue ischemia, atrophy, fibrosis, and stricture formation [95]. For example, in men undergoing radiotherapy for prostate cancer, the incidence of urethral stricture formation ranges from 2% to 32% and the incidence of distal ureteral stricture formation is approximately 6% [96, 97]. In a study of 1784 women who underwent radiotherapy for cervical cancer, McIntyre et al. found a risk of 0.15% for ureteral stricture development per year following treatment [98].

Radiation-induced ureteral strictures present several challenges due to microvascular injury and fibrosis. Endoscopic management may be less effective due to the lack of an adequate vascular supply; thus, surgical reconstruction is often required [99]. The bladder is also within the field of most pelvic irradiation treatment plans. Since many ureteral reconstruction approaches depend on bladder tissue, it is critical to assess bladder capacity and quality prior to committing to a reconstructive approach.

Urethroplasty is the most effective treatment for radiation-induced urethral strictures, with success rates ranging from 70 to 90% [95, 96, 100]. Endoscopic treatment for radiation-induced urethral strictures should be avoided due to the high rate of recurrence (40-60%) [100].

Clinical Pearls

- Endoscopic management of radiation-induced GU strictures may be less effective due to the lack of an adequate blood supply. As such, surgical reconstruction is often required.

CONGENITAL ABNORMALITIES

This section will discuss the most common congenital causes of OU, although there are many more causes less common that are not described here.

Ureteropelvic Junction Obstruction

Background

Congenital ureteropelvic junction obstruction (UPJO) can be caused by a variety of anomalies including high ureteral insertion, compression by a renal vessel crossing over the ureter, hypoplasia of a ureteral segment, and kinking of the ureter [101]. Congenital UPJO has an incidence of 1 in 1000 to 1500 births [102]. Adult patients normally present in the 3rd and 4th decades of life [103]. In addition to the congenital causes, adult UPJO may be caused by an obstructing retroperitoneal or intraluminal mass, ureteral stricture, urolithiasis, or lymphadenopathy amongst other causes.

Diagnosis

Patients may present with flank pain, recurrent UTI, nephrolithiasis, hematuria, or even renin-mediated hypertension. The most common imaging finding is hydronephrosis with an abrupt transition at the UPJ without an obstructing calculus. Initial diagnosis in pediatric patients is often made with renal ultrasound, although adults are often diagnosed with a CT scan done for renal colic. In a retrospective review of 220 pediatric patients with UPJO, Wong et al. found that color doppler ultrasound is 93.3% sensitive and 92.7% specific for identifying crossing vessels. Color doppler ultrasound outperformed magnetic resonance urography (MRU), which achieved a sensitivity and specificity of only 71.7% and 77.6%, respectively [104]. In adults, vascular ultrasound may be limited by body mass index and visceral fat. A contrast CT scan or formal CT angiography (CTA) may be needed to evaluate the presence of a crossing vessel at the UPJ [105]. MAG-3 renal scintigraphy can be used to assess functional obstruction and to provide differential renal function, which can impact clinical decision-making.

Treatment

Asymptomatic pediatric patients with low-grade hydronephrosis may be observed due to the possibility of spontaneous resolution, which ranges from 33% to 77% [106]. These patients should be followed with semi-annual RBUS to assess for improvement and interval MAG-3 scan if needed. Reconstruction is often performed if there is worsening or lack of improvement on RBUS, the patient is symptomatic, or renal scarring often secondary to recurrent UTI's [101]. Nephrectomy may be considered in symptomatic patients with very low differential renal function (< 10 – 20%) [105-107].

UPJO is a clinical diagnosis driven by the history and not solely imaging. Symptomatic adults often describe the so-called "Dietel's Crisis" during which high consumption of fluid, caffeine, alcohol, or other diuretics elicits flank pain. The degree of hydronephrosis may vary dramatically between asymptomatic periods and acute flank pain events. Nuclear renal scanning or even Whittaker testing may provide evidence for obstruction. Determining whether surgery is indicated requires shared decision-making and thorough counseling is of paramount importance.

UPJO can be treated endoscopically (endopyelotomy) or with definitive surgical reconstruction (pyeloplasty). Endopyelotomy, which can be performed in both retrograde and antegrade fashion, is relatively contraindicated in cases of a crossing vessel, poor renal function, and severe hydronephrosis. Doo et al. examined the long-term outcomes of endopyelotomy for UPJO in 77 patients and found success in 67.5% of cases at a median follow-up of 37.3 months [108]. Minimally invasive pyeloplasty (performed laparoscopically or robotically) has become the gold standard for treatment of UPJO in children and adults due to significantly higher success rates than endopyelotomy, and abbreviated recovery compared to open surgery [109]. Syzdelko et al. compared the outcomes of antegrade endopyletomy to that of laparoscopic pyeloplasty. They found that laparoscopic pyeloplasty achieved a significantly higher success rate at 95.3% versus 55.4% [110]. Although endopyelotomy is used less often as a primary treatment option for UPJO, it may still play a valuable role in the management of secondary UPJO after failure of primary pyeloplasty.

In the case of a complex UPJO, anastomosis of the ureter directly into the lower pole calyx (ureterocalicostomy) is a viable option as well, especially if there is lower pole renal parenchymal atrophy. Radford et al. examined the efficacy of ureterocalicostomy in 13 pediatric patients with complicated UPJO and described adequate drainage, function, and symptom relief in 12 of 13 patients at mean follow-up of 32 months [111].

Posterior Urethral Valves

Background

PUV are congenital membranous folds in the male posterior urethra that lead to the obstruction of urinary flow. Prolonged prenatal bladder obstruction and distention leads to bladder hypertrophy with eventual dysfunction and loss of compliance. Elevation of intravesical pressure leads to vesicoureteral reflux (VUR) causing progressive renal damage. The incidence of PUV is approximately 1:3800 live male births [112]. It occurs exclusively in males and approximately 50% of patients progress to ESRD within 10 years of diagnosis [113].

Diagnosis

Patients may present postnatally or prenatally on maternal fetal ultrasound. Findings can include oligohydramnios with bilateral hydronephrosis, bladder distention, bladder wall thickening (> 3mm), and the "keyhole sign" (prostatic urethral dilation) [114]. Postnatal patients present with obstructive voiding symptoms, palpably distended bladder, UTIs, hydronephrosis, urinary retention, and renal failure [115]. Postnatal diagnosis is made through ultrasound followed by voiding cystourethrogram (VCUG). This may be followed by renal scintigraphy for the assessment of differential renal function [114, 115].

Treatment

There currently is no consensus for prenatal treatment, which is generally limited to the third trimester [114]. Treatment options include fetal cystoscopy, fetal endoscopic valve ablation, and vesicoamniotic shunt [115]. Vesicoamniotic shunts should be performed at major pediatric centers due to the complexities of the procedure. Postnatal treatment initially involves immediate placement of urethral catheter or suprapubic tube, and ultimately endoscopic valve ablation. Many patients may suffer from VUR following valve ablation, which may require treatment with continuous antibiotics prophylaxis and/or ureteral reimplantation [116]. Preterm infants in which valve ablation is not possible may require creation of a vesicostomy initially [117, 118].

Ureterocele

Background

A ureterocele is a cystic dilatation of the distal ureter protruding into the bladder, which can lead to obstruction of urinary flow and stone formation. Ureteroceles occur in approximately 1:4000 live births and are 4-6 times more common in females than in males [119]. While ureteroceles are most frequently diagnosed in pediatric patients, they can be found incidentally in adults as well [4].

Diagnosis

Patients often present with hydronephrosis and occasionally with BOO (in the case of a bulky ureterocele extending into the bladder neck). Ureteroceles are often associated with complete ureteral duplication [120]. In pediatric patients, the initial diagnosis is made by RBUS and/or VCUG. VCUG should be performed to check for VUR. A ureterocele can be confirmed directly by cystoscopy. Renal scintigraphy can be performed to assess differential renal function [120]. In cases with complex anatomic abnormalities, MRU has proven valuable [121].

Treatment

Ureteroceles can be managed with endoscopic incision or definitive surgical excision depending on their location, size, patient age, and associated symptoms [122]. Endoscopic drainage is commonly used as the initial treatment but may result in a high rate of de novo VUR (up to 75%) [123]. If initial endoscopic incision fails, further treatment options include ureteral reimplantation, heminephrectomy in duplex systems with or without lower tract reconstruction, and total nephroureterectomy, depending on the clinical scenario [120]. Asymptomatic patients, however, can be observed when incidentally detected, especially in adults.

Ureterovesical Junction Obstruction

Background

Congenital ureterovesical junction obstruction (UVJO) can be caused by abnormal ureteral insertion into the bladder, distal ureteral atresia, or a non-peristaltic distal ureteral segment, among other causes. UVJO is often associated with severe dilatation of the ipsilateral ureter of greater than 8 mm, known as megaureter [124]. Congenital UVJO accounts for 4% of cases of fetal hydronephrosis [125]. In adults, UVJO is more commonly associated with a history of an impacted distal ureteral calculus, prior ureteroscopic instrumentation, radiation, or prior transurethral resection procedures.

Diagnosis

Patients may present with hydroureteronephrosis, UTI, or flank pain. Diagnosis in pediatric patients is often made with RBUS. Renal scintigraphy can be used to assess differential renal function. CTU can be used to assess anatomy as well.

Treatment

Definitive treatment of UVJO consists of ureteral reimplantation with tapering of the megaureter if necessary [126]. These procedures can be done via open or minimally invasive approaches. In adults, endoscopic management has been effective in some small series. Arrabal-Martin et al. treated 18 adult patients with UVJO endoscopically with cold knife incision with a success rate of 94.5% of cases at 36 month following treatment [127].

Retrocaval Ureter

Background

Retrocaval ureter (RCU) is a congenital anomaly in which the persistence of the cardinal vein anteriorly to the proximal ureter leads to ureteral tortuosity, resulting in OU. The incidence of RCUs is about 1 in 1500 individuals worldwide [128]. RCUs are predominantly right-sided with patients normally presenting in their 30's or 40's [129].

Diagnosis

Patients with RCUs generally complain of right flank pain or present asymptomatically with incidentally discovered right hydronephrosis. Microscopic or gross hematuria may also be present and there can be associated nephrolithiasis due to urinary stasis. RBUS will often show right-sided hydronephrosis. CTU is the preferred method of diagnosis as it can serve to distinguish RCU from other retroperitoneal causes of ureteral obstruction. Renal scintigraphy can be considered at diagnosis to assess for differential renal function and degree of obstruction [130].

Treatment

Asymptomatic patients with no evidence of renal compromise can be observed [131 Symptomatic patients with a functional ipsilateral kidney should be treated with surgical reconstruction by ureteral transection and re-anastomosis anterior to the vena [130].

Extrinsic Causes

Benign Prostatic Hyperplasia

Background

BPH is one of the most common etiologies of OU in men. About 50% of men have histologic evidence of BPH in the 6th decade of life [132]. BPH is the result of both epithelial and stromal hyperplasia, predominantly in the transition zone of the prostate. Progressive narrowing of the prostatic urethra results in BOO, which impedes urinary flow and ultimately leads to upper urinary tract deterioration from elevated voiding and/or storage pressures [133].

Diagnosis

The initial evaluation of BPH consists of a history, physical exam including digital rectal exam, urinalysis, and an AUA Symptom Index to assess for severity of symptoms [134]. BPH often causes bothersome LUTS. LUTS can be subdivided into irritative versus obstructive symptoms. Irritative symptoms include frequency, urgency, and nocturia. Obstructive symptoms include a weak, staccato, or slow urinary stream as well as hesitancy, incomplete bladder emptying, urinary retention, straining, and post void dribbling. Locally advanced prostate cancer can also restrict urinary flow, although this is an uncommon presenting symptom for the disease. Voiding diaries can be a useful adjunct to better understand a particular patient's symptom complex and help guide treatment.

On physical exam, patients may have bladder distention and discomfort upon suprapubic palpation. Patients with symptomatic BPH often, but not always, have an enlarged prostate on digital rectal exam [135]. It is important to remember that total prostate size, particularly on palpation, does not always correlate with symptomatic BPH or LUTS [136]. The prostate should feel smooth and relatively firm, in contrast to prostate cancer, which is generally irregular, nodular, and hard. Urinalysis should be performed to explore other potential causes of voiding dysfunction such as malignancy or infection [133]. In a study of 302 men with LUTS, a PSA of greater than 4 ng/mL was predictive of BOO in 89% of cases [137].

Several adjunct studies may be helpful in deciding treatment options. A post-void residual (PVR) urine should be checked to determine the baseline emptying of the bladder [138]. An elevated and/or increasing PVR may imply BPH refractory to medical treatment. Uroflowmetry and urodynamics can be used to further characterize the degree of BOO and detrusor contractility [139]. Determination of prostatic volume by cross-sectional or transrectal ultrasound imaging should also be considered before surgical management as prostate volume can alter surgical planning significantly [134].

Treatment

In the case of acute retention due to BPH, urgent decompression should be performed with urethral catheterization [140]. Suprapubic catheterization may be performed when urethral catheterization is either not possible or contraindicated. Long-term management of BPH can include both medical and surgical options. Alpha-1 adrenergic receptor blockers can relax prostatic smooth muscle, thus decreasing outflow resistance. The prostate volume can also be medically reduced over time with the use of 5α reductase inhibitors, although this medication often takes months to cause a clinically significant improvement in LUTS. In patients with concomitant irritative symptoms, anticholinergics may also be used; however, caution is advised in patients with a large PVR due to the risk of urinary retention. For patients with erectile dysfunction, daily type-5 phosphodiesterase inhibitors can have comparable benefits to alpha-1 blockers in LUTS while simultaneously treating erectile dysfunction, although no significant difference in uroflow parameters or PVR have been noted [141].

Table 5: Indications for surgical management of BPH

Indications
• Medically refractory LUTS
• Recurrent UTI's
• Medically refractory urinary retention
• Gross hematuria secondary to BPH
• Recurrent bladder stones
• Unwillingness to use medical treatment • Progressive renal deterioration

The indications for surgical management of BPH are listed in Table 5 [134]. A variety of surgical options exist that aim to reduce or remove outlet obstruction at the prostate level. Transurethral resection of the prostate is a common surgical approach. Outlet reduction can be performed using several different energy sources, including electrical, vapor, laser, ultrasonic, and thermal energy. Patients with large prostates (>80g) may be considered for open or minimally invasive simple prostatectomy, or laser enucleation [142]. Prostatic urethral lift

(PUL), which retracts the prostatic lobes using implants, has been shown to be efficacious with minimal sexual side effects [143].

Clinical Pearls

- A non-enlarged prostate on physical exam does not rule out BPH as a cause of outlet obstruction. Conversely, a large prostate does not necessarily lead to bothersome urinary symptoms or necessitate treatment.

Traumatic Ureteral Injury

Background

Ureteral injury can occur from laceration, transection, ligation, thermal injury, devascularization, or avulsion. Three-fourths of ureteral injuries are caused by iatrogenic injury, with the distal third of the ureter being the most affected site [144], primarily due to its vulnerability during gynecologic and colorectal procedures [145]. Ureteral injury resulting in stricture secondary to ureteroscopy occurs in 0.5 to 2.5% of cases [146]. Ureteral injury can also occur with both blunt and penetrating GU trauma at a rate of 3 ureteral injuries per 10,000 trauma admissions [147].

Diagnosis

The presentation of ureteral injury can be insidious and may initially appear asymptomatic. A low threshold for evaluation is warranted after high-risk injuries or procedures. However, some injuries can present with signs of ureteral obstruction or urine extravasation. Laboratory analysis may show elevated creatinine and BUN. Hematuria is a common but non-specific finding. Patients with abdominal drains following surgery may have excessive drainage volumes with elevated fluid creatinine when compared to serum creatinine [148]. In stable trauma patients with suspected ureteral injury, the AUA recommends a CTU [149]. If initial imaging is equivocal, RPG can be utilized, which can also facilitate treatment with stent placement [90]. In patients with suspected ureteral injury undergoing laparotomy for trauma, the AUA recommends that the ureters be visualized and investigated for signs of injury [149].

Treatment

Treatment of ureteral injury depends on a variety of factors including the length, location, time to diagnosis, and mechanism of injury. The AUA provides clear guidelines for the management of common ureteral injuries [149]. Endoscopic ureteral injuries should initially be treated with diversion of the urinary tract proximal to the injury with a ureteral stent and/or PCN placement. If sufficient drainage cannot be achieved, repair is recommended. For injuries noted intraoperatively, they should be immediately repaired or stented. A PCN should be placed if a ureteral stent cannot be placed or internal drainage is inadequate. If a small segment of the ureter is non-viable, it can be resected and repaired over a stent. More extensive ureteral injuries may require formal reconstruction following a period of drainage. Distal and mid ureteral injuries may require bladder reimplantation with possible psoas hitch and/or Boari flap reconstruction. Proximal ureteral injuries can be repaired with pyeloplasty. If repair is contraindicated, for example, due to hemodynamic instability, urinary diversion with either with a nephrostomy tube and/or a ureteral stent should be performed, with the plan for delayed reconstruction.

Clinical Pearls

- Immediate ureteral injury may be asymptomatic, but there should be a low threshold for evaluation after high-risk procedures or trauma with a suggestive mechanism.
- Excessive abdominal drain output following surgery may indicate a ureteral laceration. This can be assessed with a drain fluid creatinine.

Retroperitoneal Fibrosis

Background

RPF is caused by chronic peri-aortitis leading to inflammation of the retroperitoneum with ensuing fibrosis and compression of retroperitoneal structures. Van Bommel et al. estimated the incidence of RPF to be about 1.3 in 100,000 [150]. In a study of 204 patients with RPF, ureteral obstruction was seen in 95.6% of patients [151]. RPF is most often idiopathic but has been associated with autoimmune disease, radiation, surgery, asbestos exposure, tobacco smoke, several medications, and malignancies including pancreas, breast, stomach, prostate cancers [150, 151].

Diagnosis

Symptoms include non-colicky ipsilateral flank pain, as well as oliguria, nausea, and constitutional symptoms. Vascular and lymphatic constriction can lead to lower extremity and GU edema, as well as deep venous thrombosis [152]. Laboratory analysis may show postrenal azotemia. CRP or erythrocyte sedimentation rate can be elevated [153]. RPF will often appear as mass surrounding the anterolateral aorta and possibly the inferior vena cava on CT or MRI. Enhancement is usually present in the early active phase of the disease [154]. Ureters classically appear medially deviated and tapered due to compression with resultant hydronephrosis [154]. The differential diagnosis also includes malignant processes such as metastatic testicular cancer, lymphoma, or retroperitoneal sarcoma; biopsy may be indicated in certain clinical circumstances to establish (or refute) a malignant diagnosis.

Treatment

Treatment depends on the severity and extent of RPF. In patients presenting with OU, decompression with placement of either ureteral stents or PCN may be necessary. Long-term treatment of RPF involves immunosuppressive therapy with corticosteroids, close follow-up imaging, and monitoring of renal function and inflammatory markers [152]. Surgical treatment is generally restricted to cases failing medical management. Surgical options include open or minimally invasive ureterolysis, essentially freeing the ureter from the surrounding fibrosis and then intraperitonealization of the ureters and/or wrapping them in an omental flap. In a retrospective review of 50 patients with ureteric obstruction secondary to RPF treated with open ureterolysis and omental wrapping, 94% of patients maintained spontaneous urinary drainage without stenting one year following treatment [155].

Other Causes

Neurogenic Bladder

Background

Neurogenic bladder (NGB) is a dysfunction of the bladder, internal urethral sphincter, or external urethral sphincter due to the disruption of central or peripheral nerve pathways, leading to disordered micturition [156]. Impaired voiding and detrusor spasticity obstruct urinary flow and increase intravesical pressures, leading to upper urinary tract deterioration over time [157]. Pathophysiology involves transmission of elevated bladder pressures to the upper tract due to a loss of bladder compliance. Causes of NGB include spinal cord injury, radical pelvic surgery, multiple sclerosis, diabetes mellitus, spina bifida, cerebral palsy, Parkinson's disease, stroke, and dementia, among many others [158].

Diagnosis

Patients often present with a variety of motor and sensory urinary symptoms. The specific constellation of symptoms depends on the level of nervous system dysfunction. Video urodynamic studies (VUDS) are the mainstay in the diagnosis of neurogenic bladder. Elevated detrusor leak point pressures can be predictive of upper urinary tract deterioration when greater than 40 cm/H20 [159]. These patients are often followed with regular VUDS to measure progression of their bladder function. RBUS is commonly used in long-term surveillance to exclude development of hydronephrosis, a known risk factor for renal deterioration, and bladder stones [160].

Treatment

Treatment of NGB varies by severity of bladder pathology, symptoms experienced by the patient, and degree of upper tract deterioration. It is important to start with conservative measures such as time voiding, double voiding, and management of constipation and neurogenic bowel symptoms. Anti-cholinergic or beta-3 agonist medication can be used in patients with neurogenic detrusor overactivity [161]. Clean intermittent catheterization (CIC) can facilitate bladder emptying if patients are unable to adequately and safely do so spontaneously [160]. Indwelling urethral or suprapubic catherization can be used when urethral self-catherization is difficult due to poor hand function or contraindicated due to anatomic factors; however, indwelling catheters increases the risk of urinary tract complications when compared to CIC and it is preferable toas avoid these as a definitive treatment if possible [162].

If first-line treatment fails, surgical management can involve intravesical botulinum toxin [163]. Neuromodulation with either sacral neuromodulation (SNM) or percutaneous tibial nerve stimulation (PTNS) have also proven efficacious. SNM has been shown to improve quality of life (QOL) and provides long-term decreases in the rates of urinary retention, incontinence, frequency, and urgency [164]. PTNS has also shown promise in the treatment of NGB. In a clinical trial of 70 patient's neurogenic overactivity secondary to multiple sclerosis, PTNS resulted in significant decreases in urgency, frequency, as well as improved continence and QOL [165]. In cases refractory to medical therapy and less invasive procedures, surgical options such as augmentation cystoplasty and urinary diversion may be indicated [166].

Clinical Pearls

- Most patients with NGB present with a variety of symptoms depending on the level of their neurologic dysfunction or injury.
- Long term follow-up is important to prevent renal deterioration and mitigate other complications such as UTIs and bladder stones.

Tuberculosis

Background

Genitourinary tuberculosis (TB) is responsible for up to 40% of extrapulmonary manifestations of tuberculosis (TB) [167]. GU TB arises via lymphohematogenous spread or direct GU contact. OU results from repetitive granuloma formation with concomitant fibrosis and calcium deposition anywhere in the urinary tract. About 24% of patients with GU TB will experience renal failure [52].

Diagnosis

Symptoms include flank pain, irritative voiding symptoms, and recurrent UTI's. A history of TB exposure or pulmonary disease would raise suspicion. On physical exam, patients may have flank pain on percussion or nodularity of the testicles, epididymis, or prostate. Diagnosis is confirmed by both laboratory and radiographic testing. Laboratory testing includes mycobacterial culture of three early morning urine samples, polymerase chain reaction (PCR), and acid-fast staining [167]. The gold standard imaging modality is urography, either with IV urography or CTU [168]. Findings may include calyceal blunting, dilation, filling defects, intrarenal strictures, hydronephrosis, and renal parenchymal calcifications [52]. Patients should also be tested for HIV due to high co-incidence in patients with GU TB [169].

Treatment

Acute obstruction should be addressed via stent or PCN placement. Following initial decompression, treatment is four-drug therapy, including rifampin, isoniazid, pyrazinamide and ethambutol for the first two months followed by rifampin and isoniazid for the following 4 months [167]. Chronic obstruction may be amenable to endoscopic treatment with laser incision or balloon dilation of intrarenal and/or ureteral stricture disease [170].

Conclusion

OU can result from a variety of mechanisms and has a myriad of approaches to treatment depending on the etiology. However, the central theme of relieving the obstruction and treating the underlying etiology remains constant. Both UUO and BUO progress through predictable pathophysiological patterns with the ultimate consequence being fibrosis and deterioration of renal function. Following relief of obstruction, the recovery of renal function is dependent on several factors, including duration, patient age at onset, baseline renal function, and the condition of the contralateral kidney. Surgical management is dependent on the etiology and patient-specific factors must always be considered when deciding the optimal approach. POD is a common physiological side effect that results following the relief of bilateral urinary tract obstruction. New discoveries surrounding the pathophysiology, treatment, and prevention of obstructive uropathy are evolving.

REFERENCES

[1] Liaño F, Pascual J. Epidemiology of acute renal failure: a prospective, multicenter, community-based study. Madrid Acute Renal Failure Study Group. *Kidney Int.* 1996 Sep;50(3):811-8.

[2] Madsen MG. Urinary biomarkers in hydronephrosis. *Dan Med J.* 2013 Feb; 60(2):B4582.

[3] Moody TE, Vaughn ED Jr, Gillenwater JY. Relationship between renal blood flow and ureteral pressure during 18 hours of total unilateral uretheral occlusion. Implications for changing sites of increased renal resistance. *Invest Urol.* 1975 Nov;13(3):246-51.

[4] Peters CA, Meldrum KK, McDougal W, Wein A, Kavoussi L, Partin A. Campbell-Walsh Urology. 10th ed. Philadelphia: Saunders Elsevier; 2011. 776, 791-792p.

[5] Capelouto CC, Saltzman B. The pathophysiology of ureteral obstruction. *J Endourol.* 1993 Apr;7(2):93-103.

[6] Hegarty NJ, Young LS, Kirwan CN, O'Neill AJ, Bouchier-Hayes DM, Sweeney P, Watson RW, Fitzpatrick JM. Nitric oxide in unilateral ureteral obstruction: effect on regional renal blood flow. *Kidney Int.* 2001 Mar;59(3):1059-65.

[7] Martínez-Klimova E, Aparicio-Trejo OE, Tapia E, Pedraza-Chaverri J. Unilateral Ureteral Obstruction as a Model to Investigate Fibrosis-Attenuating Treatments. *Biomolecules.* 2019 Apr 8;9(4):141.

[8] Altheaby A, Alharbi N, Alzamil A, Alzahrani E, Alshaia AM, Aldowsary B, Aboalsamah G, Farooqui M, Bin Saad K, Arabi Z. How Does the Remaining Single Kidney Cope After Contralateral Nephrectomy of the Kidney Donor? A Single-Center Cohort Study. *Cureus.* 2020 Nov 15;12(11):e11491.

[9] Kim SW, Lee J, Park JW, Hong JH, Kook H, Choi C, Choi KC. Increased expression of atrial natriuretic peptide in the kidney of rats with bilateral ureteral obstruction. *Kidney Int.* 2001 Apr;59(4):1274-82.

[10] Halbgewachs C, Domes T. Postobstructive diuresis: pay close attention to urinary retention. *Can Fam Physician.* 2015 Feb;61(2):137-42.

[11] Frøkiaer J, Marples D, Knepper MA, Nielsen S. Bilateral ureteral obstruction downregulates expression of vasopressin-sensitive AQP-2 water channel in rat kidney. *Am J Physiol.* 1996 Apr;270(4 Pt 2):F657-68.

[12] Sophasan S, Sorrasuchart S. Factors inducing post-obstructive diuresis in rats. *Nephron.* 1984;38(2):125-33.

[13] Leslie SW, Sajjad H, Sharma S. Postobstructive Diuresis. [Updated 2020 Sep 22]. In: *StatPearls* [Internet]. Treasure Island (FL): StatPearls Publishing; 2020 Jan [Cited 2021 Feb 10]-. Available from: https://www.ncbi.nlm.nih.gov/books/NBK459387/

[14] Mauck, R, Thomas S. *Consults & Emergencies: Post Obstructive Diuresis.* American Urological Association, American Urological Association, 9 Feb. 2021[Cited 2021 Feb

10], Available from: https://university.auanet.org/modules/webapps/core/index.cfm#/corecontent/196.

[15] Shokeir AA, Provoost AP, Nijman RJ. Recoverability of renal function after relief of chronic partial upper urinary tract obstruction. *BJU Int.* 1999 Jan;83(1):11-7.

[16] Sharma U, Yadav SS, Tomar V. Factors influencing recoverability of renal function after urinary diversion through percutaneous nephrostomy. *Urol Ann.* 2015 Oct-Dec;7(4):499-503.

[17] Kukreja R, Desai M, Patel SH, Desai MR. Nephrolithiasis associated with renal insufficiency: factors predicting outcome. *J Endourol.* 2003 Dec;17(10):875-9.

[18] Hennus PM, van der Heijden GJ, Bosch JL, de Jong TP, de Kort LM. A systematic review on renal and bladder dysfunction after endoscopic treatment of infravesical obstruction in boys. *PLoS One.* 2012;7(9):e44663.

[19] Li XD, Wu YP, Wei Y, Chen SH, Zheng QS, Cai H et al. Predictors of Recoverability of Renal Function after Pyeloplasty in Adults with Ureteropelvic Junction Obstruction. *Urol Int.* 2018;100(2):209-215.

[20] Mishra S, Sinha L, Ganesamoni R, Ganpule A, Sabnis RB, Desai M. Renal deterioration index: preoperative prognostic model for renal functional outcome after treatment of bilateral obstructive urolithiasis in patients with chronic kidney disease. *J Endourol.* 2013 Nov;27(11):1405-10.

[21] Leahy AL, Ryan PC, McEntee GM, Nelson AC, Fitzpatrick JM. Renal injury and recovery in partial ureteric obstruction. *J Urol.* 1989 Jul;142(1):199-203.

[22] Komninos C, Mitsogiannis I. Obstruction-induced alterations within the urinary bladder and their role in the pathophysiology of lower urinary tract symptomatology. *Can Urol Assoc J.* 2014 Jul;8(7-8):E524-30.

[23] McGuire EJ, Woodside JR, Borden TA, Weiss RM. Prognostic value of urodynamic testing in myelodysplastic patients. *J Urol.* 1981 Aug;126(2):205-9.

[24] Leng WW, McGuire EJ. Obstructive uropathy induced bladder dysfunction can be reversible: bladder compliance measures before and after treatment. *J Urol.* 2003 Feb;169(2):563-6.

[25] Rishor-Olney CR, Hinson MR. Obstructive Uropathy. [Updated 2020 Jul 6]. In: *StatPearls* [Internet]. Treasure Island (FL): StatPearls Publishing; 2020 Jan [Cited 2021 Feb 10]-. Available from: https://www.ncbi.nlm.nih.gov/books/NBK558921/

[26] Kaufman DP, Basit H, Knohl SJ. Physiology, Glomerular Filtration Rate (GFR) [Updated 2020 Jul 26]. In: *StatPearls* [Internet]. Treasure Island (FL): StatPearls Publishing; 2020 Jan [Cited 2021 Feb 10]-. Available from: https://www.ncbi.nlm.nih.gov/books/NBK500032/

[27] Tyagi A, Aeddula NR. Azotemia. [Updated 2020 May 21]. In: *StatPearls* [Internet]. Treasure Island (FL): StatPearls Publishing; 2020 Jan [Cited 2021 Feb 10]-. Available from: https://www.ncbi.nlm.nih.gov/books/NBK538145/

[28] Assimos D, Krambeck A, Miller NL, Monga M, Murad MH, Nelson CP et al. Surgical Management of Stones: American Urological Association/Endourological Society Guideline, PART I. *J Urol.* 2016 Oct;196(4):1153-60.

[29] Patel IJ, Rahim S, Davidson JC, Hanks SE, Tam AL, Walker TG et al. Society of Interventional Radiology Consensus Guidelines for the Periprocedural Management of Thrombotic and Bleeding Risk in Patients Undergoing Percutaneous Image-Guided Interventions-Part II: Recommendations: Endorsed by the Canadian Association for

Interventional Radiology and the Cardiovascular and Interventional Radiological Society of Europe. *J Vasc Interv Radiol.* 2019 Aug;30(8):1168-1184.

[30] Kim SO, Song SH, Park K, Kwon D. Overexpression of aquaporin-1 and caveolin-1 in the rat urinary bladder urothelium following bladder outlet obstruction. *Int Neurourol J.* 2013 Dec;17(4):174-9.

[31] Kim SO, Choi D, Song SH, Ahn KY, Kwon D, Park K, et al. Effect of detrusor overactivity on the expression of aquaporins and nitric oxide synthase in rat urinary bladder following bladder outlet obstruction. *Can Urol Assoc J.* 2013 May-Jun;7(5-6):E268-74.

[32] Araki I, Du S, Kamiyama M, Mikami Y, Matsushita K, Komuro M, Furuya Y, Takeda M. Overexpression of epithelial sodium channels in epithelium of human urinary bladder with outlet obstruction. *Urology.* 2004 Dec;64(6):1255-60.

[33] İnal S, Altuntaş A, Kidir V, Özorak A, İlgin Y, Sezer MT. Utility of serum creatinine/cystatin C ratio in diagnosis of postrenal acute kidney injury. *J Res Med Sci.* 2014 Nov;19(11):1086-9.

[34] Hung SF, Chung SD, Kuo HC. Increased serum C-reactive protein level is associated with increased storage lower urinary tract symptoms in men with benign prostatic hyperplasia. *PLoS One.* 2014 Jan 15;9(1):e85588.

[35] Hansen KL, Nielsen MB, Ewertsen C. Ultrasonography of the Kidney: A Pictorial Review. *Diagnostics* (Basel). 2015 Dec 23;6(1):2.

[36] Onen A. Grading of Hydronephrosis: An Ongoing Challenge. *Front Pediatr.* 2020 Aug 27;8:458.

[37] Viazzi F, Leoncini G, Derchi LE, Pontremoli R. Ultrasound Doppler renal resistive index: a useful tool for the management of the hypertensive patient. *J Hypertens.* 2014 Jan;32(1):149-53.

[38] Jandaghi AB, Falahatkar S, Alizadeh A, Kanafi AR, Pourghorban R, Shekarchi B, Zirak AK, Esmaeili S. Assessment of ureterovesical jet dynamics in obstructed ureter by urinary stone with color Doppler and duplex Doppler examinations. *Urolithiasis.* 2013 Apr;41(2):159-63.

[39] Brisbane W, Bailey MR, Sorensen MD. An overview of kidney stone imaging techniques. *Nat Rev Urol.* 2016 Nov;13(11):654-662.

[40] Bagheri MH, Ahlman MA, Lindenberg L, Turkbey B, Lin J, Cahid Civelek A, Malayeri AA, Agarwal PK, Choyke PL, Folio LR, Apolo AB. Advances in medical imaging for the diagnosis and management of common genitourinary cancers. *Urol Oncol.* 2017 Jul;35(7):473-491.

[41] Engelsgjerd JS, LaGrange CA. Retroperitoneal Fibrosis. [Updated 2020 May 30]. In: *StatPearls* [Internet]. Treasure Island (FL): StatPearls Publishing; 2020 Jan [Cited 2021 Feb 10]-. Available from: https://www.ncbi.nlm.nih.gov/books/NBK482409/

[42] Atawurah H, Maison POM, Owusu-Ansah M, Asante-Asamani A. Retrocaval Ureter: Report of Two Cases. *Case Rep Urol.* 2019 Nov 3;2019:2815748.

[43] Williams PM, Fletcher S. Health effects of prenatal radiation exposure. *Am Fam Physician.* 2010 Sep 1;82(5):488-93.

[44] Yoon I, Slesinger TL. Radiation Exposure In Pregnancy. *StatPearls*. Treasure Island (FL): StatPearls Publishing; May 8, 2021.

[45] Wang C, Asch D, Cavallo J, Cohan R, Dillman J, Ellis J, et al. *ACR Manual on Contrast Media.* Reston, VA: American College of Radiology; 2021.

[46] Taylor AT. Radionuclides in nephrourology, part 1: Radiopharmaceuticals, quality control, and quantitative indices. *J Nucl Med.* 2014 Apr;55(4):608-15.

[47] Taylor AT. Radionuclides in nephrourology, Part 2: pitfalls and diagnostic applications. *J Nucl Med.* 2014 May;55(5):786-98.

[48] Bao J, Manatunga A, Binongo JN, Taylor AT. Key variables for interpreting 99mTc-mercaptoacetyltriglycine diuretic scans: development and validation of a predictive model. *AJR Am J Roentgenol.* 2011 Aug;197(2):325-33.

[49] von Rundstedt FC, Scovell JM, Bian SX, Lee D, Mayer WA, Link RE. Percent of Tracer Clearance at 40 Minutes in MAG3 Renal Scans Is More Sensitive Than T1/2 for Symptomatic Ureteropelvic Junction Obstruction. *Urology.* 2017 May;103:245-250.

[50] Rossleigh MA. Renal infection and vesico-ureteric reflux. *Semin Nucl Med.* 2007 Jul;37(4):261-8.

[51] Mehta SR, Annamaraju P. Intravenous Pyelogram. [Updated 2020 Jun 27]. In: *StatPearls* [Internet]. Treasure Island (FL): StatPearls Publishing; 2020 Jan [Cited 2021 Feb 10]-. Available from: https://www.ncbi.nlm.nih.gov/books/NBK559034/

[52] Merchant S, Bharati A, Merchant N. Tuberculosis of the genitourinary system-Urinary tract tuberculosis: Renal tuberculosis-Part I. *Indian J Radiol Imaging.* 2013 Jan;23(1):46-63.

[53] Whitaker RH. The Whitaker test. *Urol Clin North Am.* 1979 Oct;6(3):529-39. PMID: 505672.

[54] Lupton EW, George NJ. The Whitaker test: 35 years on. *BJU Int.* 2010 Jan;105(1):94-100.

[55] Jaffe RB, Middleton AW Jr. Whitaker test: differentiation of obstructive from nonobstructive uropathy. *AJR Am J Roentgenol.* 1980 Jan;134(1):9-15.

[56] Scales CD Jr, Smith AC, Hanley JM, Saigal CS; Urologic Diseases in America Project. Prevalence of kidney stones in the United States. *Eur Urol.* 2012 Jul;62(1):160-5.

[57] Strope SA, Wolf JS Jr, Hollenbeck BK. Changes in gender distribution of urinary stone disease. *Urology.* 2010 Mar;75(3):543-6.

[58] Daudon M, Jungers P, Bazin D, Williams JC Jr. Recurrence rates of urinary calculi according to stone composition and morphology. *Urolithiasis.* 2018 Oct;46(5):459-470.

[59] Alelign T, Petros B. Kidney Stone Disease: An Update on Current Concepts. *Adv Urol.* 2018 Feb 4;2018:3068365.

[60] Papatsoris AG, Varkarakis I, Dellis A, Deliveliotis C. Bladder lithiasis: from open surgery to lithotripsy. *Urol Res.* 2006 Jun;34(3):163-7.

[61] Thakore P, Liang TH. Urolithiasis. [Updated 2020 Nov 20]. In: *StatPearls* [Internet]. Treasure Island (FL): StatPearls Publishing; 2020 Jan [Cited 2021 Feb 10]-. Available from: https://www.ncbi.nlm.nih.gov/books/NBK559101/

[62] Minotti B, Treglia G, Pascale M, Ceruti S, Cantini L, Anselmi L et al. Prevalence of microhematuria in renal colic and urolithiasis: a systematic review and meta-analysis. *BMC Urol.* 2020 Aug 8;20(1):119.

[63] Pearle MS, Goldfarb DS, Assimos DG, Curhan G, Denu-Ciocca CJ, Matlaga BR et al. American Urological Assocation. Medical management of kidney stones: AUA guideline. *J Urol.* 2014 Aug;192(2):316-24.

[64] Nicolau C, Claudon M, Derchi LE, Adam EJ, Nielsen MB, Mostbeck G et al. Imaging patients with renal colic-consider ultrasound first. *Insights Imaging.* 2015 Aug;6(4):441-7.

[65] Valovska MI, Pais VM Jr. Contemporary best practice urolithiasis in pregnancy. *Ther Adv Urol.* 2018 Feb 8;10(4):127-138.

[66] Goldsmith ZG, Oredein-McCoy O, Gerber L, Bañez LL, Sopko DR, Miller MJ et al. Emergent ureteric stent vs percutaneous nephrostomy for obstructive urolithiasis with sepsis: patterns of use and outcomes from a 15-year experience. *BJU Int.* 2013 Jul;112(2):E122-8.

[67] Pearle MS, Pierce HL, Miller GL, Summa JA, Mutz JM, Petty BA et al. Optimal method of urgent decompression of the collecting system for obstruction and infection due to ureteral calculi. *J Urol.* 1998 Oct;160(4):1260-4.

[68] Tchey DU, Ha YS, Kim WT, Yun SJ, Lee SC, Kim WJ. Expectant Management of Ureter Stones: Outcome and Clinical Factors of Spontaneous Passage in a Single Institution's Experience. *Korean J Urol.* 2011 Dec;52(12):847-51.

[69] Furyk JS, Chu K, Banks C, Greenslade J, Keijzers G, Thom O et al. Distal Ureteric Stones and Tamsulosin: A Double-Blind, Placebo-Controlled, Randomized, Multicenter Trial. *Ann Emerg Med.* 2016 Jan;67(1):86-95.

[70] Al-Ansari A, Al-Naimi A, Alobaidy A, Assadiq K, Azmi MD, Shokeir AA. Efficacy of tamsulosin in the management of lower ureteral stones: a randomized double-blind placebo-controlled study of 100 patients. *Urology.* 2010 Jan;75(1):4-7.

[71] Campschroer T, Zhu X, Vernooij RW, Lock MT. Alpha-blockers as medical expulsive therapy for ureteral stones. Cochrane Database Syst Rev. 2018 Apr 5;4(4):CD008509.

[72] Sun Y, Lei GL, Yang L, Wei Q, Wei X. Is tamsulosin effective for the passage of symptomatic ureteral stones: A systematic review and meta-analysis. *Medicine* (Baltimore). 2019 Mar;98(10):e14796.

[73] Meltzer AC, Burrows PK, Wolfson AB, Hollander JE, Kurz M, Kirkali Z et al. Effect of Tamsulosin on Passage of Symptomatic Ureteral Stones: A Randomized Clinical Trial. *JAMA Intern Med.* 2018 Aug 1;178(8):1051-1057.

[74] McClinton S, Starr K, Thomas R, McLennan G, McPherson G, McDonald A et al. SUSPEND Study Group. Use of drug therapy in the management of symptomatic ureteric stones in hospitalized adults (SUSPEND), a multicentre, placebo-controlled, randomized trial of a calcium-channel blocker (nifedipine) and an α-blocker (tamsulosin): study protocol for a randomized controlled trial. *Trials.* 2014 Jun 20;15:238.

[75] Logothetis CJ, Assikis V, Sarriera JE. *Complications Resulting from Primary Cancer Progression*. In: Kufe DW, Pollock RE, Weichselbaum RR, et al., editors. Holland-Frei *Cancer Medicine*. 6th edition. Hamilton (ON): BC Decker; 2003. Available from: https://www.ncbi.nlm.nih.gov/books/NBK13537/

[76] Sountoulides P, Mykoniatis I, Dimasis N. Palliative management of malignant upper urinary tract obstruction. *Hippokratia.* 2014 Oct-Dec;18(4):292-7. PMID: 26052193; PMCID: PMC4453800.

[77] Oh JJ, Byun SS, Jeong CW, Kwak C, Kim HH, Ku JH. Association Between Preoperative Hydronephrosis and Prognosis After Radical Cystectomy Among Patients With Bladder Cancer: A Systemic Review and Meta-Analysis. *Front Oncol.* 2019 Mar 19;9:158.

[78] Alwaal A, Blaschko SD, McAninch JW, Breyer BN. Epidemiology of urethral strictures. *Transl Androl Urol.* 2014 Jun;3(2):209-13.

[79] Smith TG 3rd. Current management of urethral stricture disease. *Indian J Urol.* 2016 Jan-Mar;32(1):27-33.

[80] Fam XI, Singam P, Ho CC, Sridharan R, Hod R, Bahadzor Bet al. Ureteral stricture formation after ureteroscope treatment of impacted calculi: a prospective study. *Korean J Urol.* 2015 Jan;56(1):63-7.

[81] Bayne DB, Gaither TW, Awad MA, Murphy GP, Osterberg EC, Breyer BN. Guidelines of guidelines: a review of urethral stricture evaluation, management, and follow-up. *Transl Androl Urol.* 2017 Apr;6(2):288-294.

[82] Goel A, Gupta A, Dalela D. Antegrade urethrogram: A technique to visualize the proximal bulbous urethral segment in anterior urethral stricture. *Indian J Urol.* 2009 Jul;25(3):415-6.

[83] Lucas JW, Ghiraldi E, Ellis J, Friedlander JI. Endoscopic Management of Ureteral Strictures: an Update. *Curr Urol Rep.* 2018 Mar 2;19(4):24.

[84] Wessells H, Angermeier KW, Elliott S, Gonzalez CM, Kodama R, Peterson AC et al. Male Urethral Stricture: American Urological Association Guideline. *J Urol.* 2017 Jan;197(1):182-190.

[85] Steenkamp JW, Heyns CF, de Kock ML. Internal urethrotomy versus dilation as treatment for male urethral strictures: a prospective, randomized comparison. *J Urol.* 1997 Jan;157(1):98-101.

[86] Vetterlein MW, Weisbach L, Riechardt S, Fisch M. Anterior Urethral Strictures in Children: Disease Etiology and Comparative Effectiveness of Endoscopic Treatment vs. Open Surgical Reconstruction. *Front Pediatr.* 2019 Jan 31;7:5.

[87] Feng MI, Bellman GC, Shapiro CE. Management of ureteral obstruction secondary to pelvic malignancies. *J Endourol.* 1999 Sep;13(7):521-4.

[88] Kim JW, Hong B, Shin JH, Park J, Kim JH, Gwon DI, Ryu MH, Ryoo BY. A Prospective Randomized Comparison of a Covered Metallic Ureteral Stent and a Double-J Stent for Malignant Ureteral Obstruction. *Korean J Radiol.* 2018 Jul-Aug;19(4):606-612.

[89] Chung HH, Kim MD, Won JY, Won JH, Cho SB, Seo TS et al. Multicenter experience of the newly designed covered metallic ureteral stent for malignant ureteral occlusion: comparison with double J stent insertion. *Cardiovasc Intervent Radiol.* 2014 Apr;37(2):463-70.

[90] Burks FN, Santucci RA. Management of iatrogenic ureteral injury. *Ther Adv Urol.* 2014 Jun;6(3):115-24.

[91] Lee Z, Keehn AY, Sterling ME, Metro MJ, Eun DD. A Review of Buccal Mucosa Graft Ureteroplasty. *Curr Urol Rep.* 2018 Mar 1;19(4):23.

[92] Marien T, Bjurlin MA, Wynia B, Bilbily M, Rao G, Zhao LC, Shah O, Stifelman MD. Outcomes of robotic-assisted laparoscopic upper urinary tract reconstruction: 250 consecutive patients. *BJU Int.* 2015 Oct;116(4):604-11.

[93] Milhoua PM, Miller NL, Cookson MS, Chang SS, Smith JA, Herrell SD. Primary endoscopic management versus open revision of ureteroenteric anastomotic strictures after urinary diversion--single institution contemporary series. *J Endourol.* 2009 Mar;23(3):551-5.

[94] van Son MJ, Lock MTWT, Peters M, van de Putte EEF, Meijer RP. Treating benign ureteroenteric strictures: 27-year experience comparing endourological techniques with open surgical approach. *World J Urol.* 2019 Jun;37(6):1217-1223.

[95] Moltzahn F, Dal Pra A, Furrer M, Thalmann G, Spahn M. Urethral strictures after radiation therapy for prostate cancer. *Investig Clin Urol.* 2016 Sep;57(5):309-15.
[96] Hofer MD, Gonzalez CM. Management of radiation-induced urethral strictures. *Transl Androl Urol.* 2015 Feb;4(1):66-71.
[97] Bosch R, McCloskey K, Bahl A, Arlandis S, Ockrim J, Weiss J, Greenwell T. Can radiation-induced lower urinary tract disease be ameliorated in patients treated for pelvic organ cancer: ICI-RS 2019? *Neurourol Urodyn.* 2020 Jul;39 Suppl 3(Suppl 3):S148-S155.
[98] McIntyre JF, Eifel PJ, Levenback C, Oswald MJ. Ureteral stricture as a late complication of radiotherapy for stage IB carcinoma of the uterine cervix. *Cancer.* 1995 Feb 1;75(3):836-43.
[99] Asghar AM, Lee Z, Lee RA, Slawin J, Cheng N, Koster H et al. Robotic Ureteral Reconstruction in Patients with Radiation-Induced Ureteral Strictures: Experience from the Collaborative of Reconstructive Robotic Ureteral Surgery. *J Endourol.* 2020 Sep 21.
[100] Khourdaji I, Parke J, Chennamsetty A, Burks F. Treatment of Urethral Strictures from Irradiation and Other Nonsurgical Forms of Pelvic Cancer Treatment. *Adv Urol.* 2015;2015:476390.
[101] Al-Aaraj MS, Badreldin AM. Ureteropelvic Junction Obstruction. [Updated 2020 Jul 11]. In: *StatPearls* [Internet]. Treasure Island (FL): StatPearls Publishing; 2020 Jan [Cited 2021 Feb 10]-. Available from: https://www.ncbi.nlm.nih.gov/books/NBK560740/
[102] Chang CP, McDill BW, Neilson JR, Joist HE, Epstein JA, Crabtree GR et al. Calcineurin is required in urinary tract mesenchyme for the development of the pyeloureteral peristaltic machinery. *J Clin Invest.* 2004 Apr;113(7):1051-8.
[103] Lowe FC, Marshall FF. Ureteropelvic junction obstruction in adults. *Urology.* 1984 Apr;23(4):331-5. doi: 10.1016/0090-4295(84)90133-x. PMID: 6369711.
[104] Wong MCY, Piaggio G, Damasio MB, Molinelli C, Ferretti SM, Pistorio A et al. Hydronephrosis and crossing vessels in children: Optimization of diagnostic-therapeutic pathway and analysis of color Doppler ultrasound and magnetic resonance urography diagnostic accuracy. *J Pediatr Urol.* 2018 Feb;14(1):68.
[105] Borin JF. Ureteropelvic Junction Obstruction in Adults. *Rev Urol.* 2017;19(4):261-264.
[106] Passoni NM, Peters CA. Managing Ureteropelvic Junction Obstruction in the Young Infant. *Front Pediatr.* 2020 May 27;8:242.
[107] Gnech M, Berrettini A, Lopes RI, Moscardi P, Esposito C, Zucchetta P et al. Pyeloplasty vs. nephrectomy for ureteropelvic junction obstruction in poorly functioning kidneys (differential renal function <20%): a multicentric study. *J Pediatr Urol.* 2019 Oct;15(5):553.e1-553.e8.
[108] Doo CK, Hong B, Park T, Park HK. Long-term outcome of endopyelotomy for the treatment of ureteropelvic junction obstruction: how long should patients be followed up? *J Endourol.* 2007 Feb;21(2):158-61.
[109] Autorino R, Eden C, El-Ghoneimi A, Guazzoni G, Buffi N, Peters CA, et al. Robot-assisted and laparoscopic repair of ureteropelvic junction obstruction: a systematic review and meta-analysis. *Eur Urol.* 2014;65(2):430–52.
[110] Szydełko T, Kopeć R, Kasprzak J, Apoznański W, Kołodziej A, Zdrojowy R, Lorenz J. Antegrade endopyelotomy versus laparoscopic pyeloplasty for primary ureteropelvic junction obstruction. *J Laparoendosc Adv Surg Tech A.* 2009 Feb;19(1):45-51.

[111] Radford AR, Thomas DF, Subramaniam R. Ureterocalicostomy in children: 12 years experience in a single centre. *BJU Int.* 2011 Aug;108(3):434-8.

[112] Brownlee E, Wragg R, Robb A, Chandran H, Knight M, McCarthy L; BAPS-CASS. Current epidemiology and antenatal presentation of posterior urethral valves: Outcome of BAPS CASS National Audit. *J Pediatr Surg.* 2019 Feb;54(2):318-321.

[113] Casella DP, Tomaszewski JJ, Ost MC. Posterior urethral valves: renal failure and prenatal treatment. *Int J Nephrol.* 2012;2012:351067.

[114] Sharma S, Joshi M, Gupta DK, Abraham M, Mathur P, Mahajan JK, Gangopadhyay AN, Rattan SK, Vora R, Prasad GR, Bhattacharya NC, Samuj R, Rao KLN, Basu AK. Consensus on the Management of Posterior Urethral Valves from Antenatal Period to Puberty. *J Indian Assoc Pediatr Surg.* 2019 Jan-Mar;24(1):4-14.

[115] Bingham G, Rentea RM. Posterior Urethral Valve. [Updated 2020 Aug 1]. In: *StatPearls* [Internet]. Treasure Island (FL): StatPearls Publishing; 2020 Jan [Cited 2021 Feb 10]-. Available from: https://www.ncbi.nlm.nih.gov/books/NBK560881/

[116] Tourchi A, Kajbafzadeh AM, Aryan Z, Ebadi M. The management of vesicoureteral reflux in the setting of posterior urethral valve with emphasis on bladder function and renal outcome: a single center cohort study. *Urology.* 2014 Jan;83(1):199-205.

[117] Lukong CS, Ameh EA, Mshelbwala PM, Jabo BA, Gomna A, Anumah MA et al. Role of vesicostomy in the management of posterior urethral valve in Sub-Saharan Africa. *J Pediatr Urol.* 2014 Feb;10(1):62-6.

[118] Sarhan OM. Posterior urethral valves: Impact of low birth weight and preterm delivery on the final renal outcome. *Arab J Urol.* 2017 Mar 7;15(2):159-165.

[119] Schultza K, Todab LY. Genetic Basis of Ureterocele. *Curr Genomics.* 2016 Feb;17(1):62-9.

[120] Merlini E, Lelli Chiesa P. Obstructive ureterocele-an ongoing challenge. *World J Urol.* 2004 Jun;22(2):107-14.

[121] Arlen AM, Kirsch AJ, Cuda SP, Little SB, Jones RA, Grattan-Smith JDet al. Magnetic resonance urography for diagnosis of pediatric ureteral stricture. *J Pediatr Urol.* 2014 Oct;10(5):792-8.

[122] Shah H, Tiwari C, Shenoy NS, Dwivedi P, Gandhi S. Transurethral incision of ureteroceles in paediatric age group. *Turk J Urol.* 2017 Dec;43(4):530-535.

[123] Palmer BW, Greger H, Mannas DB, Kropp BP, Frimberger D. Comparison of endoscopic ureterocele decompression techniques. Preliminary experience--is the watering can puncture superior? *J Urol.* 2011 Oct;186(4 Suppl):1700-3.

[124] Hodges SJ, Werle D, McLorie G, Atala A. Megaureter. *ScientificWorldJournal.* 2010 Apr 13;10:603-12.

[125] Zaffanello M, Brugnara M, Cecchetto M, Manfredi R, Zuffante M, Fanos V. Paediatric unilateral giant hydroureteronephrosis from idiopathic ureterovesical stricture: a case report. *BMJ Case Rep.* 2009;2009:bcr08.2008.0782.

[126] Shokeir AA, Nijman RJ. Primary megaureter: current trends in diagnosis and treatment. *BJU Int.* 2000 Nov;86(7):861-8.

[127] Arrabal-Martín M, Zuluaga-Gómez A, Merino-Salas S, Nogueras-Ocaña M, Arrabal-Polo MÁ. Endoscopic treatment of ureterovesical junction obstructive pathology: A description of the oblique meatotomy technique and results. *Can Urol Assoc J.* 2013 Nov-Dec;7(11-12):E728-31.

[128] Kyei MY, Yeboah ED, Klufio GO, Mensah JE, Gepi-Atee S, Zakpaa L, Morton B, Adusei B. Retrocaval ureter: two case reports. *Ghana Med J.* 2011 Dec;45(4):177-80.
[129] Murphy BJ, Casillas J, Becerra JL. Retrocaval ureter: computed tomography and ultrasound appearance. *J Comput Tomogr.* 1987 Jan;11(1):89-93.
[130] Abdessater M, El Khoury R, Elias S, Bart S, Coloby P, Sleiman W. Diagnosis and laparoscopic management of retrocaval ureter: A review of the literature and our case series. *Int J Surg Case Rep.* 2019;59:165-175.
[131] Yen JM, Lee LS, Cheng CW. Conservative management of retrocaval Ureter: A case series. *Int J Surg Case Rep.* 2015;15:93-5.
[132] Berry SJ, Coffey DS, Walsh PC, Ewing LL. The development of human benign prostatic hyperplasia with age. *J Urol.* 1984 Sep;132(3):474-9.
[133] Roehrborn CG. Benign prostatic hyperplasia: an overview. *Rev Urol.* 2005;7 Suppl 9(Suppl 9):S3-S14.
[134] Parsons JK, Dahm P, Köhler TS, Lerner LB, Wilt TJ. Surgical Management of Lower Urinary Tract Symptoms Attributed to Benign Prostatic Hyperplasia: AUA Guideline Amendment 2020. *J Urol.* 2020 Oct;204(4):799-804.
[135] Simon RM, Howard LE, Moreira DM, Roehrborn C, Vidal AC, Castro-Santamaria R et al. Does Prostate Size Predict the Development of Incident Lower Urinary Tract Symptoms in Men with Mild to No Current Symptoms? *Results from the REDUCE Trial. Eur Urol.* 2016 May;69(5):885-91.
[136] Roehrborn CG. Pathology of benign prostatic hyperplasia. *Int J Impot Res.* 2008 Dec;20 Suppl 3:S11-8.
[137] Laniado ME, Ockrim JL, Marronaro A, Tubaro A, Carter SS. Serum prostate-specific antigen to predict the presence of bladder outlet obstruction in men with urinary symptoms. *BJU Int.* 2004 Dec;94(9):1283-6.
[138] Asimakopoulos AD, De Nunzio C, Kocjancic E, Tubaro A, Rosier PF, Finazzi-Agrò E. Measurement of post-void residual urine. *Neurourol Urodyn.* 2016 Jan;35(1):55-7.
[139] Reynard JM, Yang Q, Donovan JL, Peters TJ, Schafer W, de la Rosette JJ et al. The ICS-'BPH' Study: uroflowmetry, lower urinary tract symptoms and bladder outlet obstruction. *Br J Urol.* 1998 Nov;82(5):619-23.
[140] Ng M, Baradhi KM. Benign Prostatic Hyperplasia. [Updated 2020 Aug 10]. In: *StatPearls* [Internet]. Treasure Island (FL): StatPearls Publishing; 2020 Jan [Cited 2021 Feb 10]-. Available from: https://www.ncbi.nlm.nih.gov/books/NBK558920/
[141] Oelke M, Giuliano F, Mirone V, Xu L, Cox D, Viktrup L. Monotherapy with tadalafil or tamsulosin similarly improved lower urinary tract symptoms suggestive of benign prostatic hyperplasia in an international, randomised, parallel, placebo-controlled clinical trial. *Eur Urol.* 2012 May;61(5):917-25.
[142] Pariser JJ, Packiam VT, Adamsky MA, Bales GT. Trends in Simple Prostatectomy for Benign Prostatic Hyperplasia. *Curr Urol Rep.* 2016 Aug;17(8):57.
[143] Perera M, Roberts MJ, Doi SA, Bolton D. Prostatic urethral lift improves urinary symptoms and flow while preserving sexual function for men with benign prostatic hyperplasia: a systematic review and meta-analysis. *Eur Urol.* 2015 Apr;67(4):704-13.
[144] Dobrowolski Z, Kusionowicz J, Drewniak T, Habrat W, Lipczyñski W, Jakubik P et al.. Renal and ureteric trauma: diagnosis and management in Poland. *BJU Int.* 2002 May;89(7):748-51.

[145] McGeady JB, Breyer BN. Current epidemiology of genitourinary trauma. *Urol Clin North Am.* 2013 Aug;40(3):323-34.

[146] de la Rosette JJ, Skrekas T, Segura JW. Handling and prevention of complications in stone basketing. *Eur Urol.* 2006 Nov;50(5):991-8; discussion 998-9.

[147] Siram SM, Gerald SZ, Greene WR, Hughes K, Oyetunji TA, Chrouser K, et al. Ureteral trauma: patterns and mechanisms of injury of an uncommon condition. *Am J Surg.* 2010 Apr;199(4):566-70.

[148] Wang JH, Kung YH, King TM, Chang MC, Hsu CW. Measurement of peritoneal fluid urea nitrogen and creatinine levels is useful to detect iatrogenic urinary tract leakage in colorectal surgery. *J Chin Med Assoc.* 2015 May;78(5):283-6.

[149] Morey AF, Broghammer JA, Hollowell CMP, McKibben MJ, Souter L. Urotrauma Guideline 2020: AUA Guideline. *J Urol.* 2021 Jan;205(1):30-35.

[150] van Bommel EF, Jansen I, Hendriksz TR, Aarnoudse ALHJ. Idiopathic retroperitoneal fibrosis: prospective evaluation of incidence and clinicoradiologic presentation. *Medicine (Baltimore).* 2009 Jul;88(4):193-201.

[151] Brandt AS, Kamper L, Kukuk S, Haage P, Roth S. Associated findings and complications of retroperitoneal fibrosis in 204 patients: results of a urological registry. *J Urol.* 2011 Feb;185(2):526-31.

[152] Runowska M, Majewski D, Puszczewicz M. Retroperitoneal fibrosis - the state-of-the-art. *Reumatologia.* 2016;54(5):256-263.

[153] Pelkmans LG, Aarnoudse AJ, Hendriksz TR, van Bommel EF. Value of acute-phase reactants in monitoring disease activity and treatment response in idiopathic retroperitoneal fibrosis. *Nephrol Dial Transplant.* 2012 Jul;27(7):2819-25.

[154] Caiafa RO, Vinuesa AS, Izquierdo RS, Brufau BP, Ayuso Colella JR, Molina CN. Retroperitoneal fibrosis: role of imaging in diagnosis and follow-up. *Radiographics.* 2013 Mar-Apr;33(2):535-52.

[155] O'Brien T, Fernando A. Contemporary role of ureterolysis in retroperitoneal fibrosis: treatment of last resort or first intent? An analysis of 50 cases. *BJU Int.* 2017 Oct;120(4):556-561.

[156] Tayyeb M, Tadi P. Neurogenic Bladder. [Updated 2020 Aug 16]. In: *StatPearls* [Internet]. Treasure Island (FL): StatPearls Publishing; 2020 Jan [Cited 2021 Feb 10]-. Available from: https://www.ncbi.nlm.nih.gov/books/NBK560617/

[157] Shingleton WB, Bodner DR. The development of urologic complications in relationship to bladder pressure in spinal cord injured patients. *J Am Paraplegia Soc.* 1993 Jan;16(1):14-7.

[158] Powell CR. Not all neurogenic bladders are the same: a proposal for a new neurogenic bladder classification system. *Transl Androl Urol.* 2016 Feb;5(1):12-21.

[159] McGuire EJ, Woodside JR, Borden TA, Weiss RM. Prognostic value of urodynamic testing in myelodysplastic patients. *J Urol.* 1981 Aug;126(2):205-9.

[160] Taweel WA, Seyam R. Neurogenic bladder in spinal cord injury patients. *Res Rep Urol.* 2015 Jun 10;7:85-99.

[161] Cameron AP. Medical management of neurogenic bladder with oral therapy. *Transl Androl Urol.* 2016 Feb;5(1):51-62.

[162] Salameh A, Mohajer MA, Daroucihe RO. Prevention of urinary tract infections in patients with spinal cord injury. *CMAJ.* 2015 Aug 11;187(11):807-811.

[163] Dorsher PT, McIntosh PM. Neurogenic bladder. *Adv Urol.* 2012;2012:816274.

[164] Sanford MT, Suskind AM. Neuromodulation in neurogenic bladder. *Transl Androl Urol.* 2016 Feb;5(1):117-26.

[165] de Sèze M, Raibaut P, Gallien P, Even-Schneider A, Denys P, Bonniaud V et al. Transcutaneous posterior tibial nerve stimulation for treatment of the overactive bladder syndrome in multiple sclerosis: results of a multicenter prospective study. *Neurourol Urodyn.* 2011 Mar;30(3):306-11.

[166] Gor RA, Elliott SP. Surgical Management of Neurogenic Lower Urinary Tract Dysfunction. *Urol Clin North Am.* 2017 Aug;44(3):475-490.

[167] Abbara A, Davidson RN; Medscape. Etiology and management of genitourinary tuberculosis. *Nat Rev Urol.* 2011 Dec 9;8(12):678-88.

[168] Mthalane NBA, Dlamini NNM. Multidetector computed tomography has replaced conventional intravenous excretory urography in imaging of the kidneys: A scoping review of multidetector computed tomography findings in renal tuberculosis. *SA J Radiol.* 2018 Feb 16;22(1):1283.

[169] Figueiredo AA, Lucon AM, Júnior RF, Ikejiri DS, Nahas WC, Srougi M. Urogenital tuberculosis in immunocompromised patients. Int Urol Nephrol. 2009;41(2):327-33.

[170] Goel A, Dalela D. Options in the management of tuberculous ureteric stricture. *Indian J Urol.* 2008 Jul;24(3):376-81.

In: Issues in Kidney Disease – Acute Kidney Injury
Editors: S. Z. Fadem and A. Arslan Yousuf Awan ISBN: 978-1-68507-002-1

Chapter 7

ACUTE TUBULAR INJURY - PATHOPHYSIOLOGY AND CLINICAL IMPLICATIONS

Micah Schub[2, †], MD, Solomiia Savedchuk[2,†], MD, Sebastian Franco[1], MD and Matthew A. Sparks[2,3,*], MD

[1]Department of Medicine, Duke University School of Medicine, Durham, NC, USA
[2]Division of Nephrology, Department of Medicine, Duke University School of Medicine, Durham, NC, USA
[3]Renal Section, Durham VA Health Care System, Durham, NC, USA

ABSTRACT

Acute tubular necrosis (ATN) is the most common cause of acute kidney injury (AKI) in hospitalized patients and is associated with a high morbidity and mortality. Incidence of ATN varies widely, depending on the criteria used to define an AKI, with up to 20% in patients hospitalized and 75% in patients admitted to the intensive care unit. Since the introduction of hemodialysis over four decades ago, the mortality rates from ATN in patients hospitalized and in the ICU have stayed the same, up to 30% and 80%, respectively [1].

One of the main reasons for the lack of significant progress in the area of ATN is its complex and multifaceted pathophysiology, involving changes in glomerular hemodynamics, tubular cell metabolism, changes in microvasculature of the kidney, activation of inflammatory pathways, innate/adaptive immune system response, and fibrogenesis. Additionally, the criteria used to define AKI - rise in serum creatinine and a fall in urine output - are late consequences to kidney injury that has already occurred to the most sensitive part of the proximal tubule. Thus, leading to delayed implementation of therapeutic strategies. In the last decade, tremendous progress has been made in basic and translational research in ATN, providing new insights into pathogenesis of ATN. Novel

* Corresponding Author's Email: matthew.sparks@duke.edu.
† Co-first authors.
† Co-first authors.

strategies that hold promises as potential therapeutics have emerged from these findings and are under various stages of investigation.

In this chapter, we focus on the etiologies of ATN, innate protective mechanisms of the kidney against ATN, the underlying pathophysiological mechanisms, and morphological features of ATN. We discuss the clinical and laboratory markers of ATN, urine microscopy findings, and novel biomarkers of AKI. We then proceed to discuss evidence-based fluid management strategies for management of ATN, trials on the timing of kidney replacement therapy, and novel therapeutics under current investigations.

Keywords: AKI, ATN

INTRODUCTION

In clinical medicine, the differential diagnoses and pathophysiologic paradigms often revolve around triplets. For instance, a classical consideration of the causes of AKI is taught as "pre-renal, intra-renal, and post-renal." The etiologies of ATN mirror this paradigm. While less-considered culprits exist, the three principal causes of ATN are ischemia, sepsis, and nephrotoxins. Before leaping into these causes of ATN, however, an illumination of terms is in order. We define AKI as an abrupt decrease in kidney function as manifested by concrete numeric criteria of increase in baseline serum creatinine and/or decrease in urine output [2]. An illustrative definition of ATN is borrowed from an oft-cited prospective, multicenter The Madrid Acute Renal Failure Study Group that examined the epidemiology of AKI: "When kidney function [does] not improve after correction of possible prerenal causes and when hepatorenal syndrome, vascular, interstitial, glomerular, and obstructive etiologies [are] excluded" [3].

This definition highlights that ATN should be first and foremost conceptualized as a clinical syndrome. The suspicion for ATN is predicated on a clinical context that suggests the entitites that are known to be associated with ATN. In fact, the study from which our definition is taken goes on to subdivide ATN into etiologic groups that include nephrotoxic ATN, septic ATN, and 'medical ATN' (which they define as the presence of a precipitating factor such as volume depletion, low cardiac output, or arterial hypotension). It is true that other data may lend support to the ultimate diagnosis of ATN. Classically, urine electrolytes and examination of urine sediment are both heralded as clues to cinch the case. For example, a fractional excretion of sodium (FeNa) of greater than 2 percent is consistent with ATN, and the presence of muddy brown casts on urine microscopy is diagnostic of ATN. However, these data have flaws - either in their interpretation or lack of sensitivity [4-6]. Kidney biopsy is another approach to confirming a case of ATN, as there are characteristic histopathologic findings that point the observer towards the diagnosis. Yet, in medical practice, kidney biopsies are rarely performed when our suspicion of ATN is high and concern for other etiologies is low [7]. Ultimately, then, this leaves the diagnostician in a place in which clinical history is paramount.

With this important clinical context underscored, an understanding of the three principle etiologies of ATN (ischemia, sepsis, nephrotoxins) becomes paramount. First, let us explore ischemic insult to the kidney. Ischemia encompasses any entity that decreases perfusion to the kidneys to trigger a prolonged prerenal state. The kidney is uniquely susceptible to ischemia because the glomerulus is at a high pressure state [8]. Subsequent lack of perfusion to this functional unit of the organ can lead to downstream inflammation, the details of which are elucidated below. An important first step is to methodically consider a classical differential diagnosis of shock (e.g., hypovolemic shock to include hemorrhage, distributive shock to include anaphylaxis and neurogenic cause, and cardiogenic shock) [9]. Beyond this, renal artery occlusion, such as an embolus or dissection, can cause kidney ischemia. Finally, surgery itself is thought to cause kidney ischemia, especially intra-abdominal or cardiothoracic procedures.

Sepsis is another common cause of ATN. One might easily imagine that septic shock - "a clinical construct of sepsis with persisting hypotension requiring vasopressors to maintain mean arterial pressure (MAP) ≥65 mm Hg despite adequate volume resuscitation" (10) - could reduce perfusion to the kidneys. However, when implicating sepsis as a separate etiology of ATN, the role of kidney blood flow alterations in the pathogenesis of ATN is the subject of ongoing debate (11). Curiously, there is a disconnect between the often precipitous decrease in glomerular filtration rate seen in sepsis and the corresponding mild degree of damage identified on histology from kidney biopsy. In fact, less than a quarter of patients with sepsis-associated AKI on autopsy revealed histologic features of ATN (12). Instead, the underlying driver for injury from this etiology is thought to be triggered by molecules associated with pathogens themselves or the cells that they damage in their immediate vicinity. This, in turn, initiates downstream innate, cellular, and humoral immune systems that activate several inflammatory pathways to include complement, fibrinolytic, coagulation and cytokine cascades that relay nonspecific damage to the kidney [11]. Systemic infection, then, should always be strongly considered when investigating a cause of ATN, even in the absence of overt hypotension.

Finally, we discuss nephrotoxins. To define nephrotoxins more rigorously, we refer to [1] pharmacologic treatments and other iatrogenically administered agents, [2] occupational exposures, and [3] recreational ingestions. Many prescription medications have been implicated in causing ATN. Those most commonly cited include antimicrobials (e.g., the antifungal amphotericin, the antibacterial aminoglycosides and vancomycin) [13-15] and the chemotherapeutic cisplatin. Intravenous radiocontrast agents have also been implicated to cause ATN, however these associations are more complicated to unravel and are now termed contrast-associated AKI [16]. Next, consideration of occupational exposures will broadly include heavy metals or organic solvents. Lastly, with respect to recreational ingestions, commonly referenced offenders include cocaine, synthetic cannabinoids, and herbal remedies such as aristolochic acid [17].

Outside the principle three, endogenous toxins are also known to be culprits of ATN. These include heme pigment nephropathy, rhabdomyolysis, and hemoglobinuria. Curiously, these three phenomena are inextricably linked. The umbrella entity of heme pigment nephropathy is either caused by rhabdomyolysis or massive intravascular hemolysis leading to hemoglobinuria. Separate differential diagnosis for both muscle fiber breakdown and intravascular breakdown of red blood cells affords a comprehensive exploration of these possible causes of ATN [18].

Before moving onto the pathophysiology that underpins ATN, we should address one last important clinical consideration. An astute physician can leverage the base rates of AKI etiologies by calibrating their differential diagnosis to match their domain of practice. Specifically, in the hospital setting (to include both the floor and ICU), ATN represents 65% of cases of intrarenal AKI [3]. Thus, if a diagnostic fluid challenge (or diuresis given the right clinical context) with repeat serum creatinine excludes contribution of a prerenal state, and bladder scan with or without bilateral kidney ultrasonography excludes obstructive etiologies, then one can confidently localize the lesion to *within* the kidney. Once this preliminary step is secured, the statistical likelihood is that the case in consideration is an example of ATN.

How Are the Kidneys Protected Against Ischemia?

Under physiological conditions, the kidney is able to auto regulate glomerular perfusion in spite of wide fluctuations of blood pressure. The three major mechanisms to maintain glomerular filtration are [19]:

Tubuloglomerular Feedback

This protective mechanism is maintained by the juxtaglomerular apparatus (JGA), which is located between the afferent and efferent arterioles and an adjacent portion of distal convoluted tubule called the macula densa. It comprises: 1) macula densa cells, which are densely packed specialized tubular cells in the distal convoluted tubule abutting the afferent and efferent arteriole leading in and out of a single glomerulus 2) juxtaglomerular cells (JGC) of afferent arteriole (granular cells), that secrete renin 3) mesangial cells with tight junctions between each other. The macula densa maintains a stable glomerular filtration rate (GFR) by sensing distal sodium (Na^+) and chloride (Cl^-) delivery as well as modulating changes in the afferent arterial tone [20] (Figure 1).

1. Increased filtration at the glomerulus or decreased reabsorption of Na^+ at the proximal tubule results in the macula densa being exposed to tubular fluid with high Na^+ and Cl^- concentrations. Sodium/potassium/2 chloride ($Na^+/K^+/2Cl^-$) cotransporters on the luminal surface of macula densa cells then transport more Na^+ from the tubular fluid into the cell.
2. This increase in intracellular Na^+ concentration results in an increase in intracellular osmolarity which leads to water movement inside the macula densa cell, causing cellular swelling [21]. When the cell swells, adenosine triphosphate (ATP) escapes via stretch activated maxi-anion channels [22].
3. ATP is converted to adenosine, which binds to G protein-coupled adenosine type 1 (A_1) receptors in the afferent arteriole, activating the G_i/G_o signaling cascade. This eventually leads to release of intracellular calcium (Ca^{2+}), which spreads to neighboring cells via gap junctions.
4. Increases intracellular Ca^{2+}results in arteriolar vasoconstriction and inhibits renin release.
5. Reduced filtration at the glomerulus or increased reabsorption of Na^+ in the proximal tubule results in macula densa being exposed to tubular fluid low in Na^+ and Cl^-. $Na^+/K/2Cl^-$ channels at the luminal surface of macula densa cells therefore transport low levels of Na^+ into the cell.
6. This leads to activation of a complex signaling cascade that eventually activates prostaglandin E synthase and results in synthesis of prostaglandin E_2 (PGE_2).

7. PGE_2 acts on G protein-coupled PGE_2 type 2 (EP_2) and type 4 (EP_4) receptors in JGC and activates renin release.

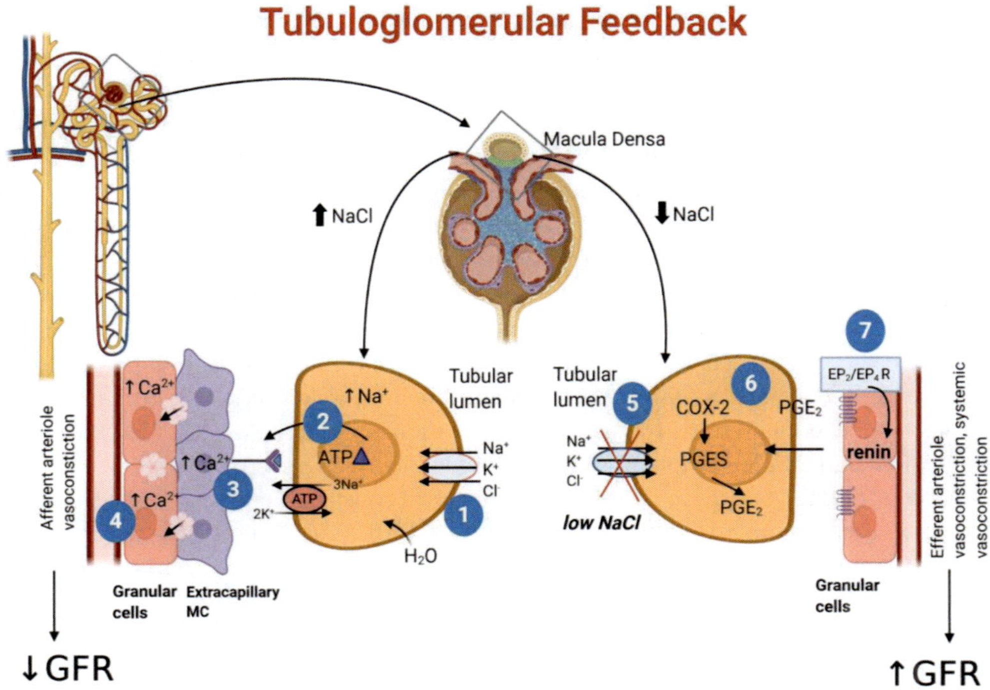

NaCl - sodium chloride, COX-2 - cyclooxygenase-2, PGES - Prostaglandin E synthase, PGE_2 - Prostaglandin E_2, EP_2/EP_4 - Prostaglandin E_2 receptor 2/ receptor 4, MC - mesangial cell.

Figure 1. Illustration of tubuloglomerular feedback in the states of low and high distal sodium delivery.

Renin-Angiotensin Aldosterone System Activation

Reduced kidney blood flow stimulates renin release from the granular cells of JGA which converts angiotensinogen to angiotensin (Ang) I, which is subsequently converted to Ang II by angiotensin-converting enzyme (ACE). Ang II causes vasoconstriction of the efferent arteriole in order to restore glomerular filtration rate [23].

Myogenic Reflex

While the aforementioned hormonal mechanisms involve the efferent arteriole vasoconstriction, afferent arteriole is the key player in the myogenic reflex. This is explained by the fact that afferent arteriole is a larger muscular vessel, as compared to efferent arteriole. The myogenic reflex refers to the contraction initiated by the myocyte itself as opposed to an external stimulus. The smooth muscle cells of the afferent arteriole react to the stretching of the muscle by opening the stretch activated ion channels, leading to the depolarization of the cell, and muscle contraction which in its turn decreases the blood flow. Alternatively, when the smooth muscles in the afferent arteriole relax, the stretch-activated ion channels remain closed, resulting in its vasodilation, thus increasing the rate of blood flow through the glomerulus [24].

In addition to the aforementioned mechanisms, there is a whole complex system of autocrine and paracrine defense mechanisms to preserve kidney function that are still poorly understood. These mechanisms are especially important in the kidney medulla, as medullary blood flow is less than 10% of the total blood flow to the kidney, resulting in the medulla being relatively hypoxic in normal physiological conditions (partial pressure of oxygen is in range from 10 to 20 mm Hg) [25]. On the other hand, increases in medullary blood flow can result in the wash out of the corticomedullary osmotic gradient and impair urinary concentrating ability, whereas decreased medullary blood flow can lead to ischemia, scarring, and potentially cortical necrosis [26, 27]. Therefore, tight regulation of medullary blood flow is crucial for normal kidney function. Kidney pericytes are thought to be involved in the medullary blood flow regulation [28]. Pericytes are contractile mesenchymal cells which possess elongated processes that encircle the endothelial wall, and are associated with glomeruli and cortical medullary peritubular capillaries and vasa recta. Crislip et al. demonstrated in rats that higher pericyte density is associated with reduced outer medullary congestion in post ischemic kidney injury (the role of medullary congestion in ATN discussed below) [29].

Important to note, that these mechanisms maintain a constant blood flow to the kidney over the range of arterial pressures from 60 to 160 mm Hg [30]. When blood pressure drops below this, these compensatory mechanisms are overwhelmed, leading to inability to maintain glomerular filtration. Therefore, AKI can ensue (Figure 2).

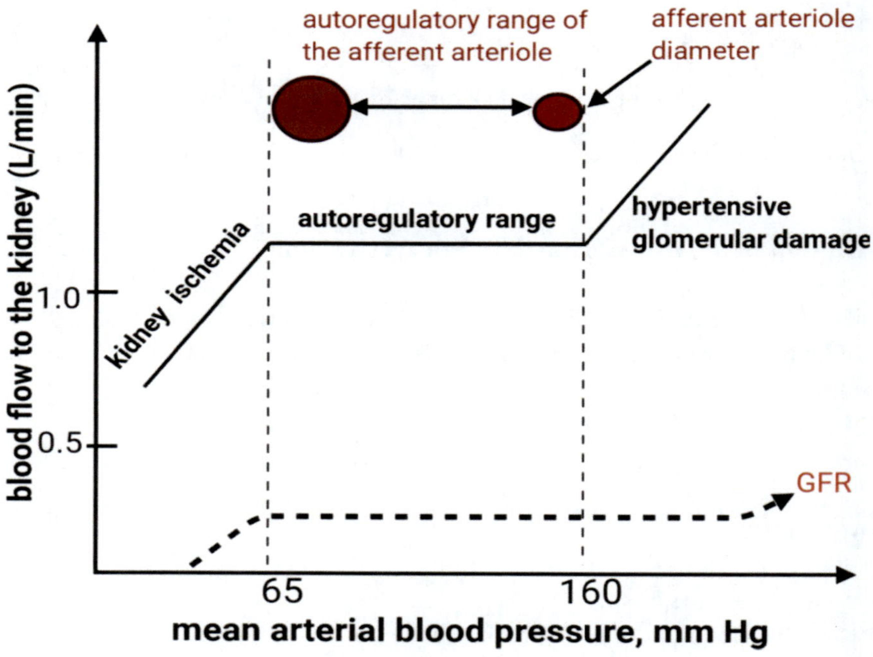

Figure 2. Kidney autoregulation. GFR- glomerular filtration rate.

Pathophysiology of ATN

The three stages of ischemic ATN include: initiation, extension and maintenance, followed by recovery [31]. Clinical correlation is denoted by italic text, which is further discussed in the *novel therapies* section.

Initiation Stage of ATN

During the initiation stage, changes are seen in both vascular and tubular autoregulatory systems [32, 33] (Figure 3).

In the glomerulus, endothelial cell injury is observed, resulting in the loss of the endothelium-dependent nitric oxide (NO) mediated relaxation, enhanced pressor sensitivity, and activation of vasoconstrictor pathways (which might be related to the resultant increase in cytosolic Ca^{2+}in the afferent arterioles, *see section on therapies*). Therefore, the normal autoregulatory response of the kidney vasculature to vasodilate in response to the decreased kidney perfusion is lost. Vasoconstriction exacerbates ongoing kidney ischemia, perpetuating a vicious cycle [34].

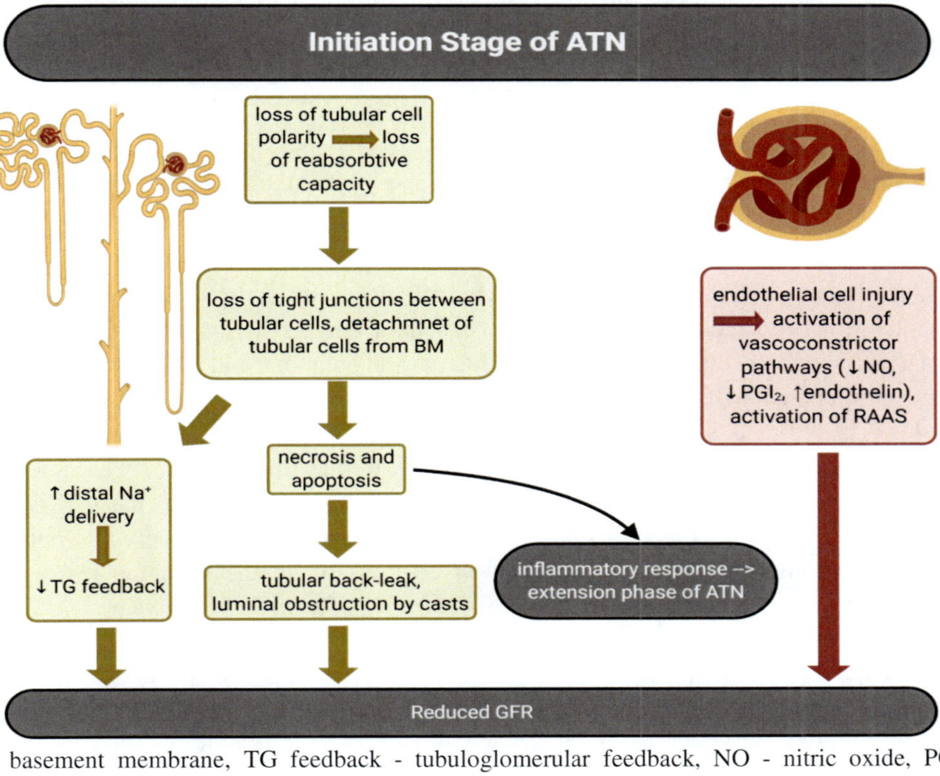

BM - basement membrane, TG feedback - tubuloglomerular feedback, NO - nitric oxide, PGI_2 - prostaglandin I_2, RAAS - renin angiotensin aldosterone system.

Figure 3. Glomerular and tubular changes during initiation stage of ATN.

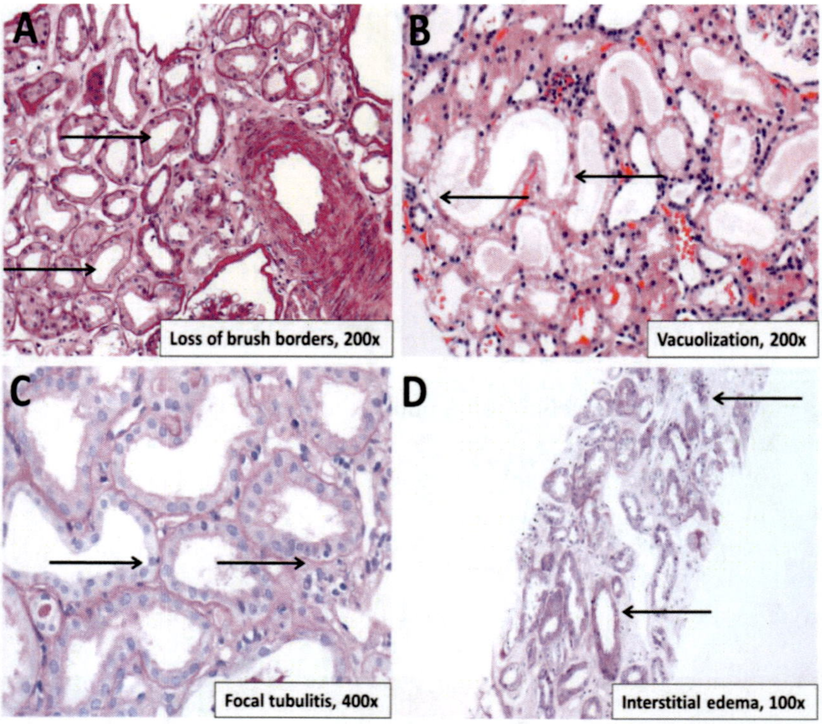

Figure 4. Morphological changes in ischemic ATN. A. Hematoxylin and eosin stained kidney cortex with arrows showing loss of proximal tubule brush borders. B. Hematoxylin and eosin stained kidney cortex with arrows showing vacuolization of proximal tubules. C. Periodic acid Schiff stained kidney cortex with arrows showing focal areas of immune cell accumulation (tubulitis). D. Periodic acid Schiff stained kidney cortex with arrows showing areas of interstitial edema. Courtesy of Tiffany Caza, MD, PhD.

In the kidney tubules, ischemia leads to cell death by at least two pathophysiologic mechanisms: necrosis and apoptosis. Necrosis is characterized by loss of membrane integrity, cytoplasmic swelling, nuclear pyknosis, cellular fragmentation, and inflammatory response. Apoptosis is characterized by cytoplasmic and nuclear shrinkage, DNA fragmentation, and breakdown of the cells into the apoptotic bodies to be removed by phagocytosis. These two forms of cell death frequently coexist and are two extremes of continuum. The mode of cell death depends primarily on the severity of the insult and resistance of the cell type [35]. Necrosis occurs after severe injury and the proximal tubules are uniquely susceptible, but apoptosis predominates after less severe injury, especially in the ischemia resistant distal nephron segments [36]. *Inhibition of apoptosis holds promise in ischemic ATN.*

Prominent morphological features in the setting of ischemic ATN are loss of proximal tubular brush border, patchy loss of tubular cells, focal areas of proximal tubular dilatation and distal tubular casts, vascular congestion in peritubular capillaries, leukocyte accumulation and peritubular capillaritis, apoptosis and areas of cellular regeneration (Figure 4) [37, 38]. Despite the name of acute tubular necrosis, frank tubular necrosis is rarely found in human intrinsic kidney injury.

Extension and Maintenance Phases

These phases are characterized by outer medullary congestion and inflammatory response. The medullary congestion worsens the already existent hypoxic environment and, thus, the hypoxic injury in S3 segment of proximal tubule and TAL of the loop of Henle [39]. Pericytes are now being increasingly recognized to play an important role in regulating blood flow in medullary vasa recta. Pericytes are stromal cells that support the vasculature, and a subset of pericytes are mesenchymal stem cells, that serve as progenitors of interstitial myofibroblasts in kidney fibrogenesis and progression to chronic kidney disease (CKD) [40]. In the setting of AKI, pericytes get activated, migrate into the kidney interstitium, leaving the endothelium of the kidney peritubular capillary bed unstable with resultant capillary rarefaction. Subsequently, pericytes transdifferentiate into myofibroblasts, which are key players in kidney fibrogenesis [41]. Moreover, studies in rats have shown that there is a correlation between pericyte density and improved recovery following kidney injury [29].

Inflammatory Response

Damaged tubular cells as well as resident macrophages attract circulatory immune system cells by releasing damage associated molecular patterns (DAMPs) and chemokines. DAMP recognition activates the immune cells to secrete proinflammatory cytokines (tumor necrosis factor (TNF)-α, interleukin (IL)-6, IL-8, monocyte chemoattractant protein-1 (MCP-1)), which in turn induces further cellular necrosis - the vicious cycle is termed necroinflammation [42, 43].

Uridine diphosphate glucose (UDP-glucose) is thought to be an early initiator and propellant of ischemia-induced AKI. UDP-glucose is one of the numerous DAMPs, and acts as potent agonist of the proinflammatory purinoceptor $P2Y_{14}$ receptor when secreted from injured cells. Battistone et al. [44] underscores the pivotal role of UDP-glucose and $P2Y_{14}$ receptor interaction in the initiation and extension phase of inflammation in AKI. $P2Y_{14}$ receptors are highly expressed in α-intercalated cells of the collecting duct. In the setting of ischemia-reperfusion injury, their expression increases dramatically. While most nucleotides are rapidly degraded after their release outside of the cell, extracellular UDP-glucose is stable in most tissues. Inflammatory receptor activation UDP-glucose/$P2Y_{14}$ receptor signaling pathway leads to produce proinflammatory chemokines, which attract circulating neutrophils, monocytes and macrophages from the blood vessels into the kidney stroma, accounting for extension and maintenance phases of AKI. *The inhibition of $P2Y_{14}$ receptors is being studied as a potential therapeutic in AKI* [44].

Due to the pro-inflammatory microenvironment, recruited macrophages develop a M1 phenotype, which contributes to the ongoing necroinflammation and kidney injury [45]. T cells and B cells are also associated with ischemic ATN. Likewise, complement system activation, primarily the alternative pathway, has been described in ischemic ATN [46, 47].

Recovery Phase

Over the course of events, which are not fully understood, macrophage phenotype changes toward anti-inflammatory effector function [48]. Activated M2 macrophages establish predominantly anti-inflammatory milieu, and this change in environment marks the transition from injury phase to the recovery phase, epithelial and tubular repair mechanisms, proliferation and fibrosis begin to predominate [49, 50]. Without this change to the anti-inflammatory micromilieu, necroinflammation leads to cell death and tissue damage.

Markers of AKI

Clinical and Laboratory Markers

Decrease in Glomerular Filtration Rate

Acute and profound decrease in glomerular filtration rate (GFR) occurs even in the absence of changes visible on light microscopy. This is explained by afferent arteriolar vasoconstriction in the setting of predominant vasoconstrictive response. Additionally, the back leakage of tubular filtrate into the interstitium in the setting of loss of tight junctions between tubular cells and the loss of epithelial cells lining the basement membrane of the tubules contributes to worsening interstitial edema. Lastly, tubular obstruction with epithelial cell casts contributes to the decrease in GFR [51]. Laboratory-wise, reduction in GFR is marked by elevated creatinine.

Urine Volume

Changes in urine volume are relatively non-sensitive for the diagnosis of AKI. However, in the setting of established AKI, oliguria has been associated with worse prognosis and earlier time to initiation of kidney replacement therapy. Studies have shown that patients with non-oliguric AKI have a lower peak serum creatinine concentration than patients with oliguric AKI. Moreover, retrospective and prospective studies have shown that patients with non-oliguric AKI have a lower incidence of requiring dialysis during the acute phase of the illness compared to patients with oliguric AKI (28 versus 84% and 46 versus 82% in different studies), a lower rate are requiring long-term dialysis >90 days, and a lower hospital mortality [52-54].

Urine Microscopy

Classic urine microscopy findings in patients with ATN include renal tubular epithelial (RTE) cells, RTE cell casts and granular casts (muddy brown casts) (Figure 5). Muddy brown granular casts in the urine are formed by release of Tamm-Horsfall protein within a thick ascending limb surrounded by sloughed epithelial cells. Urine sediment examination is a simple, fast and cheap method for the diagnosis and assessment of ATN. Urinary sediment score, which is based on the number of granular casts and RTE cells, is associated with the Acute Kidney Injury Network (AKIN) stages of AKI and with the risk of worsening AKI [55].

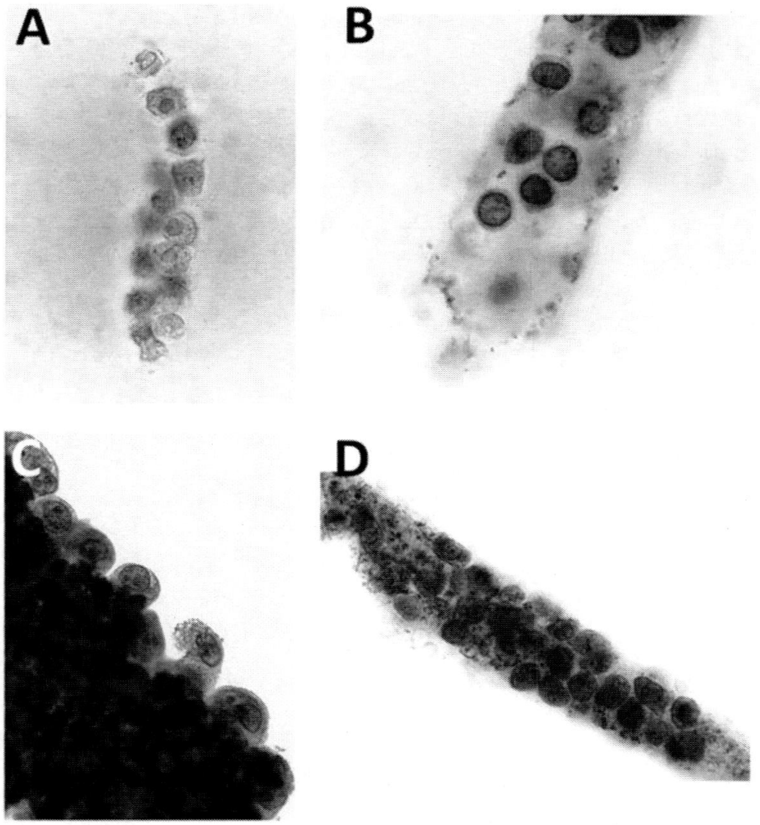

Figure 5. Urine Microscopy Findings. A. Brightfield, unstained (original magnification x1000) showing tubular epithelial cell cast. B. Brightfield, with Sternheimer-Malbin stain (original magnification x1000) C. Brightfield, unstained (original magnification x1000) C. Tubular epithelial cells along the surface of a dense granular cast - brightfield, with Sternheimer-Malbin stain (original magnification x1000) D. Brightfield, with Sternheimer-Malbin stain - (original magnification x1000). Courtesy of Jay Seltzer, MD.

Changes Reflected in Urinalysis

- Isosthenuria: Loss of urinary concentration capacity marks intrinsic kidney damage during hypoperfusion or toxic injury. Reduction in urine osmolarity indicates that prerenal azotemia which is characterized by normal or enhanced urinary concentration has been transferred to an established ATN. The loss of urinary concentrating ability is reflecting injury to the kidney medulla.
- Proteinuria: Proteinuria, tubular in origin, can be present and is typically less than 1 g/day. Urine protein to creatinine ratio in the setting of AKI should be interpreted with caution as the creatinine is not at the steady state (production is not equal to excretion in the setting of AKI), resulting in falsely high protein to creatinine ratio.

- Other data suggestive of ATN, that reflect proximal tubule dysfunction, includes blood urea nitrogen (BUN) to serum creatinine ratio of less than 20, FeNa greater than 2% (in the absence of diuretics) or fractional excretion of urea (FeUrea) greater than 50%. However, it is important to note a few diagnostic limitations of fractional excretion of sodium and urea. First, low FeNa (<1%) has been shown to be diagnostic of prerenal azotemia in oliguric patients, however in non-oliguric patients FeNa often times falls in indeterminate range between those of patients with prerenal azotemia and oliguric ATN [56]. Furthermore, there are several clinical scenarios of ATN where FeNa is low (<1%), which classically include contrast induced nephropathy, myoglobinuric ATN, septic ATN [5, 57]. Lastly, although FeUrea was found to be more sensitive and specific than FeNa in the setting of diuretic use in early studies [58], subsequent studies have shown that FeUrea lacks both sensitivity and specificity in distinguishing prerenal azotemia from ATN [59].

Current definition of AKI including RIFLE (Risk, Injury, Failure, Loss of kidney function), AKIN (Acute Kidney Injury Network) and KDIGO (Kidney Disease: Improving Global Outcomes) criteria rely on changes of creatinine and/or urine output. However, as outlined above, these criteria are not very sensitive or specific for AKI. Over the past decade there have been a large number of studies focused on discovering early markers of AKI. These are covered in the Table 1 below.

TREATMENT OF ATN

Over the last several decades there have been numerous novel therapeutics studied for the treatment of ATN. Despite numerous large scale clinical trials, a targeted pharmacologic therapy has yet to emerge as the standard of care. The current clinical approach in treating a patient with ATN is commonly referred to as "conservative treatment." This consists of fluid management, avoidance of further insults, and kidney replacement therapy when indicated. The following section outlines the current standard of care as well as novel therapeutic agents in various stages of development.

Fluid Strategies for Prevention and Treatment of ATN

In hemodynamically mediated ATN, the judicious use of fluids in order to maintain macrovascular perfusion is essential in preventing progression of kidney injury [67, 68]. However, it is still unclear exactly how much and which fluids are useful in patients at risk or with AKI. In a large randomized trial, from the Acute Respiratory Distress Syndrome (ARDS) Clinical Trial Network, comparing a conservative versus a liberal strategy of fluid management in patient with acute lung injury, showed that there was a non-significant trend toward a decrease in the incidence of kidney replacement therapy (KRT) than those in the liberal fluid arm (10% versus 14%; $P = 0.06$). Predictably, the liberal fluid arm was associated with a higher fluid balance, -136 ± 491 ml in the conservative-strategy group and 6992 ± 502 ml in the liberal-strategy group ($P < 0.001$), likely driving this need for KRT [69].

Table 1. Biomarkers of AKI

Biomarker	Major Description	Role in the Kidney	Timing	Strength	Limitations
Functional markers					
Creatinine, serum	113 Da amino acid derivative, breakdown product of creatine in muscle	Freely filtered at the glomerulus. Secreted in a proximal tubule.	Rises 24-48 hours after kidney injury	Produced at a constant rate	-Variable between individuals. -Delayed rise after injury. -Medications can affect tubular secretion (TMP-SMX, cimetidine, probenecid)
BUN, serum	60 Da amino acid derivative, produced by liver in urea cycle from protein metabolism	Freely filtered at the glomerulus Reabsorbed in a proximal tubule	Rises within 6- 12 hours	Low cost	-Varies with dietary intake -Medications can affect urea production (steroids) - Upper GI bleed raises BUN
Cystatin C, serum and urine	13 kDA protein, inhibitor of cysteine proteinases in all nucleated cells	Freely filtered at the glomerulus. Reabsorbed in proximal tubule and fully degraded locally	Detected 12-24 hours postinjury, peak levels at 24-48 hours	Produced at a constant rate. Glomerular filtration marker (serum). Biomarker of proximal tubule dysfunction (urine)	-May increase in other inflammatory conditions. - Albuminuria increases urinary excretion of cystatin [60]
Albuminuria	66 kDa blood protein	Minimally filtered at the glomerulus. Filtered albumin is reabsorbed in proximal tubule	Variable	Marker of glomerular filtration barrier injury	-Difficult to distinguish AKI vs CKD. -Variability in spot vs 24 hour collections
Markers of tubular damage - upregulated enzymes					
Kidney injury molecule-1 (KIM-1), urine and serum [61]	38 kDa membrane glycoprotein; upregulated in tubular injury. Activates immune cells Th-1, Th-2, Th-17, promotes apoptotic and necrotic cell clearance and remodeling of injured epithelium	Produced by undifferentiated proximal tubular cells	Detected 12-24 hours postinjury, peak levels at 48-72 hours	Approved by FDA for pre-clinical drug development	Expressed at high levels in patients with clear cell RCC, CKD with proteinuria, sickle-cell nephropathy
IL-18, serum and urine [62]	18 kDa proinflammatory cytokine expressed by macrophages, dendritic cells, monocytes, proximal tubular cells	Mediator of AKI	Elevated within first 6 hours after injury, peak levels 12-18 hours	Under clinical investigation	Elevated in inflammation, heart failure.

Table 1. (Continued)

Biomarker	Major Description	Role in the Kidney	Timing	Strength	Limitations
Neutrophil gelatinase - associated lipocalin (NGAL) [63]	25 kDa lipocalin protein, expressed by kidney tubular epithelial cells undergoing proliferation and regeneration, immune cells	Urine NGAL originates from damaged epithelial cells of the nephron and chelates labile iron released from damaged cells. Plasma NGAL derived from kidneys via tubular back leak and from other organs	Detected as early as 3 hours after injury, peak at 6 hours and can have sustained elevation up to 5 days	Under clinical investigation	Levels confounded by systemic infection, hydration status. Elevated in CKD, hypertension. Overall, poor diagnostic and prognostic performance
Liver fatty acid binding protein (L-FABP) [64]	15 kDa cytoplasmic protein that transports free fatty acids to mitochondria and peroxisomes. Protects against reactive oxygen species	Upregulated production in proximal tubular cells in ischemic AKI.	Detected within 1 hour after injury, peak levels within 6 hours	Approved as a diagnostic tool in Japan	Levels elevated in liver disease, ADPKD, CKD, sepsis
Prognostic biomarkers					
Tissue inhibitor of metalloproteinases 2 (TIMP-2) Insulin growth factor binding protein- 7 (IGFBP7) [65]	Cell cycle arrest proteins	TIMP2 stimulates p27 expression and IGFBP-7 increases expression of p53 and p21 which block cyclin-dependent protein kinase complexes during cell cycle, resulting in transient cell cycle arrest in AKI.	Detected within 4-8 hours after kidney injury	POC device measuring the product of these 2 biomarkers "Nephrocheck" approved by FDA in 2014 for prediction of AKI KDIGO stage 2 -3	Ongoing investigations
Furosemide stress test [66]	2-hour urine output after high dose furosemide (1mg/kg in furosemide naive patients, and 1.5 mg/kg in patients with prior exposure) predicts progression to more severe AKI.	Assessing the tubular function	Ideally performed in early AKI in clinically euvolemic patients.	<200 ml in the first 2 hours predicts progression to (AKIN) stage 3 AKI with sensitivity of 87% and specificity of 84%.	N/A

Da - dalton, kDa - kilodalton, TMP-SMX- trimethoprim-sulfamethoxazole, GI - gastrointestinal, RCC- renal cell carcinoma, ADPKD - autosomal dominant polycystic kidney disease.

Table 2. Summary of clinical trials examining normal saline and balanced solutions. IVF - intravenous fluids, L - liter

	Yunos et al	**SPLIT**	**SMART**	**SALT-ED**
Years conducted	2008-2009	2014	2016-2017	2016
Year published	2012	2015	2018	2018
Country	Australia	New Zealand	US	US
Number of centers	Single	Multiple	Single	Single
Randomization	No	Start month randomized	Start month randomized	Start month randomized
Blinding	No	Yes	No	No
Design	Non randomized, 6 months saline, washout, 6 months balanced	2 crossovers of 7 week block (total 28 weeks)	Multiple crossovers of 1 month (total 12 - 22 months)	8 crossovers of 1 month (total 16 months)
Setting	ICU	4 ICUs	5 ICUs	ED/In-patients
Balanced crystalloid	Hartmann or Plasmalyte	Plasmalyte 148	Ringer, Plasmalyte 148	95% Ringer, 5% Plasmalyte 148
Number of patients	1,533	2,278	15,802	13,347
Mean age	60 years	60.5 years	58 years (median) IQR 44-69	53 years (median) IQR 37-67
Race	n/a	65% white, 18% maori/Pacific islander	80.4% white	78% white, 19% black
Women	40%	34.5%	42.5%	51%
Baseline creatinine (mg/dl)	1	0.98	0.89 (median)	0.93 (median)
Volume of IVF per patient	3-4L	1.1L (median)	2.5L	1.6L (median)

Table modified with permission from NephJC by Dr. Swapnil Hiremath [71, 72].

Table 3. Outcomes of clinical trials examining normal saline and balanced solutions

	Yunos		SPLIT		SMART		SALT-ED	
	Saline	Balanced	Saline	Balanced	Saline	Balanced	Saline	Balanced
Death in Hospital	65 (9%)	59 (8%)	95 (8.6%)	87 (7.6%)	875 (11.1%)	818 (10.3%)	105 (1.6%)	95 (1.4%)
Need for KRT	57 (7.5%)	42 (5.4%)	38 (3.4%)	38 (3.3%)	220 (2.9%)	189 (2.5%)	31 (0.5%)	18 (0.3%)
Hospital Stay (days)	11	11	7.33	7.45	25.3	25.5	25	25
AKI	105 (14%)	65 (8.4%)	104 (10.2%)	105 (9.8%)	858 (11.5%)	807 (10.7%)	560 (8.6%)	528 (8.0%)
Change in Creatinine	0.25	0.17	0.18	0.21	0.04	0.04	0.12	0.13
MAKE	N/A	N/A	N/A	N/A	1211 (15.4%)	1139 (14.3%)	370 (5.6%)	315 (4.7%)

KRT - kidney replacement therapy, AKI - acute kidney injury, MAKE - major adverse kidney events (the composite of death, new receipt of KRT, or persistent AKI (defined as a final inpatient creatinine value ≥200% of the baseline value). Table modified with permission from NephJC by Dr. Swapnil Hiremath [71, 72].

Subsequently, a secondary analysis from the SOAP study, prospective multicenter observational study designed to evaluate the epidemiology of sepsis in European countries, assessed fluid balance on the outcome of AKI in patients admitted to the intensive care unit. This study was more applicable, including all comers to the ICU and addressed outcomes in patients with kidney failure. Mean fluid balance was significantly more positive in patients with early and late AKI than in patients without AKI throughout the first 7 days of the ICU admission (HR 1.21, 95% CI 1.13–1.28, $p < 0.001$). Also, mean fluid balance was more positive among non-survivors than among survivors [70]. All of this information supports a more judicious fluid administration strategy with a goal of maintaining euvolemia.

There is mounting evidence showing the superiority of balanced crystalloids over normal saline (NS) in the prevention of AKI. The supraphysiologic concentration of chloride (Cl^-) in NS translates to an elevated tubular Cl^- concentration. Through tubuloglomerular feedback, there is decreased renin release and a subsequent decrease in GFR [73, 74]. In 2018 the SMART trial demonstrated a benefit of balanced crystalloid over normal saline in critically ill adults (Table 3). The trial was a pragmatic, randomized, multiple-crossover trial conducted in five intensive care units with 15,802 adults receiving saline or balanced crystalloids solution. The use of balanced crystalloids was associated with a lower rate of major adverse kidney events (MAKE) within 30 days (14.3% vs 15.4%, P = 0.04) [71]. Similarly the SALT-ED trial (another pragmatic clinical trial from the same institution), conducted in non-critically ill adults in emergency departments, showed a similar lower incidence of major adverse kidney events within 30 days in the blanched crystalloid group compared to the saline (4.7% vs. 5.6%, P = 0.01) [71]. These pragmatic trials argue for the routine use of balanced crystalloid over saline in a multitude of settings.

Kidney Replacement Therapy

Ideally, tubular injury can be mitigated with timely and judicious fluid administration, maintenance of kidney perfusion and avoidance further insults. Unfortunately, progression to kidney failure and the associated life-threatening sequelae is often unavoidable. For decades, it has been clear that KRT provides life sustaining treatment for patients with critical illness, but it has not always been clear how KRT should be administered in terms of timing, dose, and modality [75]. We will focus primarily on timing of KRT in this review. Studies on modalities have not found one modality to be superior to another (intermittent KRT versus continuous KRT) and this decision is often guided by patient hemodynamics [76]. In regards to dose, the KDIGO Clinical Practice Guideline recommends delivering an effluent volume of 20 to 25 mL/kg/hr for continuous KRT in patients with AKI [77]. This is based upon several randomized clinical trials.

Timing

There have been multiple important clinical trials in the past 5 years that have shed light on when to initiate KRT, some with conflicting data (Table 4). The main question being answered in these trials is: Is there a benefit to starting KRT at initially sign of kidney injury (<12 hours), or is it better to wait until 48-72 hours without sign of recovery or let the sequelae of kidney dysfunction (hyperkalemia, acidosis, pulmonary edema) drive the decision to initiate? 2016 the Early versus Late Initiation of Renal Replacement Therapy in Critically Ill Patients with Acute Kidney Injury (ELAIN) trial [79], a single center RCT, showed a benefit in early initiation of KRT. There was a reduction in 90-day mortality (39.3% versus 54.7%, P = 0.03), kidney recovery (53.6% versus 38.7%, P = 0.02) and Duration of KRT (9 days versus 25 days, P = 0.04). Criticisms of the ELAIN Trial were its smaller size (~200 patients), single center, majority of patients from surgical ICU admissions, and inclusion of patients without AKI (inclusion of refractory pulmonary edema).

Table 4. Summary of trials comparing early vs late start KRT in AKI

	ELAIN	AKIKI	IDEAL-ICU	STARRT-AKI
Design	Single-surgical center, Germany N = 231	Multicenter France N = 620	Multicenter France N = 488	Multicenter Multinational N = 2927
AKI severity	KDIGO stage 2	KDIGO stage 3 (On ventilator or vasopressors)	RIFLE-F AKI (Early septic shock)	KDIGO stage 2 or 3 (Critically Ill)
The time in which early start group begins KRT after enrollment	8 hours	6 hours	12 hours	12 hours
% received KRT (early vs late)	100% vs 91%	98% vs 51%	97% vs 62%	97% vs 62%
Mortality (early vs late)	39% vs 54% (90 day)	49% vs 50% (60 day)	58% vs 54% (90 day)	44% vs 44% (90 day)
Unique findings	Time on KRT, Kidney recovery, and ventilator time favored early group	61% of survivors did not receive KRT & fewer catheter related complication in late group	Time on KRT, kidney recovery and ventilator time favored early group	More adverse events, KRT dependence and rehospitalizations in early group
ICU length of stay	No difference	No difference	No difference	Less in early group

Table modified with permission from NephJC by Sophia Ambruso, DO [78].

Subsequently, in 2018 both the Artificial Kidney Initiation in Kidney Injury (AKIKI) (80) and Initiation of Dialysis Early versus Late in the Intensive Care Unit (IDEAL-ICU) trial (81) found contradictory findings to ELAIN. IDEAL-ICU trial is a multi-center RCT with ~ 500 patients with sepsis and AKI that were randomized to receive either early start KRT (<12 hours after AKI) or delayed start KRT (>48 hours after AKI). The trial showed no significant difference in 90-day mortality between early and late start groups (58% vs 54%, P = 0.38) and showed a significant difference in KRT free days in favor of the delayed strategy (16 vs 12, P = 0.006). These findings were supported by the AKIKI Trial, a RCT comparing early start KRT (immediately after randomization) vs delayed start (driven by refractory signs and symptoms of kidney failure or a predetermined laboratory value). The AKIKI trial found similar findings between the two groups. There was an insignificant difference in mortality (P = 0.795) and significant difference in KRT free days between the early and delayed groups (11 vs 16, P < 0.001). The discordance of ELAIN compared with AKIKI and IDEAL-ICU trials was further addressed in the STARRT AKI trial (78). This was a large (>3000 patients) multicenter RCT where patients received an accelerated KRT strategy (<12 hours after AKI) or a standard strategy (met conventional indications or persisting >72 hours). It found no significant difference mortality at 90 days (43.9% versus 43.7%, P = 0.92), decreased reliance on continued RRT (10.4% vs. 6%) and fewer adverse events (23.0% vs. 16.5%, <0.001) in the in the delayed start group. Furthermore, there was a significant difference in the number of RRT dependent patients at 90 days (10.4% vs 6.0%, RR 1.74; 95% CI, 1.24 to 2.43). The size, scope and generalizability of IDEAL-ICU, AKIKI and STARRT-AKI trials argue for delayed start to KRT, basing decision to treat on traditional indicators (treatment refractory hyperkalemia, acidosis, pulmonary edema) and persistent AKI (>72 hours).

Novel Therapies for ATN

Angiotensin

Modulation of the RAS, both agonistically and antagonistically, has been explored in the treatment of ATN. This is mechanistically appealing due to angiotensin affecting peripheral vasoconstriction helping preserve mean arterial pressure (MAP), preferential vasoconstriction of the efferent arteriole, and modulation of water and sodium homeostasis through release of aldosterone and vasopressin [67]. The most promising and arguably most researched therapeutic RAS modulator is angiotensin (Ang) II. Studies have shown the upregulation of angiotensinogen, Ang I and Ang II in both the blood and the urine are associated with severity of kidney injury [82, 83]. The largest trial assessing the efficacy of Ang II is the Angiotensin II for the Treatment of High-Output Shock (ATHOS)-3 trial. This trial established that in patients with catecholamine resistant vasodilatory shock (CRVS), administration of continuous intravenous Ang II was associated with improvement in mean arterial pressure as well as a reduction in vasopressor requirements (84). It was then postulated that hemodynamic improvements in perfusion in CVRS may show an improvement in kidney outcomes. A post hoc analysis of ATHOS-3 aimed to evaluate the effect of Ang II on AKI [85]. This subgroup analysis showed that not only was survival higher (53% vs. 30%, P = 0.012) in patients treated with Ang II and placebo respectively, but also increased discontinuation of KRT by day 7 (38% vs 15%, P = 0.007). However, it should be noted that the trial was not powered for the outcomes of survival and kidney recovery. In the future, larger studies may help further elucidate the benefits of Ang II in the setting of CRVS. Currently, there is not enough data to advocate for the routine use of Ang II in this population.

Steroids

Tubular inflammation is implicated in the extension and maintenance phases of ATN. For this reason, there has been much interest in the role of corticosteroids for treating and preventing ATN. Sepsis is a particularly appealing context for steroid use due to the potential dual benefit of decreasing inflammation and raising mean arterial pressure, thereby improving kidney perfusion. The Adjunctive Corticosteroid Treatment in Critically Ill Patients with Septic Shock (ADRENAL) trial, a multicenter double-blind RCT, randomized patients with septic shock who were undergoing mechanical ventilation to receive hydrocortisone or placebo for 7 days [86]. Between the two groups, there was no difference in mortality at 90 days (27.9% vs 28.8%, P = 0.50), use of KRT (30.6% vs 32.7%, P = 0.18), and days spent alive and KRT free (42.6 vs 40.4, P = 0.29).

Trials addressing the use of steroids in patients on cardiopulmonary bypass undergoing cardiac surgery have demonstrated mixed results. In a post hoc analysis of severe AKI in the Dexamethasone for Cardiac Surgery (DECS) trial, a large multicenter RCT, a significant difference was found in in the use of KRT favoring the dexamethasone group (0.4% vs 1.0%, P = 0.02) [87]. In stratified analyses, the strongest signal for potential benefit of dexamethasone was in patients with an eGFR<15 mL/min/1.73 m^2 (7.0% vs 23.7%, P = 0.03). The major criticism of this trial was the low number of events leading to low statistical power, which is more pronounced in the stratified analysis [88]. The Steroids In Cardiac Surgery (SIRS) trial, a double-blind RCT, found results contradictory to the DECS trial. The SIRS trial found no significant difference between methylprednisolone and placebo for the primary outcome of death at 30 days (4% vs 5%, P = 0.19) and new kidney failure defined as KDIGO stage 3 AKI or greater (4.0% vs 4.0%, P = 0.21) [89]. The SIRS trial was higher powered and used a broader definition of kidney injury, leading to a much higher event rate that DECS. In both sepsis and cardiopulmonary bypass, steroids provide no clear benefit in the treatment or prevention of AKI.

Adenosine

As previously described, the nephron regulates glomerular flow in part through the tubuloglomerular feedback mechanism (Figure 1). For these reasons, manipulating this mechanism has been the study of novel therapies for ischemia mediated ATN [90]. The most promising target to date has been the secondary messenger adenosine and its receptors. The largest trial to date is the PROTECT trial, which studied the adenosine A_1 receptor antagonist Rolofylline's effect on kidney function in patients with acute heart failure and AKI. Trial results were negative showing no difference between Rolofylline and placebo in recovery from AKI (13.7% vs. 15.0%, P = 0.44) [91].

SGLT2 Inhibitors

Sodium glucose co-transporter-2 (SGLT2) inhibitors were initially developed for the treatment of type 2 diabetes. They work by inhibiting SGLT2 in the kidney, increasing blood glucose excretion, thereby lowering blood glucose levels. In addition, large scale clinical trials have shown the benefit of these medications in the treatment of heart failure and CKD. In regards to AKI, there was initially concern from case reports for an increased risk of AKI, and the Food and Drug Administration issued safety warnings about the risk AKI after the initiation of the SGLT2 inhibitors- canagliflozin and dapagliflozin. However, a population-based retrospective cohort study reviewing 39,000 patients compared the use of SGLT2 inhibitors and dipeptidyl peptidase-4 (DPP4) inhibitors for the association with AKI. Relative to new use of a DPP4 inhibitor, the initiation of a SGLT2 inhibitor was associated with a lower 90-day risk of a hospital encounter with AKI (1.10% vs 1.99%; RR 0.79, 95% CI 0.64-0.98) [92]. Similarly, retrospective cohort data from 2 large health care systems showed a decreased incidence in AKI when comparing users of SGLT-2 inhibitors compared for cross matched controls (3.8% vs 9.7%, P = 0.01 and 2.2% vs 4.6%, P < 0.01) [93]. It is unclear why this improvement is seen, but these findings argue for use of these medications in patients with indications, regardless of kidney injury risk. These studies address AKI more broadly so it is unclear whether there is a benefit for ATN specifically. Further studies are necessary in evaluating the role of SGLT-2 inhibitors in treatment of ATN and potential benefit of continuing these medicines in the setting of ATN.

Hemoperfusion

Hyperperfusion is a form of extracorporeal organ support in which the blood is circulated through a sorbent-containing column, which non-selectively removes larger molecules, usually targeting cytokines, endotoxin, or pathogens. Interest in hemoperfusion has increased in light of the coronavirus infectious disease 2019 (COVID-19) pandemic and increasing recognition that inflammatory mediators are implicated in the pathogenesis and maintenance of ATN [94]. A recent randomized, controlled, open-label, multicenter trial aimed at assessing the efficacy of hemoperfusion, showed significant IL-6 elimination in the hemoperfusion. Unfortunately this failed to translate to clinical benefit. There were no detectable differences in systemic plasma IL-6 levels between the two groups and no difference in 60 day mortality [95]. As there has yet to be a large scale clinical trial addressing the efficacy of hemoperfusion for improving kidney outcomes, there is currently no role for hemoperfusion outside of clinical trials in the treatment of ATN.

Stem Cell Therapy

In the setting of AKI, there is increased mesenchymal stem cell (MSC) migration to the site of injury. It is thought that these MSCs promote injured epithelial cells to pursue cell division and recovery rather than apoptosis and fibrosis [96]. Pre-clinical data appeared promising in mouse models studying multiple etiologies of AKI including ischemia reperfusion and cisplatin nephrotoxicity [97]. A recent multicenter phase 2 RCT was performed to address the safety and efficacy of allogeneic MSCs in reducing the time to recovery from AKI after cardiac surgery. Overall, the results of the trial were negative, showing no significant difference in time to recovery of kidney function to baseline creatinine (15 vs. 12 days, P = 0.32) or dialysis at 30 days (10.6% vs. 7.4% with placebo) [98]. Furthemore, the study medicine (MSCs) needed to be administered via an intra-aortic catheter, limiting its applicability. Despite the appeal and promise of MSCs in ATN, there has yet to be a clinical trial demonstrating benefit.

Studies Based on the Use of Early Biomarkers

Over the past decade, numerous studies have evaluated the utility of several different biomarkers in early diagnosis and risk stratification of ATN. In 2014, following the publication of three multicenter cohort studies (Sapphire, Opal and Topaz), combination of urine tissue inhibitor of metalloproteinase 2 and insulin like growth factor binding protein 7, known as [TIMP-2]*[IGFBP-7] became approved by FDA for clinical use in the USA [65, 99, 100]. [TIMP-2]*[IGFBP-7] are cell cycle arrest proteins that are expressed by renal tubular epithelial (RTE) cells in the setting of cellular stress or injury and lead to cell cycle arrest in G1 stage, protecting the cell from replicating with damaged genetic material. However, if the RTE cells do not re-initiate the cell cycle and remain arrested at G1, fibrotic phenotype ensues [101]. [TIMP-2]*[IGFBP7] are markers of cellular stress, and become elevated as early 4-8 hours after the insult, and therefore represent an ongoing kidney injury rather than already established kidney injury, manifested by rise in creatinine and drop in urine output. Implementing interventions early on "at the stage of cellular stress" holds theoretical promises. We will here describe p53 inhibition as a potential therapeutic as well as the results of the randomized controlled trial on prevention of cardiac surgery-associated AKI by implementing the KDIGO guidelines in high risk patients identified by biomarkers.

p53

The initiation phase of ATN is characterized in part by apoptosis. In AKI, p53 was shown to regulate several genes involved in cell cycle regulation and cell death making it an appealing target for therapies (102). A small interfering RNA (siRNA) targeting p53 (QPI-1002) has shown promising results in phase 2 clinical trial in patients undergoing cardiac surgery [103]. Preliminary data shows a reduction in the incidence of major adverse kidney events (MAKE) in the 90 days following cardiac surgery, reduction in the incidence of AKI in the 5 days following cardiac surgery, reduction in the severity and duration of AKI as well as trends towards overall survival and dialysis free survival. It is currently under phase 3 trial to further evaluate safety and efficacy (ClinicalTrials.gov Identifier: NCT02610283).

PREVENTION OF AKI

The prevention of cardiac surgery-associated AKI by implementing the KDIGO guidelines in high risk patients identified by biomarkers (PrevAKI) [104] trial assess the use of early biomarkers to prophylactically implement strategies to reduce AKI. In this randomized controlled trial, conducted at Muenster University Hospital, Germany, 276 patients undergoing cardiac surgery were enrolled on the basis of elevated [TIMP-2]*[IGFBP7] >0.3, signifying high risk for progression of AKI. They were randomized to control and intervention group, where intervention group involved implementation of KDIGO guidelines (optimization of volume status and hemodynamic parameters based on functional hemodynamic monitoring, avoidance of hyperglycemia, discontinuation of nephrotoxins, avoidance of radio contrast agent and angiotensin-converting enzyme inhibitor/angiotensin receptor blocker) and control group received standard of care (MAP > 65 mm Hg, CVP between 8-10, discontinuation of nephrotoxins, avoidance of radio contrast agent and angiotensin-converting enzyme inhibitor/angiotensin receptor blocker). Primary outcome was the occurrence of AKI within 72 hours after cardiac surgery and secondary outcomes included 30-, 60-, 90- day all-cause mortality, need for KRT, MAKE, and length of stay. Primary outcome occurred in 55.1% of patients in the intervention group compared to 71.7% of patients in the control group (P = 0.004, OR 0.48 (95%CI, 0.29-0.76)). There were no significant differences in any of the secondary outcomes. Although this study is promising given its positive result, its major limitation is the fact that it was a single-center study. Currently, multicenter prevAKI trial is in progress, involving the same patient population and methods.

Clinical Pearls

- ATN is the most common cause of AKI in hospitalized patients, with an incidence of up to 20% in patients non-critically ill, and up to 70% in patients admitted to the ICU.
- Clinically the diagnosis of ATN is based on ruling out pre-renal and post-renal etiologies of AKI, and microscopic examination of urine for the evidence of tubular damage (renal tubular epithelial cells, muddy brown casts).
- Three most common causes of ATN are kidney ischemia, sepsis, and nephrotoxins.
- Recognize the limitations of FeNa and FeUrea in patients with nonoliguric AKI.
- Urine output is neither a sensitive or specific marker of AKI, however patients with nonoliguric AKI have been shown to have lower incidence of KRT and lower in-hospital mortality.
- The furosemide stress test is an inexpensive and simple way to assess the presence of residual tubular function in ATN, and predicts progression to more severe stages of AKI.
- Balanced crystalloids are associated with lower incidence of major adverse kidney events, as compared to normal saline, in both patients' presenting to the emergency room and ICU.
- There is no benefit to early initiation of KRT as opposed to delayed start based on traditional indications (treatment refractory hyperkalemia, metabolic acidosis, diuretic resistant volume overload, uremia). In fact, delayed start of KRT based on these indications leads to decreased reliance on continued KRT and fewer adverse events (based on STARRT AKI trial).
- So far, no pharmacologic intervention have shown positive results in treatment of established ATN.
- Identifying patients at high risk for ATN, based on biomarkers, and implementing therapeutic strategies early before ATN is established, might be promising in preventing ATN progression.

Conclusion

ATN is the most common type of AKI in hospitalized patients. Implications of ATN extend way beyond the hospital stay, leading to decreased survival and increased progression of underlying_CKD, and therefore posing a major public health problem. The pathophysiology of ATN is complex and involves multiple pathophysiologic mechanisms that interplay and amplify each other. Diminishing the incidence and severity of ATN will also require a comprehensive approach, including identifying it early (before the damage has been established), and implementing a multifaceted therapeutic approach that is based on understanding of its complex pathophysiology. Ongoing clinical trials on novel strategies that emerged from recent findings from basic and translational research on ATN, hold promise for proactive treatment of ATN.

ACKNOWLEDGMENT

We thank Ritika Revoori for help in reviewing and formatting manuscript. Figures 1, 2, 3 were made with biorender.com.

REFERENCES

[1] Gill N, Nally JV, Jr., Fatica RA. Renal failure secondary to acute tubular necrosis: epidemiology, diagnosis, and management. *Chest.* 2005;128(4):2847-63.

[2] Kellum JA, Lameire N, Group KAGW. Diagnosis, evaluation, and management of acute kidney injury: a KDIGO summary (Part 1). *Crit Care*. 2013;17(1):204.

[3] Liano F, Pascual J. Epidemiology of acute renal failure: a prospective, multicenter, community-based study. Madrid Acute Renal Failure Study Group. *Kidney Int.* 1996;50(3):811-8.

[4] Corwin HL, Schreiber MJ, Fang LS. Low fractional excretion of sodium. Occurrence with hemoglobinuric- and myoglobinuric-induced acute renal failure. *Arch Intern Med.* 1984;144(5):981-2.

[5] Fang LS, Sirota RA, Ebert TH, Lichtenstein NS. Low fractional excretion of sodium with contrast media-induced acute renal failure. *Arch Intern Med.* 1980;140(4):531-3.

[6] Zarich S, Fang LS, Diamond JR. Fractional excretion of sodium. Exceptions to its diagnostic value. *Arch Intern Med.* 1985;145(1):108-12.

[7] Esson ML, Schrier RW. Diagnosis and treatment of acute tubular necrosis. *Ann Intern Med.* 2002;137(9):744-52.

[8] Lameire N, Van Biesen W, Vanholder R. Acute renal failure. *Lancet.* 2005;365(9457): 417-30.

[9] Vincent JL, De Backer D. Circulatory shock. *N Engl J Med.* 2013;369(18):1726-34.

[10] Shankar-Hari M, Phillips GS, Levy ML, Seymour CW, Liu VX, Deutschman CS, et al. Developing a New Definition and Assessing New Clinical Criteria for Septic Shock: For the Third International Consensus Definitions for Sepsis and Septic Shock (Sepsis-3). *JAMA*. 2016;315(8):775-87.

[11] Shum HP, Yan WW, Chan TM. Recent knowledge on the pathophysiology of septic acute kidney injury: A narrative review. *J Crit Care*. 2016;31(1):82-9.

[12] Langenberg C, Bagshaw SM, May CN, Bellomo R. The histopathology of septic acute kidney injury: a systematic review. *Crit Care*. 2008;12(2):R38.

[13] Bamgbola O. Review of vancomycin-induced renal toxicity: an update. *Ther Adv Endocrinol Metab*. 2016;7(3):136-47.

[14] Lopez-Novoa JM, Quiros Y, Vicente L, Morales AI, Lopez-Hernandez FJ. New insights into the mechanism of aminoglycoside nephrotoxicity: an integrative point of view. *Kidney Int.* 2011;79(1):33-45.

[15] Safdar A, Ma J, Saliba F, Dupont B, Wingard JR, Hachem RY, et al. Drug-induced nephrotoxicity caused by amphotericin B lipid complex and liposomal amphotericin B: a review and meta-analysis. *Medicine* (Baltimore). 2010;89(4):236-44.

[16] Mehran R, Dangas GD, Weisbord SD. Contrast-Associated Acute Kidney Injury. *N Engl J Med.* 2019;380(22):2146-55.

[17] Levey AS, James MT. Acute Kidney Injury. *Ann Intern Med.* 2017;167(9):ITC66-ITC80.

[18] Panizo N, Rubio-Navarro A, Amaro-Villalobos JM, Egido J, Moreno JA. Molecular Mechanisms and Novel Therapeutic Approaches to Rhabdomyolysis-Induced Acute Kidney Injury. *Kidney Blood Press Res.* 2015;40(5):520-32.

[19] Loutzenhiser R, Griffin K, Williamson G, Bidani A. Renal autoregulation: new perspectives regarding the protective and regulatory roles of the underlying mechanisms. *Am J Physiol Regul Integr Comp Physiol.* 2006;290(5):R1153-67.

[20] Peti-Peterdi J, Harris RC. Macula densa sensing and signaling mechanisms of renin release. *J Am Soc Nephrol.* 2010;21(7):1093-6.

[21] Komlosi P, Fintha A, Bell PD. Unraveling the relationship between macula densa cell volume and luminal solute concentration/osmolality. *Kidney Int.* 2006;70(5):865-71.

[22] Bell PD, Lapointe JY, Sabirov R, Hayashi S, Peti-Peterdi J, Manabe K, et al. Macula densa cell signaling involves ATP release through a maxi anion channel. *Proc Natl Acad Sci USA.* 2003;100(7):4322-7.

[23] Schnermann J, Briggs JP. Tubular control of renin synthesis and secretion. *Pflugers Arch.* 2013;465(1):39-51.

[24] Gilmore JP, Cornish KG, Rogers SD, Joyner WL. Direct evidence for myogenic autoregulation of the renal microcirculation in the hamster. *Circ Res.* 1980;47(2):226-30.

[25] Brezis M, Heyman SN, Epstein FH. Determinants of intrarenal oxygenation. II. Hemodynamic effects. *Am J Physiol.* 1994;267(6 Pt 2):F1063-8.

[26] Brezis M, Rosen S. Hypoxia of the renal medulla--its implications for disease. *N Engl J Med.* 1995;332(10):647-55.

[27] Pallone TL, Zhang Z, Rhinehart K. Physiology of the renal medullary microcirculation. *Am J Physiol Renal Physiol.* 2003;284(2):F253-66.

[28] Kennedy-Lydon TM, Crawford C, Wildman SS, Peppiatt-Wildman CM. Renal pericytes: regulators of medullary blood flow. *Acta Physiol* (Oxf). 2013;207(2):212-25.

[29] Crislip GR, O'Connor PM, Wei Q, Sullivan JC. Vasa recta pericyte density is negatively associated with vascular congestion in the renal medulla following ischemia reperfusion in rats. *Am J Physiol Renal Physiol.* 2017;313(5):F1097-F105.

[30] Carlstrom M, Wilcox CS, Arendshorst WJ. Renal autoregulation in health and disease. *Physiol Rev.* 2015;95(2):405-511.

[31] Rosen S, Stillman IE. Acute tubular necrosis is a syndrome of physiologic and pathologic dissociation. *J Am Soc Nephrol.* 2008;19(5):871-5.

[32] Devarajan P. Update on mechanisms of ischemic acute kidney injury. *J Am Soc Nephrol.* 2006;17(6):1503-20.

[33] Goligorsky MS. Whispers and shouts in the pathogenesis of acute renal ischaemia. *Nephrol Dial Transplant.* 2005;20(2):261-6.

[34] Molitoris BA, Sutton TA. Endothelial injury and dysfunction: role in the extension phase of acute renal failure. *Kidney Int.* 2004;66(2):496-9.

[35] Lieberthal W, Koh JS, Levine JS. Necrosis and apoptosis in acute renal failure. *Semin Nephrol.* 1998;18(5):505-18.

[36] Brezis M, Shanley P, Silva P, Spokes K, Lear S, Epstein FH, et al. Disparate mechanisms for hypoxic cell injury in different nephron segments. Studies in the isolated perfused rat kidney. *J Clin Invest.* 1985;76(5):1796-806.

[37] Lameire NH, Vanholder R. Pathophysiology of ischaemic acute renal failure. *Best Pract Res Clin Anaesthesiol*. 2004;18(1):21-36.

[38] Schrier RW, Wang W, Poole B, Mitra A. Acute renal failure: definitions, diagnosis, pathogenesis, and therapy. *J Clin Invest.* 2004;114(1):5-14.

[39] Mason J, Torhorst J, Welsch J. Role of the medullary perfusion defect in the pathogenesis of ischemic renal failure. *Kidney Int*. 1984;26(3):283-93.

[40] Armulik A, Genove G, Betsholtz C. Pericytes: developmental, physiological, and pathological perspectives, problems, and promises. *Dev Cell*. 2011;21(2):193-215.

[41] Fligny C, Duffield JS. Activation of pericytes: recent insights into kidney fibrosis and microvascular rarefaction. *Curr Opin Rheumatol*. 2013;25(1):78-86.

[42] Mulay SR, Holderied A, Kumar SV, Anders HJ. Targeting Inflammation in So-Called Acute Kidney Injury. *Semin Nephrol.* 2016;36(1):17-30.

[43] Mulay SR, Linkermann A, Anders HJ. Necroinflammation in Kidney Disease. *J Am Soc Nephrol.* 2016;27(1):27-39.

[44] Battistone MA, Mendelsohn AC, Spallanzani RG, Allegretti AS, Liberman RN, Sesma J, et al. Proinflammatory P2Y14 receptor inhibition protects against ischemic acute kidney injury in mice. *J Clin Invest.* 2020;130(7):3734-49.

[45] Kundert F, Platen L, Iwakura T, Zhao Z, Marschner JA, Anders HJ. Immune mechanisms in the different phases of acute tubular necrosis. *Kidney Res Clin Pract.* 2018;37(3):185-96.

[46] Akcay A, Nguyen Q, Edelstein CL. Mediators of inflammation in acute kidney injury. *Mediators Inflamm.* 2009;2009:137072.

[47] Kinsey GR, Li L, Okusa MD. Inflammation in acute kidney injury. *Nephron Exp Nephrol.* 2008;109(4):e102-7.

[48] Lee S, Huen S, Nishio H, Nishio S, Lee HK, Choi BS, et al. Distinct macrophage phenotypes contribute to kidney injury and repair. *J Am Soc Nephrol.* 2011;22(2):317-26.

[49] Ricardo SD, van Goor H, Eddy AA. Macrophage diversity in renal injury and repair. *J Clin Invest.* 2008;118(11):3522-30.

[50] Wen Y, Crowley SD. The varying roles of macrophages in kidney injury and repair. *Curr Opin Nephrol Hypertens*. 2020;29(3):286-92.

[51] Wangsiripaisan A, Gengaro PE, Edelstein CL, Schrier RW. Role of polymeric Tamm-Horsfall protein in cast formation: oligosaccharide and tubular fluid ions. *Kidney Int.* 2001;59(3):932-40.

[52] Anderson RJ, Linas SL, Berns AS, Henrich WL, Miller TR, Gabow PA, et al. Nonoliguric acute renal failure. *N Engl J Med.* 1977;296(20):1134-8.

[53] Leedahl DD, Frazee EN, Schramm GE, Dierkhising RA, Bergstralh EJ, Chawla LS, et al. Derivation of urine output thresholds that identify a very high risk of AKI in patients with septic shock. *Clin J Am Soc Nephrol.* 2014;9(7):1168-74.

[54] Morgan DJ, Ho KM. A comparison of nonoliguric and oliguric severe acute kidney injury according to the risk injury failure loss end-stage (RIFLE) criteria. *Nephron Clin Pract*. 2010;115(1):c59-65.

[55] Chawla LS, Dommu A, Berger A, Shih S, Patel SS. Urinary sediment cast scoring index for acute kidney injury: a pilot study. *Nephron Clin Pract.* 2008;110(3):c145-50.

[56] Miller TR, Anderson RJ, Linas SL, Henrich WL, Berns AS, Gabow PA, et al. Urinary diagnostic indices in acute renal failure: a prospective study. *Ann Intern Med.* 1978;89(1):47-50.

[57] Vaz AJ. Low fractional excretion of urine sodium in acute renal failure due to sepsis. *Arch Intern Med.* 1983;143(4):738-9.

[58] Carvounis CP, Nisar S, Guro-Razuman S. Significance of the fractional excretion of urea in the differential diagnosis of acute renal failure. *Kidney Int.* 2002;62(6):2223-9.

[59] Pepin MN, Bouchard J, Legault L, Ethier J. Diagnostic performance of fractional excretion of urea and fractional excretion of sodium in the evaluations of patients with acute kidney injury with or without diuretic treatment. *Am J Kidney Dis.* 2007;50(4):566-73.

[60] Nejat M, Hill JV, Pickering JW, Edelstein CL, Devarajan P, Endre ZH. Albuminuria increases cystatin C excretion: implications for urinary biomarkers. *Nephrol Dial Transplant.* 2012;27 Suppl 3:iii 96-103.

[61] Liangos O, Perianayagam MC, Vaidya VS, Han WK, Wald R, Tighiouart H, et al. Urinary N-acetyl-beta-(D)-glucosaminidase activity and kidney injury molecule-1 level are associated with adverse outcomes in acute renal failure. *J Am Soc Nephrol.* 2007;18(3):904-12.

[62] Liu Y, Guo W, Zhang J, Xu C, Yu S, Mao Z, et al. Urinary interleukin 18 for detection of acute kidney injury: a meta-analysis. *Am J Kidney Dis.* 2013;62(6):1058-67.

[63] Shang W, Wang Z. The Update of NGAL in Acute Kidney Injury. *Curr Protein Pept Sci.* 2017;18(12):1211-7.

[64] Xu Y, Xie Y, Shao X, Ni Z, Mou S. L-FABP: A novel biomarker of kidney disease. *Clin Chim Acta.* 2015;445:85-90.

[65] Bihorac A, Chawla LS, Shaw AD, Al-Khafaji A, Davison DL, Demuth GE, et al. Validation of cell-cycle arrest biomarkers for acute kidney injury using clinical adjudication. *Am J Respir Crit Care Med.* 2014;189(8):932-9.

[66] Koyner JL, Davison DL, Brasha-Mitchell E, Chalikonda DM, Arthur JM, Shaw AD, et al. Furosemide Stress Test and Biomarkers for the Prediction of AKI Severity. *J Am Soc Nephrol.* 2015;26(8):2023-31.

[67] Chen H, Busse LW. Novel Therapies for Acute Kidney Injury. *Kidney Int Rep.* 2017;2(5):785-99.

[68] Poukkanen M, Wilkman E, Vaara ST, Pettila V, Kaukonen KM, Korhonen AM, et al. Hemodynamic variables and progression of acute kidney injury in critically ill patients with severe sepsis: data from the prospective observational FINNAKI study. *Crit Care.* 2013;17(6):R295.

[69] National Heart L, Blood Institute Acute Respiratory Distress Syndrome Clinical Trials N, Wiedemann HP, Wheeler AP, Bernard GR, Thompson BT, et al. Comparison of two fluid-management strategies in acute lung injury. *N Engl J Med.* 2006;354(24):2564-75.

[70] Payen D, de Pont AC, Sakr Y, Spies C, Reinhart K, Vincent JL, et al. A positive fluid balance is associated with a worse outcome in patients with acute renal failure. *Crit Care.* 2008;12(3):R74.

[71] Semler MW, Self WH, Wanderer JP, Ehrenfeld JM, Wang L, Byrne DW, et al. Balanced Crystalloids versus Saline in Critically Ill Adults. *N Engl J Med.* 2018;378(9):829-39.

[72] Self WH, Semler MW, Wanderer JP, Wang L, Byrne DW, Collins SP, et al. Balanced Crystalloids versus Saline in Noncritically Ill Adults. *N Engl J Med.* 2018;378(9):819-28.

[73] Young P, Bailey M, Beasley R, Henderson S, Mackle D, McArthur C, et al. Effect of a Buffered Crystalloid Solution vs Saline on Acute Kidney Injury Among Patients in the Intensive Care Unit: The SPLIT Randomized Clinical Trial. *JAMA.* 2015;314(16):1701-10.

[74] Yunos NM, Bellomo R, Hegarty C, Story D, Ho L, Bailey M. Association between a chloride-liberal vs chloride-restrictive intravenous fluid administration strategy and kidney injury in critically ill adults. *JAMA.* 2012;308(15):1566-72.

[75] Leaf DE, Waikar SS. IDEAL-ICU in Context. *Clin J Am Soc Nephrol.* 2019;14(8):1264-7.

[76] Tandukar S, Palevsky PM. Continuous Renal Replacement Therapy: Who, When, Why, and How. *Chest.* 2019;155(3):626-38.

[77] Khwaja A. KDIGO clinical practice guidelines for acute kidney injury. *Nephron Clin Pract.* 2012;120(4):c179-84.

[78] Investigators S-A, Canadian Critical Care Trials G, Australian, New Zealand Intensive Care Society Clinical Trials G, United Kingdom Critical Care Research G, Canadian Nephrology Trials N, et al. Timing of Initiation of Renal-Replacement Therapy in Acute Kidney Injury. *N Engl J Med.* 2020;383(3):240-51.

[79] Zarbock A, Kellum JA, Schmidt C, Van Aken H, Wempe C, Pavenstadt H, et al. Effect of Early vs Delayed Initiation of Renal Replacement Therapy on Mortality in Critically Ill Patients With Acute Kidney Injury: The ELAIN Randomized Clinical Trial. *JAMA.* 2016;315(20):2190-9.

[80] Gaudry S, Hajage D, Schortgen F, Martin-Lefevre L, Verney C, Pons B, et al. Timing of Renal Support and Outcome of Septic Shock and Acute Respiratory Distress Syndrome. A Post Hoc Analysis of the AKIKI Randomized Clinical Trial. *Am J Respir Crit Care Med.* 2018;198(1):58-66.

[81] Barbar SD, Clere-Jehl R, Bourredjem A, Hernu R, Montini F, Bruyere R, et al. Timing of Renal-Replacement Therapy in Patients with Acute Kidney Injury and Sepsis. *N Engl J Med.* 2018;379(15):1431-42.

[82] Alge JL, Karakala N, Neely BA, Janech MG, Tumlin JA, Chawla LS, et al. Association of elevated urinary concentration of renin-angiotensin system components and severe AKI. *Clin J Am Soc Nephrol.* 2013;8(12):2043-52.

[83] Bellomo R, Wunderink RG, Szerlip H, English SW, Busse LW, Deane AM, et al. Angiotensin I and angiotensin II concentrations and their ratio in catecholamine-resistant vasodilatory shock. *Crit Care.* 2020;24(1):43.

[84] Khanna A, English SW, Wang XS, Ham K, Tumlin J, Szerlip H, et al. Angiotensin II for the Treatment of Vasodilatory Shock. *N Engl J Med.* 2017;377(5):419-30.

[85] Tumlin JA, Murugan R, Deane AM, Ostermann M, Busse LW, Ham KR, et al. Outcomes in Patients with Vasodilatory Shock and Renal Replacement Therapy Treated with Intravenous Angiotensin II. *Crit Care Med.* 2018;46(6):949-57.

[86] Venkatesh B, Finfer S, Cohen J, Rajbhandari D, Arabi Y, Bellomo R, et al. Adjunctive Glucocorticoid Therapy in Patients with Septic Shock. *N Engl J Med.* 2018;378(9):797-808.

[87] Jacob KA, Leaf DE, Dieleman JM, van Dijk D, Nierich AP, Rosseel PM, et al. Intraoperative High-Dose Dexamethasone and Severe AKI after Cardiac Surgery. *J Am Soc Nephrol.* 2015;26(12):2947-51.

[88] Parikh CR, Schaub JA. Acute kidney injury: Steroids for prevention of AKI after cardiopulmonary bypass. *Nat Rev Nephrol.* 2015;11(9):509-10.

[89] Whitlock RP, Devereaux PJ, Teoh KH, Lamy A, Vincent J, Pogue J, et al. Methylprednisolone in patients undergoing cardiopulmonary bypass (SIRS): a randomised, double-blind, placebo-controlled trial. *Lancet.* 2015;386(10000):1243-53.

[90] Vallon V, Muhlbauer B, Osswald H. Adenosine and kidney function. *Physiol Rev.* 2006;86(3):901-40.

[91] Voors AA, Dittrich HC, Massie BM, DeLucca P, Mansoor GA, Metra M, et al. Effects of the adenosine A1 receptor antagonist rolofylline on renal function in patients with acute heart failure and renal dysfunction: results from PROTECT (Placebo-Controlled Randomized Study of the Selective Adenosine A1 Receptor Antagonist Rolofylline for Patients Hospitalized with Acute Decompensated Heart Failure and Volume Overload to Assess Treatment Effect on Congestion and Renal Function). *J Am Coll Cardiol.* 2011;57(19):1899-907.

[92] Iskander C, Cherney DZ, Clemens KK, Dixon SN, Harel Z, Jeyakumar N, et al. Use of sodium-glucose cotransporter-2 inhibitors and risk of acute kidney injury in older adults with diabetes: a population-based cohort study. *CMAJ.* 2020;192(14):E351-E60.

[93] Nadkarni GN, Ferrandino R, Chang A, Surapaneni A, Chauhan K, Poojary P, et al. Acute Kidney Injury in Patients on SGLT2 Inhibitors: A Propensity-Matched Analysis. *Diabetes Care.* 2017;40(11):1479-85.

[94] Clark EG, Hiremath S, McIntyre L, Wald R, Hundemer GL, Joannidis M. Haemoperfusion should only be used for COVID-19 in the context of randomized trials. *Nat Rev Nephrol.* 2020;16(12):697-9.

[95] Schadler D, Pausch C, Heise D, Meier-Hellmann A, Brederlau J, Weiler N, et al. The effect of a novel extracorporeal cytokine hemoadsorption device on IL-6 elimination in septic patients: A randomized controlled trial. *PLoS One.* 2017;12(10):e0187015.

[96] Togel F, Weiss K, Yang Y, Hu Z, Zhang P, Westenfelder C. Vasculotropic, paracrine actions of infused mesenchymal stem cells are important to the recovery from acute kidney injury. *Am J Physiol Renal Physiol.* 2007;292(5):F1626-35.

[97] Monsel A, Zhu YG, Gennai S, Hao Q, Liu J, Lee JW. Cell-based therapy for acute organ injury: preclinical evidence and ongoing clinical trials using mesenchymal stem cells. *Anesthesiology.* 2014;121(5):1099-121.

[98] Swaminathan M, Stafford-Smith M, Chertow GM, Warnock DG, Paragamian V, Brenner RM, et al. Allogeneic Mesenchymal Stem Cells for Treatment of AKI after Cardiac Surgery. *J Am Soc Nephrol.* 2018;29(1):260-7.

[99] Kashani K, Al-Khafaji A, Ardiles T, Artigas A, Bagshaw SM, Bell M, et al. Discovery and validation of cell cycle arrest biomarkers in human acute kidney injury. *Crit Care.* 2013;17(1):R25.

[100] Varghese SA, Powell TB, Janech MG, Budisavljevic MN, Stanislaus RC, Almeida JS, et al. Identification of diagnostic urinary biomarkers for acute kidney injury. *J Investig Med.* 2010;58(4):612-20.

[101] Wang WG, Sun WX, Gao BS, Lian X, Zhou HL. Cell Cycle Arrest as a Therapeutic Target of Acute Kidney Injury. *Curr Protein Pept Sci.* 2017;18(12):1224-31.

[102] Zhang D, Liu Y, Wei Q, Huo Y, Liu K, Liu F, et al. Tubular p53 regulates multiple genes to mediate AKI. *J Am Soc Nephrol.* 2014;25(10):2278-89.

[103] Demirjian S, Ailawadi G, Polinsky M, Bitran D, Silberman S, Shernan SK, et al. Safety and Tolerability Study of an Intravenously Administered Small Interfering Ribonucleic Acid (siRNA) Post On-Pump Cardiothoracic Surgery in Patients at Risk of Acute Kidney Injury. *Kidney Int Rep*. 2017;2(5):836-43.

[104] Meersch M, Schmidt C, Hoffmeier A, Van Aken H, Wempe C, Gerss J, et al. Prevention of cardiac surgery-associated AKI by implementing the KDIGO guidelines in high risk patients identified by biomarkers: the PrevAKI randomized controlled trial. *Intensive Care Med*. 2017;43(11):1551-61.

In: Issues in Kidney Disease – Acute Kidney Injury
Editors: S. Z. Fadem and A. Arslan Yousuf Awan
ISBN: 978-1-68507-002-1

Chapter 8

ACUTE INTERSTITIAL NEPHRITIS

George M. Dolson**, MD
Selzman Institute for Kidney Health, Section of Nephrology, Department of Medicine, Baylor College of Medicine, Houston, TX, USA

ABSTRACT

Acute interstitial nephritis (AIN) refers to renal damage due to inflammation of the renal interstitial space, and can result from adverse medication reactions, infectious agents, chemical toxins, ionizing radiation, or immunological processes. Prescription and over the counter medications are the most common etiology for AIN. Frequently, cases of AIN may be labeled acute tubular necrosis or just acute kidney injury (AKI) without identifying the presence of AIN. Diagnosis of AIN requires high index of suspicion, and a careful medical history and review of systems for possible systemic immunological diseases or medications associated with AIN. Early diagnosis and treatment are essential to prevent renal damage and ultimately renal failure. This chapter will review the anatomy and physiology of the renal interstitium, many of the etiologies that cause AIN, and briefly review the various therapies available for treatment.

Keywords: interstitial nephritis, acute interstitial nephritis, tubulointerstitial nephritis, analgesic nephropathy

INTRODUCTION

Acute kidney injury (AKI) results from damage to any region of the kidney. Acute interstitial nephritis (AIN) refers to renal damage due to inflammation of the renal interstitial space and can be due to hypersensitivity reactions to common medications, chemical toxins, ionizing radiation, or immunological processes. AIN was anatomically described in 1898 by the pathologist William Councilman who noted cellular infiltrates in the interstitial renal spaces

* Corresponding Author's E-mail: gdolson@bcm.edu.

in patients with kidney damage associated with "scarlatina" [1]. Advancements in Pathology and Laboratory medicine through the twentieth century led to increased recognition of AIN [2]. However, the incidence of AIN is likely underreported because definitive diagnosis requires a kidney biopsy which generally is not performed [3]. A review of 259 kidney biopsies performed between 1991 and 1998 in patients over age 60 with acute kidney failure revealed 40.3% of the patients had AIN [4]. These data indicate that many cases of AIN may be labeled acute tubular necrosis (ATN), or just AKI without identifying the presence of AIN. This chapter reviews the anatomy and physiology of the renal interstitium, clinical presentation of AIN in general, and the course of AIN due to various etiologies.

Anatomy, Physiology and Clinical Significance of the Renal Interstitium

The clinical presentation of AIN results from the renal interstitial changes that occur with inflammation. The renal interstitium comprises the extravascular intertubular space which contains cellular elements and extracellular substances. Cells normally found in the renal interstitium include fibroblasts, lipid laden cells, perivascular cells, and "non-resident cells" such as macrophages. Noncellular components of the interstitium include fibrillary structures, proteoglycans, glycoproteins, and fluid. Tubule and vasculature basement membranes border the interstitium vasculature, and lymphatics course through this space [5]. Interstitial volume and the contents of the space varies from cortex to the medulla and is greater in the medulla [6]. The anatomic relationships among tubules, vasculature, and the lymphatic matrix enable water and solute transport by the kidneys [7]. On a normal renal biopsy, the renal interstitial space appears small, as the tubules, glomeruli, and vessels are tightly nested together. The capillaries and lymphatic channels that traverse the interstitial space are immersed in filtrate from tubules. Solute and water collect in the interstitium and move between tubules and the capillaries. Differential permeability between tubule basement membranes and the capillaries facilitates medullary concentration gradients [8]. The establishment of the hypertonic medulla provides the osmotic gradient for water absorption and allows the concentration of the final urine to be varied over a wide range under the influence of antidiuretic hormone. Alterations in the interstitial anatomy and types of cells has been hypothesized as a cause of essential hypertension [9].

The interstitial space contains dendritic cells, macrophages, lymphocytes, and lymphatic endothelial cells [10]. The dendritic cells, in conjunction with macrophages and lymphocytes, facilitate adaptive (acquired) immunity [11]. Dendritic cells in the renal interstitium, continuously bathed in fluids, survey their microenvironment for markers of inflammation or infection. The ability of dendritic cells to migrate throughout the body, and their localization within peripheral organs such as the kidneys, are crucial for adaptive immunity and tolerance. Renal dendritic cells can capture small molecular weight antigens from within the tubule lumen, giving these interstitial cells the ability to monitor and react to systemic inflammatory processes [12]. Therefore, dendritic cells can exhibit a robust inflammatory response to local and systemic infectious agents and other inflammatory processes within the renal interstitium.

Renal fibroblasts are spindle-shaped, flattened cells, which form a continuous network within the renal cortex and medulla [10]. Fibroblasts, normally quiescent, can transform into a more active state which synthesizes erythropoietin (EPO), a hormone which regulates erythropoiesis by the bone marrow. These EPO-synthesizing cells, primarily located in the renal cortex, sense oxygen tension in the renal interstitium. EPO generated in the renal interstitium is the central regulator of red blood cell (RBC) production by the bone marrow. Given the kidneys' high blood flow rate, the interstitial oxygen levels will closely resemble those of the blood, making the renal interstitium an ideal location for monitoring oxygenation. In contrast, chronic renal damage by interstitial fibrosis decreases EPO synthesis and results in the anemia of chronic renal disease.

Besides EPO, synthetic renal interstitial fibroblasts are involved in regulation of renal hemodynamics through generation of adenosine [13]. In the kidney, adenosine vasodilates post glomerular efferent arteriole and vasoconstricts the pre-glomerular afferent arteriole, lowering the glomerular filtration rate (GFR). Further, adenosine inhibits renin release in juxtaglomerular cells. Thus, adenosine will lower sodium chloride (NaCl) concentration of tubular fluid if it is too high, providing an important control of the tubular glomerular feedback system [10]. With chronic renal disease and interstitial fibrosis, EPO synthesis is decreased, and the tubular glomerular feedback system becomes inoperative. Patients subsequently develop anemia and a chronically low GFR.

In conclusion, the brief anatomy and physiology review described previously illustrates the role of the renal interstitium in regulating renal function, as well as systemic regulation of vascular volume, blood pressure, and hemoglobin levels. Thus, acute interstitial nephritis not only affects the kidneys but the entire body, as well.

General Clinical Presentation of Acute Interstitial Nephritis

Patients with AIN may not have chief complaints related to their kidneys. Rather they will present because of non-specific complains such as lethargy, fever, or nonspecific aches and pains [14]. Diagnosis of AIN requires high index of suspicion, as well as a careful medical history and review of systems for possible systemic immunological diseases or medications associated with AIN.

Table 1 summarizes common clinical findings and lab studies often used for the diagnosis of AIN [3]. These patients all had AIN and acute renal failure. Forty percent required dialysis. A minority of patients presented with the classic AIN triad of fever, rash, and eosinophilia. Nephrotic range proteinuria was rare, so this finding should steer the clinician toward evaluation of glomerulonephritis. Table 2 illustrate the difficulty clinicians face when evaluating a patient for AIN. For example, at least one of the findings in Table 2 could be found in most patients with AIN, but all the findings are relatively nonspecific, and a definitive diagnosis cannot be made from the findings listed in this table.

Thus, the definitive diagnosis of AIN requires a renal biopsy. However, the procedure is invasive, carries the risk of serious complications, and is expensive. A review of all biopsies performed over a 7-year period at a major metropolitan medical center found that approximately 73% of 1,065 renal biopsies were performed as part of evaluation for nephrotic syndrome, acute renal insufficiency, or progressive renal failure [4]. The subset of patients with acute kidney insufficiency who underwent biopsy is summarized in Table 3.

Table 1. Clinical and laboratory features of patients at presentation with AIN (100% with acute kidney injury)

Non-nephrotic proteinuria	93%
Leukocyturia	82%
Microhematuria	67%
Arthralgias	45%
Fever	36%
Eosinophilia	35%
Skin rash	22%
Gross hematuria	5%
Nephrotic range proteinuria	2%

Adapted from M. Praga [3]

Table 2. Chemistry, urinalysis findings AIN

Urinary eosinophils	Usually negative, not specific for AIN
Sterile pyuria	Common in AIN but not specific
Urinary WBC casts	Usually negative, and if present not specific for AIN
Hematuria	Not common in AIN
Proteinuria	Non nephrotic range in AIN, but not specific
Elevated serum creatinine	Commonly seen in all forms renal disease, but nonspecific for AIN
Hyperkalemia	Seen in AIN and acute kidney injury, therefore non-specific
Systemic leukocytosis	Sepsis, possibly pyelonephritis which is class of AIN

Adapted from Martinez-Valenzuela et al. [15]

Table 3. Findings from 1,065 renal biopsies primarily performed for evaluation of nephrotic syndrome

Renal Biopsies in Cases of Acute Renal Insufficeincy	
Glomerular diseases	45.80%
Tubulointerstitial disease, not AIN	21.70%
AIN	18.60%
Vascular diseases	12.30%
Multiple lesions without single diagnosis	1.60%

Adapted from Haas et al. [4].

Since the common causes of AIN, as reviewed below, improve when offending agent is discontinued, renal biopsy is reserved for those patients who do not improve with a therapeutic intervention, or when immunotherapy is contemplated. Renal biopsy often identifies eosinophilic infiltration of the interstitium in AIN, but such patients rarely are found to have elevated eosinophil counts systemically or in the urine. Renal ultrasound studies are widely available and frequently performed on patients with renal abnormalities. The ultrasound hallmarks of AIN, inflammation, cellular infiltration, and widening of the interstitial space are subtle and require significant physician expertise to correctly describe changes in the interstitium. The use of renal ultrasound and CT scanning when evaluating patients with acute flank pain can be useful for detecting urinary obstruction, stones, hemorrhage, and masses but provides limited information regarding AIN [16, 17].

Renal biopsy will provide a definitive diagnosis of AIN. However, the procedure is invasive, carries the risk of serious complications, and is expensive. A review of all biopsies performed over a seven-year period at a major metropolitan medical center is shown in Table 3. These biopsies were performed as part of evaluation for nephrotic syndrome, acute renal insufficiency, or progressive renal failure [4].

AIN was found in only 18.6%. Since the common causes of AIN, as reviewed below, improve when offending agent is discontinued, renal biopsy is reserved for those patients who do not improve with a therapeutic intervention, or when immunotherapy is contemplated.

In summary, a good history, physical, and complete review of systems with high suspicion for AIN is the most practical method for making the diagnosis of AIN. Consideration of the timing of kidney exposure to drugs or compounds known to cause AIN and evaluation of laboratory data will allow the clinician to tentatively identify the etiology of the offending agent.

Etiologies and Treatment of AIN

Medications

Medications account for 71% of AIN cases [18]. Of the offending medications, antibiotics, and proton pump inhibitors account for 70%. Thus, the discussion of AIN etiology and treatment will start with those medications. Table 4 summarizes the groups of medications that are known to cause AIN. Vancomycin and other aminoglycoside antibiotics, and amphotericin B are not in the list because they commonly cause acute tubular damage rather than AIN.

Antibiotics

Antibiotics are the most common medications associated with AIN, in part because they are so commonly used in modern medicine.

Methicillin, the prototypical beta lactam antibiotic, is filtered at the glomerulus, transported into tubules, and secreted in the urine. During renal excretion of these beta lactam antibiotics, they reach high concentrations the renal interstitium where antibiotic-albumin conjugates are formed and stimulate the patients' lymphocytes and T cell clones. The subsequent immunological reaction sets off an inflammatory process in the interstitial space, causing renal damage [19].

Fluoroquinolone antibiotics (such as ciprofloxacin) are widely used and associated with a twofold increased risk of acute kidney injury. Ciprofloxacin has the highest incidence of AKI in this class of meds (but has been used the longest) and is one of the most widely used medications worldwide. The estimated risk of AKI for ciprofloxacin is 2.76 (95% confidence ratio), followed by moxifloxacin and levofloxacin.

Table 4. Asterisk indicates most common causes of AIN. Medications are discussed in text that follows

Medications Associated with AIN	
Antibiotics	Methicillin and β-lactam antibiotics*, fluoroquinolones*, TB Medications (rifampin ethambutol) *, sulfur-based medicines*, minocycline, erythromycin
Analgesics	non-steroidal anti-inflammatory drugs* (eg, diclofenac), selective COX-2 inhibitors (eg, celecoxib)
Gastrointestinal medicines	proton pump inhibitors* (e.g., omeprazole), h2-receptor antagonists (e.g., ranitidine)
Antiviral medicines	acyclovir, abacavir, indinavir, atazanavir (Note: these medications cause crystalluria and might secondarily lead to AIN)
Antiepileptic medicines	phenytoin*, phenobarbital, carbamazepine
Other medicines	allopurinol*, 5-aminosalicylates* (eg, mesalamine, sulfasalazine), anti-angiogenesis medicines (tyrosine kinase inhibitors [e.g., sunitinib]),), immune checkpoint inhibitors (ipilimumab, others)

Adapted from "Keeping it Renal: Drug-Induced Acute Interstitial Nephritis (medsafe.govt.nz)".

This class of antibiotics are thought to induce acute interstitial nephritis by an acute hypersensitivity reaction. Alternatively, some cause granulomatous interstitial nephritis and/or crystal deposits [20]. Volume depletion and concurrent use of renin–angiotensin-system blockers might increase the risk of acute kidney injury, presumably due to artificial intelligence (AI), widely used to promote medical development; i.e., early detection, disease diagnosis, and management.

Rifampin treatment of tuberculosis has been associated with renal failure after 21 to 71 days of therapy. Renal biopsies revealed interstitial infiltrates, which improved when the medication was stopped. The pathology findings and improvement when medication was stopped is compatible with an immunologically mediated AIN [21].

Ethambutol induced renal failure is very rare. One case report submitted as a letter to the editor noted acute kidney failure in a patient with active pulmonary tuberculosis who recovered when the medication was withdrawn. AIN was noted on biopsy. In conclusion, both drugs are widely used and do not appear to cause significant renal failure.

Erythromycin and other Macrolides do not cause direct nephrotoxicity in general but can influence kidney function secondary to interactions with other drugs. The macrolide class of medications are strong inhibitors of CYP3A4 enzymes which metabolize medications and other compounds. CYP3A inhibition thus leads to accumulation of drugs, potentially causing toxicity. For example, in renal transplant patients, erythromycin will decrease clearance of cyclosporin, possibly causing cyclosporine to rise to renal toxic levels [22].

Sulphur-based medications include the sulfa antibiotics (sulfamethoxazole), thiazide, and loop diuretics such as furosemide, and COX 2 inhibitors. These meds have benzene rings and substitution of the ring by different moieties results in nitroso-SMX which can act as a hapten, triggering a T-cell reaction. These reactions, occurring in the renal interstitium, result in an inflammatory state causing infiltration by immune cells, and fibrocyte formation. If the immune reaction is prolonged, renal fibrosis with chronic kidney disease may develop [23]. A case report and review indicate that AIN due to sulfa drugs can resolve if medication is stopped early in the course [24]. As an aside, the hyperkalemia sometimes noted with high dosages of sulfamethoxazole-trimethoprim is due to the inhibitory effects of trimethoprim on sodium-potassium (Na/K) exchange in the principal cell located in the collecting duct, and not a result of AIN.

Minocycline was found to cause acute kidney failure shortly after administration of regular doses of the drug. Allergic symptoms plus a raised level of serum IgE or eosinophilia were observed. Renal biopsies revealed tubulitis with interstitial edema as the common characteristic findings [25]. The allergic symptoms, IgE levels, and eosinophilia point to an immune reaction. But tissue studies found tubulitis with interstitial edema. Thus, it is difficult to determine if the medication-induced kidney disease resulted from AIN or direct tubule damage causing acute tubular necrosis (ATN).

Analgesics (See Table 4)

Non-steroidal anti-inflammatory drugs (NSAIDS) block either or both COX-1 and COX-2 throughout the body. The selective COX-2 inhibitors block the mediators of inflammation in selective cells, and in the kidneys. The nonselective COX-1 and COX-2 blockers modify the effects of prostaglandins in all organs, especially the vascular, cardiovascular, GI, and renal systems. NSAIDs thus can have widespread effects on blood pressure (worsen hypertension), renal functions (GFR regulation), sodium, potassium, water balance, acid base balance, platelet function, and even reproductive functions in both men and women [26].

NSAIDs are among the most widely prescribed medications in the world today [27]. It is estimated that greater than 111 million prescriptions and 30 billion over-the-counter doses are administered in the United States each year. Perhaps 2.5 million Americans suffered NSAID-mediated renal damage. Risk factors that predispose patients to NSAID-induced renal functional changes include age >65 years, history of CV disease, diabetes, and GFR < 60 ml/minute [28]. A study looking at US patients with chronic kidney disease found that 5% took NSAIDs every day, and 66% of these patients had been taking it daily for at least a year. Given the widespread use of these medications, physicians should routinely question patients about NSAID use, especially if the patient is hypertensive and has abnormal kidney function or hyperkalemia. Acute changes in kidney function may resolve quickly if a patient's NSAID use is identified, and the medication stopped. The longer a patient has been using NSAIDS, the less likely a full recovery will occur. Corticosteroids are less likely to be efficacious if renal function remains abnormal after NSAIDS are stopped [29].

Gastrointestinal Medicines

Proton pump inhibitors (PPIs) are widely used and are a major cause of AIN. All the PPI can cause AIN, although omeprazole was the most common, possibly because it was the most widely used when the survey was performed [30]. Onset of AIN can occur within hours or months of taking the medications. The dosage of PPI does not seem to affect the onset of AIN or recovery. If a patient has an allergic reaction to one PPI, then he or she will likely have reactions to all the medications in this class [23].

Antiviral Medicines

The antiviral medications acyclovir, abacavir, indinavir, and atazanavir may precipitate drug crystals in the collecting duct of the kidney causing obstructive renal failure. The likelihood of crystal deposition depends on the patient's hydration status, the dose of medication, and the patient's renal function. These medications are more soluble in acid solutions with pH < 3.5 and they tend to precipitate at more alkaline urine pH levels [20]. Interstitial renal changes may be seen and may be due to an inflammatory process triggered by the abundance of medication crystal [31].

Antiepileptic Medicines

Allopurinol-induced **d**rug **r**eaction with **e**osinophilia and **s**ystemic **s**ymptoms (DRESS) is a rare hypersensitivity reaction with severe skin eruptions, exfoliative dermatitis, fever, eosinophilia, and lung-liver-kidney involvement. Severe AIN develops in as many as 30% of patients with DRESS. Patients improve if drug withdrawal is rapid, and corticosteroids are given. Recurrence may occur as corticosteroids are withdrawn [32].

Other Medicines

5-Aminosalicylates (e.g., mesalazine) are commonly used in the treatment of inflammatory bowel disease. Incidence of AIN is estimated at 1 in 200-500 patients who take these medications, with 19% of affected patients developing renal failure. Interestingly, AIN has been reported in patients with inflammatory bowel disease who have never taken the 5-Aminosalicylate medications. It is possible that AIN may be expressed as part of the inflammatory bowel disease (IBD) syndrome [33].

Check Point inhibitors are monoclonal antibodies that target specific receptors on both T-cells and tumor cells. These compounds prevent the T cells from recognizing the tumor as "self", initiating an immunological cascade that results in the destruction of the target cell. These immune reactions are complicated by several rare reactions in different organs, including the kidneys. Patients may develop acute renal failure due to acute tubulointerstitial nephritis. Treatment consists of discontinuing the medication and giving steroids [34, 35].

AIN due to Systemic Immunological Disease

Lupus Nephritis

Kidney involvement is common and is usually diagnosed when findings of glomerulonephritis are discovered. The renal disease is often initiated by the deposition of immune complexes (anti-nuclear, anti C1q, antiglomerular antibodies, others) in glomeruli.

Other histological findings include lupus podocytopathy, thrombotic microangiopathy, and acute AIN with tubule involvement [36]. Over the past 50 years, the diagnosis of Lupus (also called SLE, systemic lupus erythematosus) is being made earlier, which improves prognosis and treatment outcome. This has changed the epidemiology of the renal disease, as patients may now receive treatment before extensive renal damage has occurred [37]. As lupus progresses, direct renal immunological damage increases, and secondary systemic diseases, such as hypertension and vasculitis, impact the kidneys. Improvements in lupus therapy during past half century have resulted in earlier treatment and fewer steroid and cytotoxic agent complications. Overall earlier diagnosis and treatment, and refinement in long-term therapy have resulted in an improved prognosis for these patients.

Sjogren Syndrome

Sjogren's syndrome is an autoimmune disease characterized by inflammation and destruction of exocrine glands. Patients with an "overlap" syndrome will also have other glands and organs involved, including the kidneys. If the kidneys are affected, the lesion is often AIN [38]. The AIN may be asymptomatic or exhibit renal functional changes, including proximal and distal rental tubular acidosis. With time, untreated chronic acidemia results in osteoporosis, hypercalciuria and hypokalemia, and calcium deposition in the kidneys. In advanced disease, interstitial fibrosis and tubular atrophy leads to chronic renal failure. Treatment with glucocorticoids and immunosuppressive agents is recommended, but in advanced cases patients may not show improvement.

Systemic Sclerosis (Scleroderma)

Systemic sclerosis is an immune-mediated rheumatic disease characterized by fibrosis of skin, blood vessels, visceral organs, and the kidneys [36]. Renal disease results from progressive sclerosis of the renal vessels with inflammatory changes in the interstitium. Urine findings may include proteinuria, hematuria, and urinary casts indicating damage to the tubules and glomerulus. Vascular sclerosis of renal vessels progressively damages the interstitium, and leads to hypertension, which in turn accelerates progressing of renal failure. Treatment of systemic sclerosis focuses on control of hypertension and damage to vasculature. Blood pressure control is difficult in these patients, and multi-drug strategies are required. Not only are patients severely hypertensive, but they may also have cardiovascular, neurovascular, and renal vascular damage. Malignant hypertension during scleroderma crisis is a medical emergency and must be treated aggressively [39].

Wasp Stings

Acute Kidney Injury (AKI) from wasp sting venom is a rare complication reported mostly from Asia [40]. Generally, stings cause a painful local reaction that resolves spontaneously.

Repeat stings in a previously sensitized host, or multiple envenomation by swarms of wasps has resulted in AKI in 21% of patients with severe reactions who required hospitalization.

Venom-induced systemic reactions included anaphylaxis, rhabdomyolysis, and hemolysis with disseminated intravascular coagulation, hepatic damage, respiratory distress, and cardiovascular collapse. Patients with the most severe reactions required renal replacement therapy and suffered a mortality as high as 50%. Reported renal effects of the stings included nephrotic syndrome, proximal renal tubular acidosis, and acute kidney failure. Renal biopsies showed acute tubular injury and AIN [41]. In severe cases, therapy consisted of hospitalization, respiratory, and cardiovascular support, including corticosteroid therapy, and occasionally renal replacement therapy. Use of continuous veno-venous hemofiltration (CVVH) or continuous veno-venous hemodialysis (CVVHD) may improve outcomes, possibly due to the ability of these dialysis modalities to remove larger molecules from the circulation [42].

IgG4 Related Tubulointerstitial Nephritis

IgG4 immunoglobulin disease is a fibroinflammatory disorder that is now known to affect any organ [43]. The main histologic feature of the disease is a multiorgan lymphoplasmacytic tissue infiltrate rich in IgG4 positive plasma cells. Observed kidney lesions include membranous glomerulonephritis and AIN with tubule damage.

Hypocomplementemia, C3 and C4 has been observed [44]. Once diagnosis is made, most patients receive steroid treatment for two to 4 weeks with gradual tapering of dosage. Rituximab has been used in steroid sparing protocols or as adjuvant therapy in patients with refractory disease. Steroid and or immunosuppressant therapy results in improvement, but usually not normalization of renal function.

Tubulointerstitial Nephritis and Uveitis (TINU) Syndrome

TINU is an idiopathic immune- mediated process, which typically presents with uveitis. Etiology is unclear but likely involves a variety of the HLA antigens [45]. TINU appears to be an idiopathic immune-mediated process, but there are reports of prior respiratory infections, as well as Tuberculosis, Toxoplasma, and Varicella.

Pathogenesis of this disease is unknown but is suspected to be initiated in a susceptible individual by an environmental factor. Both T and B cell immune systems are thought to be involved in the disease process. Ocular disease may develop before or up to 14 months after TIN onset. Steroid therapy is the mainstay of treatment, but the optimum length of treatment is unclear.

Clinical Pearls

- The renal interstitium is a dynamic region of the kidney, continuously exposed to the circulating body fluids, and has a central role in maintaining the internal milieu.
- Diseases of the renal interstitium may initially present with a combination of alterations in blood pressure, changes in fluid and electrolyte balance, systemic hematologic changes, and nonspecific alterations in the urinalysis. Renal failure may not be an initial finding.
- The most common etiology for AIN involves a reaction to medications.
- AIN patients may initially present with few symptoms or abnormal values.. Diagnosis requires a high degree of suspicion and a thorough history and physical (H&P), including a history of prescribed and over-the-counter medication use.
- General approach to therapy of medication-induced AIN.
  1. When AIN is diagnosed by clinical criteria, stop the offending medications. This may cure the problem.
  2. If kidney abnormalities do not resolve within 1 to 2 weeks, give a short oral course of corticosteroids.
  3. If corticosteroids have minimal or no effect, consider a renal biopsy to determine the renal abnormality.
  4. Once a renal biopsy diagnosis is made, initiate specific treatment.

REFERENCES

[1] Eknoyan G. The early modern kidney--nephrology in and about the nineteenth century. Part 1. *Semin Dial.* 2013; 26: 73–84.

[2] Raghavan R, Eknoyan G. Acute interstitial nephritis - a reappraisal and update. *Clin Nephrol.* 2014; 82: 149–62.

[3] Praga M, González E. Acute interstitial nephritis. *Kidney Int.* 2010; 77: 956–61.

[4] Haas M, Spargo BH, Wit EJ, Meehan SM. Etiologies and outcome of acute renal insufficiency in older adults: a renal biopsy study of 259 cases. *Am J Kidney Dis.* 2000; 35: 433–47.

[5] Lemley KV, Kriz W. Anatomy of the renal interstitium. *Kidney Int.*1991; 39: 370–81.

[6] Knepper MA, Danielson RA, Saidel GM, Post RS. Quantitative analysis of renal medullary anatomy in rats and rabbits. *Kidney Int.*1977; 12: 313–23.

[7] Williams JC Jr, Schafer JA. Cortical interstitium as a site for solute polarization during tubular absorption. *Am J Physiol.* 1988; 254: F813–23.

[8] Aukland K, Bogusky RT, Renkin EM. Renal cortical interstitium and fluid absorption by peritubular capillaries. *Am J Physiol.* 1994; 266: F175–84.

[9] Sadowski J, Bądzyńska B. Altered renal medullary blood flow: A key factor or a parallel event in control of sodium excretion and blood pressure? *Clin Exp Pharmacol Physiol.* 2020; 47: 1323–32.

[10] Zeisberg M, Kalluri R. Physiology of the Renal Interstitium. *Clin J Am Soc Nephrol.* 2015; 10: 1831–40.

[11] Kurts C, Ginhoux F, Panzer U. Kidney dendritic cells: fundamental biology and functional roles in health and disease. *Nat Rev Nephrol.* 2020; 16: 391–407.

[12] Lukacs-Kornek V, Burgdorf S, Diehl L, Specht S, Kornek M, Kurts C. The kidney-renal lymph node-system contributes to cross-tolerance against innocuous circulating antigen. *J Immunol*. 2008; 180: 706–15.

[13] Nishiyama A, Rahman M, Inscho EW. Role of interstitial ATP and adenosine in the regulation of renal hemodynamics and microvascular function. *Hypertens Res*. 2004; 27: 791–804.

[14] Caravaca-Fontán F, Fernández-Juárez G, Praga M. Acute kidney injury in interstitial nephritis. *Curr Opin Crit Care.* 2019; 25: 558–64.

[15] Martinez Valenzuela L, Draibe J, Fulladosa X, Torras J. New Biomarkers in Acute Tubulointerstitial Nephritis: A Novel Approach to a Classic Condition. *Int J Mol Sci.* 2020; 21: E4690.

[16] Goel RH, Unnikrishnan R, Remer EM. Acute Urinary Tract Disorders. *Radiol Clin North Am*. 2015; 53: 1273–92.

[17] Hammond NA, Nikolaidis P, Miller FH. Infectious and inflammatory diseases of the kidney. *Radiol Clin North Am*. 2012; 50: 259–70, vi. (vi.).

[18] Eddy AA. Drug-induced tubulointerstitial nephritis: hypersensitivity and necroinflammatory pathways. *Pediatr Nephrol*. 2020; 35: 547–54.

[19] Whitaker P, Naisbitt D, Peckham D. Nonimmediate β-lactam reactions in patients with cystic fibrosis. *Curr Opin Allergy Clin Immunol*. 2012; 12: 369–75.

[20] Morales-Alvarez MC. Nephrotoxicity of Antimicrobials and Antibiotics. *Adv Chronic Kidney Dis.* 2020; 27: 31–37.

[21] Neugarten J, Gallo GR, Baldwin DS. Rifampin-induced nephrotic syndrome and acute interstitial nephritis. *Am J Nephrol*. 1983; 3: 38–42.

[22] Ma TK, Chow KM, Choy AS, Kwan BC, Szeto CC, Li PK. Clinical manifestation of macrolide antibiotic toxicity in CKD and dialysis patients. *Clin Kidney J.* 2014; 7: 507–12.

[23] Raghavan R, Shawar S. Mechanisms of Drug-Induced Interstitial Nephritis. *Adv Chronic Kidney Dis.* 2017; 24: 64–71.

[24] Moledina DG, Perazella MA. Drug-Induced Acute Interstitial Nephritis. *Clin J Am Soc Nephrol.* 2017; 12: 2046–49.

[25] Joh K, Aizawa S, Yamaguchi Y, et al. Drug-induced hypersensitivity nephritis: lymphocyte stimulation testing and renal biopsy in 10 cases. *Am J Nephrol*. 1990; 10: 222–30.

[26] Rahman S, Malcoun A. Nonsteroidal antiinflammatory drugs, cyclooxygenase-2, and the kidneys. *Prim Care*. 2014; 41: 803–21.

[27] Harris RC. An update on cyclooxygenase-2 expression and metabolites in the kidney. *Curr Opin Nephrol Hypertens*. 2008; 17: 64–69.

[28] Plantinga L, Grubbs V, Sarkar U, et al. Nonsteroidal anti-inflammatory drug use among persons with chronic kidney disease in the United States. *Ann Fam Med.* 2011; 9: 423–30.

[29] Clarkson MR, Giblin L, O'Connell FP, et al. Acute interstitial nephritis: clinical features and response to corticosteroid therapy. *Nephrol Dial Transplant*. 2004; 19: 2778–83.

[30] Brewster UC, Perazella MA. Acute kidney injury following proton pump inhibitor therapy. *Kidney Int.* 2007; 71: 589–93.

[31] Mizokami F, Mizuno T. Acute kidney injury induced by antimicrobial agents in the elderly: awareness and mitigation strategies. *Drugs Aging*. 2015; 32: 1–12.

[32] Praga M, Sevillano A, Auñón P, González E. Changes in the aetiology, clinical presentation and management of acute interstitial nephritis, an increasingly common cause of acute kidney injury. *Nephrol Dial Transplant.* 2015; 30: 1472–79.

[33] Izzedine H, Simon J, Piette AM, et al. Primary chronic interstitial nephritis in Crohn's disease. *Gastroenterology*. 2002; 123: 1436–40.

[34] Santos MLC, de Brito BB, da Silva FAF, Botelho ACDS, de Melo FF. Nephrotoxicity in cancer treatment: An overview. *World J Clin Oncol*. 2020; 11: 190–204.

[35] Shingarev R, Glezerman IG. Kidney Complications of Immune Checkpoint Inhibitors: A Review. *Am J Kidney Dis*. 2019; 74: 529–37.

[36] Ponticelli C, Doria A, Moroni G. Renal disorders in rheumatologic diseases: the spectrum is changing (Part 1: connective tissue diseases). *J Nephrol*. 2020. https://doi.org/10.1007/s40620-020-00772-7.

[37] Christopher-Stine L, Siedner M, Lin J, et al. Renal biopsy in lupus patients with low levels of proteinuria. *J Rheumatol*. 2007; 34: 332–35.

[38] Jasiek M, Karras A, Le Guern V, et al. A multicentre study of 95 biopsy-proven cases of renal disease in primary Sjögren's syndrome. *Rheumatology*. (Oxford) 2017; 56: 362–70.

[39] Shah M, Patil S, Patel B, et al. Trends in Hospitalization for Hypertensive Emergency, and Relationship of End-Organ Damage With In-Hospital Mortality. *Am J Hypertens*. 2017; 30: 700–06.

[40] Gong J, Yuan H, Gao Z, Hu F. Wasp venom and acute kidney injury: The mechanisms and therapeutic role of renal replacement therapy. *Toxicon*. 2019; 163: 1–7.

[41] Sharma A, Wanchu A, Mahesha V, Sakhuja V, Bambery P, Singh S. Acute tubulo-interstitial nephritis leading to acute renal failure following multiple hornet stings. *BMC Nephrol.* 2006; 7: 18.

[42] Zhang L, Yang Y, Tang Y, et al. Recovery from AKI following multiple wasp stings: a case series. *Clin J Am Soc Nephrol*. 2013; 8: 1850–56.

[43] Zhang P, Cornell LD. IgG4-Related Tubulointerstitial Nephritis. *Adv Chronic Kidney Dis*. 2017; 24: 94–100.

[44] Raissian Y, Nasr SH, Larsen CP, et al. Diagnosis of IgG4-related tubulointerstitial nephritis. *J Am Soc Nephrol* .2011; 22: 1343–52.

[45] Amaro D, Carreño E, Steeples LR, Oliveira-Ramos F, Marques-Neves C, Leal I. Tubulointerstitial nephritis and uveitis (TINU) syndrome: a review. *Br J Ophthalmol.* 2020; 104: 742–47.

In: Issues in Kidney Disease – Acute Kidney Injury
Editors: S. Z. Fadem and A. Arslan Yousuf Awan
ISBN: 978-1-68507-002-1

Chapter 9

CONTRAST INDUCED ACUTE KIDNEY INJURY

Sehrish Ali**, DO and Venkat Ramanathan, MD
Selzman Institute for Kidney Health, Section of Nephrology, Department of Medicine,
Baylor College of Medicine, Houston, TX, USA
Michael E. DeBakey VA Medical Center, Houston, TX, USA

ABSTRACT

Contrast induced acute kidney injury (CI-AKI), also known as CIN, is one of the leading causes of acute kidney injury for hospitalized patients worldwide. The pathophysiology involves ischemic tubular injury in addition to decreased renal perfusion caused by high viscosity of contrast agents. Patients with pre-existing chronic kidney disease are more susceptible to develop CI-AKI. Older contrast agents with higher ionicity and osmolality have an increased incidence of causing injury. Additionally, procedures that involve intra-arterial contrast agent administration are associated with an increased risk of developing CI-AKI. Various risk models are present to predict the likelihood of developing CI-AKI, but to minimize the risk, iso-osmolar or selected low osmolar contrast media is advised with the smallest amount of volume. Pre and post procedure volume expansion with isotonic intravenous fluids is also advised. Management of CI-AKI is supportive.

Keywords: contrast induced nephropathy, CIN, contrast induced acute kidney injury, acute kidney injury, CI-AKI

INTRODUCTION

Conventional contrast agents used to visualize the vasculature typically contain iodine which absorb x-ray photons and make them a widely popular tool for clear visualization, pathological diagnosis, and procedural intervention. However, the benefits in diagnosis come with several adverse effects that can be attributed to contrast media agents including nausea, vomiting, hypersensitivity reactions, thyroid dysfunction, laryngeal edema, bronchospasm, and

* Corresponding Author's E-mail: Sehrish.ali2@bcm.edu.

anaphylaxis [1]. Contrast induced acute kidney injury (CI-AKI), also known as CIN, is an adverse effect related to contrast media that is associated with more than 10% of cases of hospital acquired AKI and is the third leading cause of iatrogenic AKI in hospitalized patients [2].

The first incidence of CI-AKI was reported in case reports in 1954 and 1957 depicting anuric AKI resulting from intravenous (IV) pyelography in a patient with multiple myeloma [3, 4]. Since then, there have been significant strides in minimizing this risk on the kidneys. Today CI-AKI is most commonly associated with AKI following contrast media exposure with computerized tomography (CT) scans or coronary and non-coronary angiography. There is a variable incidence of CI-AKI that results from procedural differences, clinical settings and the presence of risk factors. Despite these variations, there is an increased morbidity and mortality with CI-AKI, making management and prevention of CI-AKI that much more important.

Pathophysiology

Contrast agents cause acute kidney injury by direct and indirect mechanisms. In addition to direct injury to tubular epithelium, contrast agents can cause ischemic injury related to vasoconstriction within the kidney mediated by adenosine, angiotensin II, reduced nitric oxide. At baseline, the outer renal medulla has poor blood flow and reduced tissue oxygen saturation, making it even more susceptible to hypoxic injury during periods of compromised perfusion [6, 7]. Additionally, increased blood viscosity and tubular fluid viscosity worsens renal perfusion, and tubular obstruction, respectively. Finally, iodinated contrast agents increase oxidative stress, which can lead to the formation of reactive oxygenated species and cause direct cytotoxic injury and tubular cell death [6, 7].

Clinical Features and Diagnosis

The diagnosis of CI-AKI is made when either there is a rise in serum creatinine by 25% or an absolute increase by 0.5mg/dl within 48 hours after iodinated IV contrast media exposure. It is important to note that serum creatinine can continue to rise for up to five days after contrast exposure and can take up to 7-10 days for it to return to baseline [8]. Serum cystatin C (CysC) levels have also been studied as a diagnostic marker for CI-AKI. An increase of CysC greater than 10% within 24 hours following contrast media exposure indicates higher likelihood of having CI-AKI [9].

Patients that have CI-AKI usually have non-oliguria and the urinalysis is bland without any proteinuria. The urine microscopy can have muddy brown casts, similar to what is seen with acute tubular necrosis. The fractional excretion of sodium is typically less than 1% due to vasoconstriction. The diagnosis of CI-AKI is usually clinical, and a kidney biopsy is not necessary unless the diagnosis is unclear.

Factors

Co-Morbidities

There are various risk factors that have been associated with higher incidences of CI-AKI. Contrast media half-life is 1-2 hours in patients with normal renal function and is excreted by the kidneys within 24 hours of administration. Having pre-existing kidney disease is one of the most important and independent risk factors for developing CI-AKI, as the excretion of the agent is delayed in these patients [10]. Previously, patients with eGFR< 60 ml/min/ 1.73 m2 were associated to be at a higher risk for developing CI-AKI. However, with newer evidence KDIGO guidelines associate a higher risk of CI-AKI with those patients that have eGFR< 45 ml/min/ 1.73 m2 [11, 12]. The chance of developing CI-AKI increases in proportion to the severity of underlying kidney disease. Patients with kidney disease that have concurrent proteinuria or diabetes have an even higher risk for CI-AKI [10].

Other co-morbidities associated with increased incidences of CI-AKI include multiple myeloma and congestive heart failure. Older age, hyperglycemia independent of having the diagnosis of diabetes mellitus, concurrent use of nephrotoxic agents (i.e., NSAIDs), hemodynamic instability or having volume depletion also increases the risk to develop CI-AKI [10] (Table 1).

Few controversial studies have reported an association of CI-AKI in patients that have cirrhosis, have a history of kidney transplant, or are on renin-angiotensin aldosterone system blockade [13, 14] (Table 1).

Table 1. Risk factors associated with CI-AKI

Highest Risk Factors	**Chronic Kidney Disease**
	Chronic Kidney Disease + Diabetes
	Chronic Kidney Disease + Proteinuria
	High Contrast Volume
Other Risk Factors	Old Age
	Congestive Heart Failure
	Concurrent use of nephrotoxic Agents
	Hemodynamic Instability
	Volume Depletion
	Hyperglycemia
	Multiple Myeloma
Controversial Risk Factors	Cirrhosis
	Renin-Angiotensin Aldosterone Blockade
	History of Kidney Transplant

Contrast Agent Characteristic

The incidence of developing CI-AKI is also dependent on the type of contrast media as well as the dose of contrast media volume administered. The higher the volume of contrast media used, the higher the risk for AKI. Therefore, the volume of contrast media administered should be as minimal as possible. Contrast agents can be identified by their ionicity and their osmolality. The first generation, high osmolar contrast agents were ionic (monomeric structures) and had high osmolality (approximately four times the osmolality of blood). These characteristics gave them a higher viscosity, which induced hypoxemia and tubular stress making them highly nephrotoxic. These agents were replaced by nonionic and ionic (dimeric structure) low osmolar contrast agents (approximately twice the osmolality of blood), which were associated with decreased incidences of nephrotoxicity. The latest generation iso-osmolar contrast agents are nonionic and iso-osmolar to plasma, which were developed to further attenuate the risk of nephrotoxicity. However, these iso-osmolar contrast agents have a dimeric structure and have increased viscosity. A meta-analysis compared both of these contrast agents in patients with chronic kidney disease stage III and did show iso-osmolar agents to be less nephrotoxic than low osmolar contrast agents [15, 16, 17].

Procedures at Highest Risk

Multiple studies previously have attributed the route of contrast agent administration and type with the development of CI-AKI. Intra-arterial contrast agent administration was associated with a higher risk of CI-AKI in comparison to IV contrast agent administration because they have a higher peak iodine concentration in the vasculature. Recent studies have suggested that higher rates of AKI after catheter angiography can be attributed to differences in their comorbid conditions making them more prone to hemodynamic compromise, contrast media volumes, and procedural techniques/complications increasing their risk for cholesterol crystals, thrombi dislodging or microembolization rather than actual nephrotoxicity related to intra-arterial contrast media exposure [12, 17, 18].

Risk Model

Different risk models have been developed to predict the likelihood of developing CI-AKI in patients undergoing percutaneous coronary angiography. A well-known risk model calculator is the Mehran risk score, a post procedure risk system that takes into account the risk factors listed above to risk stratify patients and predict their risk of developing CI-AKI and/or risk of needing renal replacement therapy [19] (Table 2A, Table 2B).

Prevention

If contrast media is to be administered current recommendations advise the use of iso-osmolar or selected low osmolar contrast media with the smallest amount of volume. Moreover, the administration of additional contrast media should be avoided for over 48 to 72 hours after the initial administration.

Table 2A. Mehran Post-PCI risk score points

Hypotension (SBP* < 80 mmHg for ≥ 1 hour requiring inotropic support)	5
Intra-aortic Balloon Pump within 24 hours periprocedure	5
Congestive Heart Failure: Class III/IV	5
Age> 75 years	4
Anemia (Hct** < 39% for men or < 46% for women)	3
Diabetes Mellitus	3
Contrast Media Volume (≥ 100ml)	1 point per 100ml contrast
eGFR, mL/min/1.73 m^2	
40 to < 60	2
20 to < 40	4
< 20	6

SBP*: Systolic Blood Pressure, Hct**: Hematocrit

Adapted from: Mehran R, Aymong ED, Nikolsky E, et al. A simple risk score for prediction of contrast-induced nephropathy after percutaneous coronary intervention: development and initial validation. *J Am Coll Cardiol.* 2004;44(7):1393-1399. doi:10.1016/j.jacc.2004.06.068

Table 2B. Mehran Post-PCI Risk score interpretation

Calculated Risk Score Points	Risk of CI-AKI	Risk of RRT*
≤ 5	7.50%	0.04%
6-10	14.00%	0.12%
11-15	26.10%	1.09%
≥ 16	57.30%	12.60%

RRT*: Renal Replacement Therapy

Adapted from: Mehran R, Aymong ED, Nikolsky E, et al. A simple risk score for prediction of contrast-induced nephropathy after percutaneous coronary intervention: development and initial validation. *J Am Coll Cardiol.* 2004;44(7):1393-1399. doi:10.1016/j.jacc.2004.06.068

Fluid Administration

Volume expansion is thought to play a role in reversing the pathophysiology that is associated with CI-AKI by inhibition of the renin-angiotensin-aldosterone system (RAS). Angiotensin II attenuates vasoconstriction and helps improve medullary perfusion and hypoxia. Volume expansion also dilutes the contrast media associated with cellular damage, reducing the tubular viscosity [20].

In patients that are at high risk for developing CI-AKI pre-procedural volume expansion via intravenous fluids is recommended to minimize their risk [10]. Currently there is not sufficient data to support the use of oral hydration or oral salt loading for volume expansion over intravenous fluids [21].

The selection of intravenous fluids has evolved over time. Isotonic solutions are considered to be superior to hypotonic solutions in reducing the risk of CI-AKI because they are more effective in volume expansion [21]. Bicarbonate solution was previously thought to be associated with higher reduction in CI-AKI given its association with alkalization of the renal tubular fluid and reducing the production of reactive oxygen species [22]. However, there have been conflicting data on its benefits and a recent meta-analysis was unable to reproduce this data [23, 24]. Additionally, sodium bicarbonate infusions are expensive and have an increased risk of compounding error. Hence, isotonic normal saline solutions are favored.

It is recommended that isotonic intravenous fluids be administered at the rate of 1-1.5ml/kg/hr from 3-12 hours before until 6-24 hours after contrast administration, with goal urine flow rate of 150 ml/hour [25]. However, if a patient has history or is at risk for heart failure exacerbation, the rate of infusion may be reduced to prevent hypervolemia.

N-Acetylcysteine

N-actetylcysteine is a tripeptide that on a cellular level increases intracellular glutathione levels. In animal models, N-acetylcysteine has been associated with antioxidant properties limiting renal ischemia in addition to reducing vasoconstriction. Given its low cost, lack of severe adverse effects, and ease of administration it was previously used as the standard of care as prophylaxis for CI-AKI. However, its efficacy has not been reproducible in human clinical studies, and recent meta-analyses along with the PRESERVE trial have demonstrated its lack of prophylactic benefit [26, 27, 28, 29]. Hence, prophylaxis with N-acetylcysteine is no longer recommended for prevention of CI-AKI.

Other Agents

Theophylline is a nonselective adenosine receptor antagonist which was proposed to reduce the risk of vasoconstriction noted with contrast media. However, the data from meta-analyses was inconclusive and given its association with increased risk of ventricular arrhythmias, seizures and shock, the use of theophylline is not recommended [30, 31].

HMG-CoA reductase inhibitors, also known as statins, are a class of drugs that are associated with antioxidant and anti-inflammatory properties. It has been proposed that administration of statins prophylactically, may reduce the risk for CI-AKI [29, 32]. However, more research is needed to prove this benefit. If a patient is on statin prior to his administration of contrast media, it is recommended to continue it. Conversely, without the support of additional evidence, the initiation of statins specifically to mitigate the risk of CI-AKI is not advised.

Many other pharmacologic agents have undergone investigation to be administered prophylactically to reduce the risk of CI-AKI such as ascorbic acid, mannitol, atrial natriuretic peptide, fenoldopam and calcium antagonists. However, these agents have not been successful in trials and are not advised [32, 33].

Peri-Procedural Hemofiltration/Hemodialysis

Contrary to popular belief peri-procedural hemodialysis or hemofiltration is not advised for prevention for patients at high risk for CI-AKI. Although a single session of intermittent hemodialysis has been proven to remove 60-90% of the contrast media it has not shown to reduce the incidence of CI-AKI. Furthermore, high flux membrane used in hemofiltration can also effectively remove the contrast media, however it has not been able to reduce the risk of CI-AKI [34, 35]. Consequently, for a patient that is dialysis dependent but has residual renal function, caution must be advised with administration of contrast media. Additionally, if a patient has end stage kidney disease, post-contrast dialysis may be delayed for 24 to 48 hours unless a patient is at risk for hypervolemia.

Renin Angiotensin Aldosterone System (RAAS) Blockade

There are two conflicting theories on the use of angiotensin-converting enzyme inhibitors (ACE-I) and angiotensin receptor blockers (ARBs) with contrast media. Because there is a decrease in the glomerular filtration rate, ACE-I and ARBs may be associated with possible increased risk of CI-AKI. Alternatively, ACE-I and ARBs counteract contrast media's afferent arteriolar vasoconstrictive effect and therefore can help reduce the medullary hypoxia. Thus, there is conflicting data on the use of ACE-I/ARBs with contrast media. Hence, withholding ACE-I/ARBs prophylactically before contrast media administration is not recommended unless a patient has evidence of hypovolemia. Initiating a patient on ACE-I or ARBs, that are not currently taking them, is also not recommended [14, 36, 37].

Remote Ischemic Preconditioning (RIPC)

RIPC is a technique where a brief incident of ischemia and reperfusion in one organ reduces the risk of ischemia and injury in another organ through the release of bradykinin and adenosine. The release of these molecules has been proposed to induce antioxidant and anti-inflammatory effect that improve blood flow and reduce free radical formation. While the mechanisms appear promising, the current data have mixed results, precluding its use as prevention for CI-AKI [38, 39].

Management and Prognosis

The current management of patients that develop CI-AKI involves supportive care and prevention of future insults to the kidney. No treatment is available to reverse CI-AKI but most of the patients see a recovery in their kidney function within 3-7 days of supportive care. Monitoring for need for renal replacement therapy is prudent, however, dialysis is not usually required for CI-AKI.

Many studies suggest an increased risk for morbidity and mortality in patients that have CI-AKI [4]. Several have shown that patients that undergo cardiac angiography are at an even higher risk for adverse events in comparison to those that undergo other contrast media exposure. These adverse events include in-hospital, short term and long-term mortality, prolonged hospitalization, an increased risk for CKD progression, and other cardiovascular events. However, it is important to recognize that this study along with others have patients with other risk factors and co-morbidities that may confound the adverse event data [40].

Clinical Pearls

- CI-AKI is the third leading cause of iatrogenic AKI in hospitalized patients.
- Pathophysiology of CI-AKI involves two major theories: renal vasoconstriction leading to medullary hypoxia and renal tubular injury leading to cell death.
- Diagnosis: a rise in serum creatinine by 25% or an absolute increase by 0.5mg/dl within 48 hours post iodinated IV contrast media exposure. Most patients have non-oliguria Serum creatinine can continue to rise for up to five days after contrast exposure and can take up to 7-10 days to return to baseline.
- Co-morbidities associated with CI-AKI include pre-existing CKD +/- proteinuria or diabetes mellitus, multiple myeloma, congestive heart failure, older age, hyperglycemia, concurrent use of nephrotoxic agents, hemodynamic instability, or having volume depletion.
- Preventative measures include the use of minimum volume of low-osmolar or iso-osmolar contrast agents, volume expansion with isotonic solutions. (preferably normal saline), avoiding the administration of additional contrast media over 48 to 72 hours after the initial administration.
- N-acetycysteine is no longer recommended as prophylaxis.
- RAAS blockade is not necessary prior to contrast exposure.
- Management is supportive.

REFERENCES

[1] Bottinor W, Polkampally P, Jovin I. Adverse reactions to iodinated contrast media. *Int. J. Angiol*. 2013;22(3):149-154.

[2] Nash K, Hafeez A, Hou S. Hospital-acquired renal insufficiency. *Am. J. Kidney Dis*. 2002;39(5):930-936.

[3] Bartels E D, Brun G C, Gammeltoft A, et al. Acute anuria following intravenous pyelography in a patient with myelomatosis. *Acta Med. Scand.* 1954;150:297–302.

[4] Killmann S A, Gjorup S, Thaysen J H. Fatal acute renal failure following intravenous pyelography in a patient with multiple myeloma. *Acta Med. Scand*. 1957;158:43–6.

[5] Persson P B, Hansell P, Liss P. Pathophysiology of contrast medium-induced nephropathy. *Kidney Int*. 2005;68(1):14-22.

[6] Persson P B, Tepel M. Contrast medium-induced nephropathy: the pathophysiology. *Kidney Int Suppl*. 2006;(100):S8-S10.

[7] Solomon R J, Natarajan M K, Doucet S, et al. Cardiac Angiography in Renally Impaired Patients (CARE) study: a randomized double-blind trial of contrast-induced nephropathy in patients with chronic kidney disease. *Circulation*. 2007;115(25):3189-3196.

[8] Briguori C, Visconti G, Rivera N V, et al. Cystatin C and contrast-induced acute kidney injury. *Circulation*. 2010;121(19):2117-2122.

[9] Mehran R, Nikolsky E. Contrast-induced nephropathy: definition, epidemiology, and patients at risk. *Kidney Int. Suppl*. 2006: S11–15.

[10] Kidney Disease: Improving Global Outcomes (KDIGO) Acute Kidney Injury Work Group. KDIGO Clinical Practice Guideline for Acute Kidney Injury. *Kidney Int Suppl.* 2012; 2: 1–138.

[11] Filomia R, Maimone S, Caccamo G, et al. Acute kidney injury in cirrhotic patients undergoing contrast-enhanced computed tomography. *Medicine (Baltimore)*. 2016;95 (38):e4836.

[12] Rudnick M R, Leonberg-Yoo A K, Litt H I, Cohen R M, Hilton S, Reese PP. The Controversy of Contrast-Induced Nephropathy With Intravenous Contrast: What Is the Risk? *Am. J. Kidney Dis*. 2020;75(1):105-113.

[13] Toprak O. Conflicting and new risk factors for contrast induced nephropathy. *J. Urol.* 2007; 178: 2277–2283.

[14] Sterling K A, Tehrani T, Rudnick M R. Clinical significance and preventive strategies for contrast-induced nephropathy. *Curr. Opin. Nephrol. Hypertens.* 2008;17:616–23.

[15] Eng J, Wilson R F, Subramaniam R M, et al. Comparative Effect of Contrast Media Type on the Incidence of Contrast-Induced Nephropathy: A Systematic Review and Meta-analysis. *Ann. Intern. Med*. 2016;164(6):417-424.

[16] Pandya B, Chalhoub J M, Parikh V, et al. Contrast media use in patients with chronic kidney disease undergoing coronary angiography: A systematic review and meta-analysis of randomized trials. *Int. J. Cardiol*. 2017;228:137-144.

[17] Wichmann J L, Katzberg R W, Litwin S E, et al. Contrast-Induced Nephropathy. *Circulation.* 2015;132(20):1931-1936.

[18] McDonald J S, Leake C B, McDonald R J, et al. Acute Kidney Injury After Intravenous Versus Intra-Arterial Contrast Material Administration in a Paired Cohort. *Invest Radiol*. 2016;51(12):804-809.

[19] Mehran R, Aymong E D, Nikolsky E, et al. A simple risk score for prediction of contrast-induced nephropathy after percutaneous coronary intervention: development and initial validation. *J. Am. Coll. Cardiol*. 2004;44(7):1393-1399.

[20] Erley C M. Does hydration prevent radiocontrast-induced acute renal failure? *Nephrol Dial Transplant* 1999; 14:1064–1066.

[21] Weisbord SD, Palevsky PM. Prevention of contrast-induced nephropathy with volume expansion. *Clin. J. Am. Soc. Nephrol*. 2008;3(1):273-280.

[22] Merten G J, Burgess W P, Gray L V, et al. Prevention of Contrast-Induced Nephropathy With Sodium Bicarbonate: A Randomized Controlled Trial. *JAMA*. 2004;291(19): 2328–2334.

[23] Kooiman J, de Vries J P M, Van der Heyden J, et al. Randomized trial of one-hour sodium bicarbonate vs standard periprocedural saline hydration in chronic kidney disease patients undergoing cardiovascular contrast procedures. *PLoS One*. 2018;13(2):e0189372.

[24] Zapata-Chica C A, Bello Marquez D, Serna-Higuita L M, Nieto-Ríos J F, Casas-Arroyave FD, Donado-Gómez JH. Sodium bicarbonate versus isotonic saline solution to prevent contrast-induced nephropathy: a systematic review and meta-analysis. *Colomb. Med. (Cali)*. 2015;46(3):90-103.

[25] Stevens M A, McCullough P A, Tobin K J, et al. A prospective randomized trial of prevention measures in patients at high risk for contrast nephropathy: results of the P.R.I.N.C.E. Study. Prevention of Radiocontrast Induced Nephropathy Clinical Evaluation. *J. Am. Coll. Cardiol.* 1999; 33: 403–411.

[26] Palli E, Makris D, Papanikolaou J, et al. The impact of N-acetylcysteine and ascorbic acid in contrast-induced nephropathy in critical care patients: an open-label randomized controlled study. *Crit. Care*. 2017;21(1):269.

[27] Loomba R S, Shah P H, Aggarwal S, Arora R R. Role of N-Acetylcysteine to Prevent Contrast-Induced Nephropathy: A Meta-analysis. *Am. J. Ther*. 2016;23(1):e172-e183.

[28] Weisbord S D, Gallagher M, Jneid H, et al. Outcomes after Angiography with Sodium Bicarbonate and Acetylcysteine. *N. Engl. J. Med*. 2018;378(7):603-614.

[29] Subramaniam R M, Suarez-Cuervo C, Wilson R F, et al. Effectiveness of Prevention Strategies for Contrast-Induced Nephropathy: A Systematic Review and Meta-analysis. *Ann. Intern. Med.* 2016;164(6):406-416.

[30] Bagshaw S, Ghali W. Theophylline for the prevention of contrast-induced nephropathy: a systemic review and meta-analysis. *Arch. Intern. Med.* 2005; 165:1087 – 1093.

[31] Dai B, Liu Y, Fu L, Li Y, Zhang J, Mei C. Effect of theophylline on prevention of contrast-induced acute kidney injury: a meta-analysis of randomized controlled trials. *Am. J. Kidney Dis.* 2012;60(3):360-370.

[32] Vanmassenhove J, Vanholder R, Lameire N. Statins for the prevention of contrast-induced acute kidney injury. *Curr. Opin. Nephrol. Hypertens.* 2016;25(6):508-517.

[33] Naeem M, McEnteggart G E, Murphy T P, Prince E, Ahn S, Soares G. Fenoldopam for the prevention of contrast-induced nephropathy (CIN)-do we need more trials? A meta-analysis. *Clin. Imaging.* 2015;39(5):759-764.

[34] Cruz D N, Perazella M A, Bellomo R, et al. Extracorporeal blood purification therapies for prevention of radiocontrast-induced nephropathy: a systematic review. *Am. J. Kidney Dis.* 2006;48(3):361-371.

[35] Cruz D N, Goh C Y, Marenzi G, Corradi V, Ronco C, Perazella M A. Renal replacement therapies for prevention of radiocontrast-induced nephropathy: a systematic review. *Am. J. Med.* 2012;125:66–78.e3.

[36] Rim M Y, Ro H, Kang W C, Kim A J, Park H, Chang J H, Lee H H, Chung W, Jung J Y. The effect of renin-angiotensin-aldosterone system blockade on contrast-induced acute kidney injury: a propensity-matched study. *Am. J. Kidney Dis.* 2012;60:576–582.

[37] Zhou S, Wu C, Song Q, Yang X, Wei Z. Effect of Angiotensin-Converting Enzyme Inhibitors in Contrast-Induced Nephropathy: A Meta-Analysis. *Nephron.* 2016;133:1–14.

[38] Er F, Nia A M, Dopp H, et al. Ischemic preconditioning for prevention of contrast medium-induced nephropathy: randomized pilot RenPro Trial (Renal Protection Trial). *Circulation.* 2012;126(3):296-303.

[39] Deftereos S, Giannopoulos G, Tzalamouras V, et al. Renoprotective effect of remote ischemic post-conditioning by intermittent balloon inflations in patients undergoing percutaneous coronary intervention. *J. Am. Coll. Cardiol.* 2013;61(19):1949-1955.

[40] James M T, Samuel S M, Manning M A, et al. Contrast-induced acute kidney injury and risk of adverse clinical outcomes after coronary angiography: a systematic review and meta-analysis. *Circ. Cardiovasc. Interv.* 2013;6(1):37-43.

In: Issues in Kidney Disease – Acute Kidney Injury
Editors: S. Z. Fadem and A. Arslan Yousuf Awan
ISBN: 978-1-68507-002-1

Chapter 10

ACUTE KIDNEY INJURY IN ACUTE GLOMERULONEPHRITIS

Kiran Chintam, MD and Kartik Kalra*, MD
Department of Nephrology, Geisinger Medical Center, Danville, PA, USA

ABSTRACT

Glomerulonephritis is a relatively less common cause of acute kidney injury when compared to ATN. If diagnosed early, goal-directed therapy towards underlying GN like ANCA vasculitis or underlying disease like infection-related GN can help reduce the risk of end stage renal disease requiring dialysis or progression of acute kidney injury (AKI) to CKD in these patients. Having a high index of suspicion for GN as a cause of AKI is the key. Ongoing recent clinical trials in the management of various GN is the basis of recent treatment guidelines. This chapter has attempted to describe the characteristics, diagnosis, and treatment strategies of different glomerulonephritis.

Keywords: AKI, RPGN, AAV, MPO, Anti-GBM, IgA Nephropathy, SLE, Cryo, SVR

INTRODUCTION

Acute kidney injury (AKI) is one of the common kidney problems we encounter, particularly in hospitalized patients [1]. It affects both structure and function of the kidney. AKI imposes a heavy clinical burden on patients and a financial burden on the healthcare system. Early detection and treatment of AKI can improve outcomes for the patients. Acute glomerulonephritis is the second most common cause (6-10%) of acute kidney injury's intrinsic etiology.

* Corresponding Author's E-mail: kkalra@geisinger.edu.

Glomerulonephritis is associated with intrarenal vascular injury and causes decreased perfusion and glomerular injury secondary to proliferative inflammation leading to decreased glomerular filtration. The incidence of glomerulonephritis (GN) and GN causing AKI varies with geographic location [2, 3]. Specific therapies that may reduce the chance of AKI associated glomerulonephritis are discussed in this chapter.

Acute Glomerulonephritis

Acute glomerulonephritis (GN) can be divided based on the extent of involvement of the glomerulus. Such divisions include focal versus diffuse, crescentic versus non-crescentic, drug-induced vasculitis, and paraneoplastic glomerulonephritis [4].

Rapidly Progressive Glomerulonephritis (RPGN)

Most common GNs are granulomatous with polyangiitis (GPA, previously known as Wegener's granulomatosis), microscopic polyangiitis (MPA), and anti-glomerular basement membrane (anti-GBM) disease.

RPGN is one of the leading causes of AKI secondary to GN. All GN could progress rapidly and cause AKI, but classically RPGN is considered secondary to vasculitis caused by antineutrophil cytoplasmic antibodies (ANCA) and anti-GBM disease. RPGN is characterized by the crescent formation and a rapid decline in renal function. A crescent is made up of proliferating epithelial cells that line Bowman's capsule and infiltrating macrophages.

Anti-GBM disease is an uncommon, small vessel vasculitis involving capillaries of glomeruli and lung capillaries. It is classified as immune-complex vasculitis in the Revised International Chapel Hill Consensus Conference Nomenclature of Vasculitides. The prime target of the autoimmune response is the non-collagenous (NC1) domain of the α3 chain of type IV collagen (α3[IV]NC1) [5]. GBM contains type IV collagen, which itself consists of triple-helical α3, α4, α5. The exposure of underlying autoantigens and autoantibody (belongs to IgG class, with IgG1 and IgG3 predominating) formation results from an interplay between genetic and environmental factors [9].

ANCA-associated vasculitis (AAV) is a significant cause of RPGN. Distinctive histopathology of AAV is pauci-immune necrotizing vasculitis affecting small vessels (Chapel Hill Consensus Conference Nomenclature of Vasculitides 2012, CHCC 2012). Based on serology, histopathology, and clinical manifestations, AAV is classified into four groups (CHCC 2012): 1. Microscopic polyangiitis associated with proteinase-3 ANCA (PR3-ANCA MPA); 2. Granulomatosis polyangiitis associated with myeloperoxidase ANCA (MPO-ANCA GPA) (Wegener); 3. Eosinophilic granulomatosis polyangiitis (EGPA) (Churg-Strauss); 4. Renal-limited vasculitis (RLV). The first step in AAV is neutrophil priming by cytokines. The primed neutrophils activate alternative complement pathway and also presents ANCA antigens to the surface. These ANCA-associated neutrophils attach and penetrate blood vessels. C5a, the alternative complement pathway product, causes further amplification of inflammation by attracting more neutrophils. After a few days, the result of damage to plasma blood vessels causes them to release and activate coagulation factors. This leads to fibrinoid necrosis and scarring begins in the necrosed area due to macrophages and lymphocyte infiltration [11].

IgA Nephropathy

Immunoglobulin A Nephropathy (IgAN), also known as Berger's disease, is the most common GN. Progressive chronic kidney disease (CKD) is a common manifestation, but a rapidly advanced course is also well established and associated with > 50% crescents [7]. Pathogenesis of IgAN is the result of the interaction between genetic and environmental factors. It is described as a "multi-hit model." Patients with IgAN have a genetic predisposition of circulating aberrantly glycosylated IgA1 (Gd-IgA1). This mucosal IgA production by plasma cells could be T cell-dependent or independent processes, and anti-Gd-IgA1 autoantibodies form an immune complex [8]. Circulating immune complex activates alternative complement pathway. Circulating Immune complex and complement products deposit in kidney. The revised MEST -C (M- Mesangium, E- Endocapillary epithelium proliferation, S-Segmental glomerulosclerosis, T- tubular atrophy & interstitial fibrosis, C- Crescents) or Oxford scoring helps one to understand the pathology of IgAN. IgA can be associated with vasculitis (IgA vasculitis); or it can be related to viral diseases (HIV, Hepatitis), autoimmune diseases (inflammatory bowel disease, autoimmune hepatitis/ cirrhosis), and IgA predominant postinfectious glomerulonephritis (PIGN).

Infection Related Glomerulonephritis (PIGN: Post-Infectious GN)

Infection related GN (IRGN) is another cause of AKI. IRGN is divided based on etiology, including bacterial, viral, and other causes [10]. This chapter discusses mostly IRGN as a cause of AKI.

Bacterial IRGN

With liberal use of antibiotics, classic post-streptococcal GN is becoming infrequent in the adult population. Most cases of IRGN are often coexisting with the inciting infection. Staphylococcus species and gram-negative bacteria and occasional incidence of other bacteria associated with infection-related glomerulonephritis [6]. Patients with diabetes, cirrhosis, alcoholism, malnutrition, IV drug use, and other immunosuppressive states are prone to IRGN. Shunt nephritis is an immune-complex-mediated glomerulonephritis (GN) associated with chronically infected ventriculoatrial shunts inserted for treatment of hydrocephalus. Factors that initiate an immunologic process to cause glomerulonephritis caused by staphylococcus and other bacteria are still not completely understood. Post-streptococcal GN, for example, streptococcal pyrogenic endotoxin B (SpeB) appears to be the precipitating cause.

Viral Associated GN

Most of the time, viruses cause chronic kidney disease. Few of the viruses can cause acute kidney injury in various ways involving the glomerulus (Table 1).

Table 1. Viral causes of AKI causing GN

Virus type	Predominant glomerular histology
Dengue	ICGN, MsPGN
Hanta virus	HFRS, MsPGN
Varicella Zoster Virus	DPGN
Parvovirus	ICGN,PAN, MPA, TMA, IgA
HAV	ICGN, MsPGN
HBV	DPGN
HCV	Type 1 MPGN (by forming type 2 MC), PAN
HIV	HIVAN
CMV	cFSGS, MN, IgA, TMA, ICGN, MPGN
EBV	ICGN, MN, MsPGN
Coxsackie B	RPGN
COVID-19	Etiopathology evolving

ICGN: immune complex glomerulonephritis, MsPGN: mesangial proliferative glomerulonephritis, HFRS: hemorrhagic fever and renal syndrome, DPGN: diffuse proliferative GN, PAN: Poly arteritis nodosa, cFSGS: Collapsing Focal Segmental Glomerulosclerosis, HSP: Henoch Schoenlein purpura, TMA: Thrombotic microangiopathy, MPGN: Membranoproliferative glomerulonephritis, MC: Mixed cryoglobulins, HIVAN: HIV- associated nephropathy, HAV: hepatitis A virus, HBV: Hepatitis B virus, HCV: Hepatitis C virus.

Cryoglobulinemia

Cryoglobulins are immunoglobulins that precipitate when the serum is cooled to below 37 degrees Celsius and dissolve with rewarming [12]. Type I cryoglobulins consist of a single monoclonal immunoglobulin (usually of IgG or IgM class) and are associated with plasma cell dyscrasias or other lymphoproliferative disorders. Type II cryoglobulins are mixed cryoglobulins containing monoclonal immunoglobulin (usually IgM kappa) with rheumatoid factor activity for polyclonal immunoglobulin (usually IgG) [13]. This type is seen most commonly associated with hepatitis C virus infection and is most frequently implicated in glomerulonephritis. Other causes of type II cryoglobulinemia include dysproteinemia, other chronic infections, and autoimmune disease. Type III cryoglobulins are mixed cryoglobulins composed of polyclonal immunoglobulins (often IgG and IgM, and less frequently IgA). This form is often seen in association with infections and autoimmune disease [14] (Table 2).

Table 2. Classification of Cryoglobulins

Type	Composition	Notes
I	Isolated monoclonal immunoglobulin	Single monoclonal immunoglobulin paraprotein (usually IgM) contributing, commonly caused by Waldenström macroglobulinemia, multiple myeloma, or chronic lymphocytic leukemia.
II	Monoclonal component and a polyclonal component	The monoclonal component is usually IgM that has rheumatoid factor activity and binds to either intact polyclonal IgG or a component of IgG fragment to form IgM-IgG complexes. Associated with hepatitis C infection.
III	Polyclonal IgG and IgM	Also has rheumatoid factor activity. May be associated with an autoimmune disorder or persistent infection such as hepatitis C.

MEMBRANOPROLIFERATIVE GLOMERULONEPHRITIS

Membranoproliferative glomerulonephritis (MPGN) is characterized by the diffuse proliferation of mesangial cells with the extension of the mesangial matrix into the peripheral capillary wall, giving rise to a thickened and reduplicated appearance [15]. This in turn gives rise to the double contour or "tram-track" appearance of the GBM. The mixed mesangial and endothelial cell proliferation results in a lobular distortion of the glomerulus (lobular accentuation). Historically, MPGN was categorized based on pathologic features. However, the current classification of MPGN is based on the pathogenesis of the disease and whether it is mediated by immune complexes, complement, or endothelial dysfunction. The immunofluorescence (IF) pattern in the biopsy provides clues to the pathogenesis and help to define the following subtypes: 1. Immunoglobulin-positive, complement-positive (these can be monoclonal immunoglobulin as in plasma cell dyscrasia; or polyclonal as in hepatitis C) 2. Immunoglobulin-negative, complement-positive (disorders of complement, as with dense deposit disease or C3 glomerulonephritis).3. Immunoglobulin-negative, complement-negative (as in thrombotic microangiopathy).

Etiologies of immune complex MPGN include autoimmune diseases such as lupus nephritis (LN). However, LN usually demonstrates IgA and C1q in addition to IgG, IgM, C3, kappa, and lambda by IF, often referred to as a "full house pattern." MPGN related to hepatitis C (with or without cryoglobulins) is associated with the deposition of polyclonal immune complexes and shows granular deposition of IgM, C3, and relatively equal kappa and lambda; IgG deposition is variable. MPGN related to chronic bacterial infection and bacterial endocarditis would also produce polyclonal immune complex deposition rather than a monoclonal pattern by IF. Deposition of a monoclonal immunoglobulin can also result in an immunoglobulin-positive, complement-positive MPGN-pattern of inflammation [16].

C3 glomerulopathy has subendothelial dense deposits that resemble type I MPGN on electron microscopy (EM) but has only C3 staining without Ig on IF. Patients typically present with proteinuria, often in the nephrotic range (sometimes with nephrotic syndrome), hematuria, variable degrees of hypertension, and kidney failure C3 glomerulopathies are characterized by dysregulation of the alternative complement pathway. The abnormal function of factor H, an inhibitor of the alternative pathway, can lead to unregulated complement activation, leading to C3 glomerulopathy. This disorder is characterized by C3 deposition without other significant immune deposition. Diagnosis of C3 Glomerulopathy is largely based on the presence of C3 immunofluorescence in renal biopsy in the absence of immunoglobulins.

Clinical presentation can be very varied from indolent mild proteinuria to RPGN. Dense deposit disease (DDD) and C3 glomerulonephritis are the two types of C3 glomerulopathy. Diagnosis of DDD is based on dense basement membrane deposits on EM. One may look for C3 nephritic factor mutation, factor H deficiency/mutations, or characterization of complement factor H-related (CFHR) gene variations to rule out monoclonal protein as the etiology of C3GN, especially in older patients [17].

LUPUS NEPHRITIS

The current classification of lupus nephritis (LN) was revised by the International Society of Nephrology and the Renal Pathology Society (ISN/RPS) and is based on the findings from the kidney biopsy in patients with systemic lupus erythematosus (SLE). The presence of subendothelial and mesangial immune complex formation found in LN is postulated to be due to: 1) sequential deposition of endogenous antigen and circulating autoantibodies; and 2) entrapment of preformed immune complexes from the circulation. IgG dominant "full house" (positive IgG, IgA, IgM, C1q) glomerular deposits on immunofluorescence (IF) are seen in LN (but not specific only to LN) [18, 19].

- Class I: Minimal Mesangial Lupus Nephritis - Presentation (varies): preserved renal function, normal urinalysis or minimal hematuria/proteinuria, and no HTN. Biopsy findings: standard light microscopy (LM), immune complex deposits in the mesangium by IF, and electron microscopy (EM).
- Class II: Mesangial Lupus Nephritis - Presentation (varies): preserved renal function, microscopic hematuria, non-nephrotic proteinuria, and no HTN. Biopsy findings: mesangial expansion/hypercellularity (mononuclear cells), mesangial deposits on IF.
- Class III: Focal Lupus Nephritis- Presentation (varies): normal to elevated serum creatinine, microscopic hematuria, and proteinuria (active urinary sediment), and possible hypertension (HTN). Biopsy Findings: active or inactive lesions in <50% of glomeruli, subendothelial and mesangial deposits on IF and EM. This class has been typically further sub classified as Active (A), Active/Chronic lesions (A/C), or Chronic (healed/scarred lesions). It has been proposed that this further classification is not needed, but an overall index of activity and chronicity is suggested to be assigned.
- Class IV: Diffuse Lupus Nephritis - Presentation (varies): normal to elevated serum creatinine, microscopic hematuria and proteinuria (active urinary sediment, can be nephrotic range proteinuria), and HTN. Biopsy findings: active lesions in >50% of glomeruli, subendothelial and mesangial deposits typically seen on IF and EM. This class has been typically subdivided into segmental (S) and global (G) lesions, with activity and chronicity (A, A/C, C). Similar to Class III, it has been proposed that this

further classification is not needed, but an overall index of activity and chronicity is suggested to be assigned.

- Class V: Membranous Lupus Nephritis (a non-inflammatory form of LN) - can be seen in combination with Class III, IV, or VI. Presentation (varies): in pure class V, patients have proteinuria, which can be in the nephrotic range but with preserved renal function, no HTN, may have hematuria but normal complements. Biopsy findings: no inflammation (if pure class V), thickened capillary walls, sufficient granular immune deposits (on IF) corresponding to subepithelial electron-dense deposits on EM. Recent literature suggests that exostosin (EXT) 1/2 is the target antigen in SLE patients.
- Class VI: Advanced Sclerosing Lupus Nephritis - Defined by ≥ 90% global sclerosis without signs of activity.

Monoclonal Gammopathy with Renal Significance

Diagnosis of monoclonal gammopathy with renal significance (MGRS) requires exclusion of multiple myeloma (MM) or other lymphoproliferative disorders. Simplistically, it is monoclonal gammopathy of undetermined significance (MGUS) with renal involvement. The serum protein electrophoresis (SPEP) and immunofixation electrophoresis (IFE) can detect a light chain clone at concentrations of > 500 mg/l and > 150 mg/l, respectively [20]. Urinary protein electrophoresis (UPEP) and urine immunofixation electrophoresis (UIFE) can identify an abnormal clone of light chain in the urine to a concentration of 10 mg/l [21]. The sensitivity of free light chain (FLC) for Bence Jones protein (BJP) test is 98%. Serum or urine monoclonal protein may not be detected. Peripheral flow cytometry or PET scan can be helpful in such cases to find an underlying lymphoproliferative disorder. If no monoclonal serum/urine protein and no lymphoproliferative disorder can be found, treatment options are not well defined and can be challenging.

Clinical Approach to the Diagnosis and Treatment of AKI in Glomerulonephritis

In general, patients with glomerulonephritis have decreased kidney function, symptoms include fatigue, decreased appetite, decreased urine output, and electrolyte abnormality. Moreover, these patients may have a fever, arthralgias, malaise, micro or macroscopic hematuria, or proteinuria. Patients with vasculitis quite often have cutaneous manifestations, including vasculitic rash. Other organ systems are also involved in these patients and manifest as pulmonary hemorrhage, respiratory failure, encephalopathy, hepatitis, and myocarditis. IgAN presents as microscopic hematuria and progressive kidney disease. Patients with AKI secondary to IgA can have gross hematuria after upper respiratory tract infection or without hematuria caused by a crescentic form of IgAN. In these patients, a prompt kidney biopsy is essential to confirm the diagnosis.

Poor prognostic signs of IgaN are hypertension, proteinuria, and low eGFR at the time of diagnosis [22]. Anti-GBM disease manifests as AKI with rapid progression. 40- 60% of the time will have concurrent lung hemorrhage. Clinical manifestations of microscopic polyangiitis (MPA) and granulomatosis with polyangiitis (GPA) overlap and usually present with nonspecific symptoms and systemic inflammation signs such as fever, fatigue, myalgia, arthralgia, loss of appetite, and weight loss. Compared to MPA and eosinophilic granulomatosis with polyangiitis (EGPA), GPA is associated with more frequent upper and lower respiratory tract symptoms like nasal septal perforation, rhinitis, sinusitis, and hemoptysis. Pulmonary injury can be granulomatous in GPA. Lower extremity purpura is a common cutaneous manifestation. Purpura can affect any part of the body [23]. IRGN associated AKI presentation can be wide range, including minimal symptoms to RPGN, microscopic to gross hematuria, or nephritic to nephrotic range proteinuria.

Evaluation of the patient with AKI suspected to have glomerulonephritis should start with a good history obtained from the patient and physical examination. Obtaining a complete metabolic panel, urine analysis, and a microscope is one of the vital evaluations. The presence of hematuria caused by the glomerular origin bleeding and proteinuria are specific for the glomerular involvement of these diseases. The presence of dysmorphic RBC (Acanthocytes) > 5% of urine RBC is 95% specific for glomerular hematuria. Nephritic sediment, the presence of increased red cells (> 5/high-power field), and red cell casts are also evidence of the glomerular origin of bleeding. Cellular casts also indicate a more severe form of the disease. The other essential laboratory tests, which would help to make a diagnosis, are C3, C4, ANA, ANCA, RF, Anti-GBM assay, hepatitis, and HIV serology. In addition, SPEP, light chain assay, serum LDH, blood cultures, and streptozyme assay are based on patient history. A kidney biopsy is a standard gold test to confirm the diagnosis (KDIGO GN guidelines for IgA), classification, and prognostication of the disease. KDIGO 2020 guidelines recommend prognostication of diseases like IgAN.

An urgent identification of anti-GBM antibodies in serum is the first step in the evaluation of RPGN. Approximately 10% of the patients do not have identifiable circulating antibodies [24]. Kidney biopsy and direct immunofluorescence are the gold standards in the diagnosis.

Immunofluorescence shows a strong linear ribbon-like appearance, which signifies a deposit of autoantibody deposition in the basement membrane. The uniform age crescent is a typical histopathologic marker of the anti-GBM disease. The uniform age crescent also differentiates anti-GBM disease from ANCA vasculitis. AAV should be screened by the ANCA panel (EIA for MPO and PR3). ANCA is 80-90% sensitive, but specificity depends on the patient population, quality, and other associated inflammatory conditions [25]. Characteristic pathology is pauci-immune segmental fibrinoid necrosis of the small vessels.

Pathologically, IRGN is a proliferative glomerular disease. It is usually associated with exudative, endocapillary, and mesangial immune complex deposition. Infective endocarditis-associated IRGN shows evidence of crescents in more than 50% of the patients. Shunt nephritis can be associated with MPGN pattern. Immunofluorescence staining is positive for C3 and includes IgA-dominant deposition due to IRGN usually caused by staphylococcus species, E Coli, and Klebsiella. Infective endocarditis causing GN and shunt nephritis can present as ANCA vasculitis.

Management

Rules of general management of AKI include monitoring electrolytes, treating hyperkalemia, encouraging a low sodium diet, lifestyle modification, and avoiding further nephrotoxic agents; these apply to AKI treatment secondary to GN. Other guidelines include maintaining hemodynamic stability and treating hypertension. Treatment directed towards specific underlying etiology will help to reverse AKI or halt further worsening of kidney function. Untreated RPGN typically progresses to end-stage kidney disease over days to weeks to a few months. However, patients with fewer crescents (< 50 percent of glomeruli affected by crescents on initial biopsy) may have a more protracted, not so rapidly progressive course [26].

Various forms of GN may present as AKI. Although GN as a cause of AKI in a particular case may be suspected on clinical grounds, it often requires recourse to the invasive procedure of renal biopsy, which currently represents the gold standard test for diagnosing the medical conditions of the kidney. The frequency of GN underlying AKI varies widely in various studies.

IgA Nephropathy -AKI (IgAN-AKI)

IgAN-AKI associated with IgAN should be treated conservatively, always exclude reversible causes. Renin-angiotensin system (RAS) blockade shows promising evidence to decrease proteinuria. Management includes initiating RAS blockade once AKI is resolved or stabilized.

Statins showed some evidence to reducing proteinuria in less severe cases. Weight loss and smoking cessation have been beneficial. The use of steroids and other immunosuppressive therapy is validated in progressive kidney disease caused by IgAN. If the patient presents with rapidly progressive IgAN, management includes treating the patient with cyclophosphamide and corticosteroids akin to ANCA vasculitis guidelines.

Anti-GBM Disease

Time is of the essence in the treatment of RPGN, especially in the case of anti-GBM disease. Per Kidney Disease Improving Global Outcomes (KDIGO) guidelines, treatment should be started if there is a strong suspicion of anti-GBM disease even though the diagnosis is not confirmed. Treatment consists of plasma exchange until no antibody is detected, then simultaneously treat with steroids (taper and use lowest possible dose for six months) plus oral cyclophosphamide (for three months). No maintenance therapy is necessary for isolated anti-GBM disease. Recurrence of anti-GBM after transplant is a remote possibility provided antibodies are not detected at the time of transplant (most transplant centers recommend six months seronegativity before transplant).

AAV treatment traditionally included induction with high dose steroids and cyclophosphamide (CYCLOPS study). With the evidence of adverse effects of high dose steroids and cyclophosphamide, targeted B cell therapy emerged as an alternative to cyclophosphamide. Rituximab, which targets CD20 on B cells, is becoming the mainstay of

AAV treatment (RAVE, RITUXIVAS study). A recent well-famed PEXIVAS study, the largest randomized controlled trial in the field of vasculitis to date, proved the use of low dose steroids in AAV treatment with non-inferior results and low side effects compared to standard high dose steroids. Plasmapheresis was included as the first-line intervention of AAV induction therapy (MEPEX study). The PEXIVAS study also evaluated the minimal role of plasmapheresis in induction therapy. All patients who receive induction therapy will be continued on maintenance therapy with Rituximab or Azathioprine.

Infection Related Glomerulonephritis

Aim for infection control if infection coexists with GN at the time of presentation, conservative management- volume, hypertension control, and dialysis if having difficulty controlling volume and uremia.

Virus-induced GN and AKI treatment depends on the treatment of viremia and conservative care. Immune-mediated GN is treated with steroids, rituximab, and plasmapheresis.

C3 Glomerulopathy

For C3 glomerulopathy, treatment can be conservative (with ACE/ARB blockade) in mild disease. Treatment with Eculizumab has shown good response but is expensive [17]. Treatment with plasma infusion or exchange can be applied if genetic deficiency or mutation in C3 or Factor H or if C3 nephritic factor is identified. Treatment with rituximab can be attempted, but there is no good evidence to support that [27] Rituximab (preferred for IgM) or Cytoxan therapy, in addition to steroids, can be used in severe or progressive disease. Besides proliferative glomerulonephritis, MGRS can present as other renal disorders similar to myeloma (other than cast nephropathy) such as immune deposition disease, amyloidosis, and proximal tubular dysfunction. Treatment for MGRS should be considered even after ESRD if the patient is a candidate for transplant due to the high rate of recurrence [15].

Treatment of Cryoglobulinemia depends on the severity of disease and the underlying cause. If Hep C +, immunosuppressive therapy should be initiated first; after disease, stabilization then antiviral therapy can be introduced. The exception to this might be patients with life-threatening disease in which both could be started simultaneously. In patients with persistent hepatitis C virus (HCV)-related cryoglobulinemia, immunological improvement may lag behind viral clearance and the sustained viral response (SVR). A monoclonal population of autoreactive memory B-cells may persist after viral eradication has been achieved. Persistent immunological activity after a SVR should prompt a kidney to assess the need for immunosuppressive therapy. Plasmapheresis is indicated in patients with life threatening disease, hyperviscosity syndrome, high cryocrit levels > 10% and severe cutaneous vasculitis [28, 29].

Lupus Nephritis (LN)

Management of lupus nephritis starts with ISN/RPS (International Society of Nephrology/Renal Pathology Society) classification of LN and associated clinical correlations. It will guide treatment choice. The patients with class I and class II LN are considered to have a good prognosis as long as their disease is stable. Usually, treatment of extra kidney manifestation is sufficient for these patients. Treatment of class III (A&A/C), class IV(A&A/C), and class V are divided into induction and maintenance phases. The aim of induction therapy is to achieve remission of the disease, which is reducing the protein creatinine ratio below 0.7 mg/g, reducing hematuria, and obtaining normalization or stabilization of GFR. After achieving remission, the patient needs to be on maintenance therapy. KDIGO and EULAR/ERA developed independent guidelines (Figure 1)

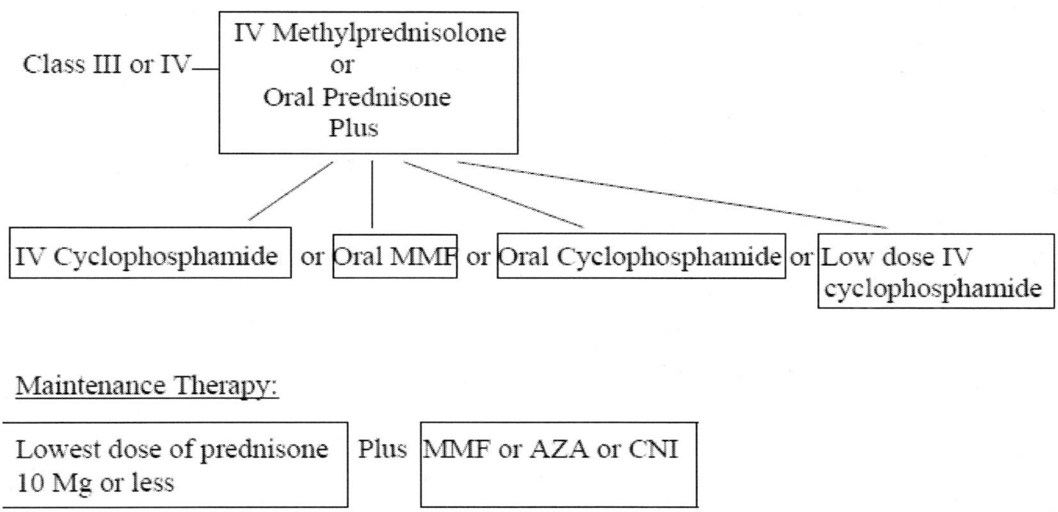

MMF: Mycophenolate, AZA: Azathioprine, CNI: Calcineurin inhibitors.

Figure 1. Induction Therapy Schematic Diagram – Lupus Nephritis.

Management of class V LN depends on the degree of proteinuria (Nephrotic vs. Non-nephrotic), presence or absence of abnormal kidney function. Use RAAS inhibitors to control proteinuria. Use immunosuppression if proteinuria more than 1g/d.

New randomized control studies showed promising results with Belimumab (BLISS-LN) in the treatment of LN [30]. FDA approved Voclosporin in the treatment of LN; it is an analogue of cyclosporine [31].

AKI in Patients with Nephrotic Syndrome

Acute kidney injury can develop in patients with nephrotic syndrome, for example, in minimal change disease. Most of the time, these patients have significant proteinuria. The patient also develops AKI due to the use of nephrotic agents, over diuresis, and increased diuresis. Patients can present with AKI, hematuria, and symptoms of kidney infarction if they have renal thrombosis. Significant hypoalbuminemia, particularly in membranous nephropathy, is a risk factor for renal vein thrombosis.

PROGNOSIS

Patients with acute kidney injury are more likely to develop chronic kidney disease in the future. They are also at higher risk of end-stage renal disease and premature death [32]. Patients who have an acute kidney injury episode should be monitored for the development or worsening of chronic kidney disease. Untreated RPGN at any age typically runs a rapidly fatal course. Despite improved treatment, the disease in patients of all ages is still associated with about 20% mortality in the first year of diagnosis and results in ESRD in up to 25% of surviving patients within 4 years [33]. Unfavorable prognostic factors include age > 60 years, oliguric renal failure, higher serum creatinine level, crescents in > 75% of glomeruli. Patients with double-antibody disease appear to have renal prognoses somewhat better than patients with only anti-GBM antibody disease and worse than patients with pauci-immune disease. About 30% of patients with pauci-immune RPGN do not respond to treatment; among non-responders, about 40% require dialysis, and 33% die within 4 years. In contrast, among patients who respond to treatment, < 20% of patients require dialysis, and about 3% die. Death is usually due to infectious or cardiac causes. Kidney transplantation is effective for all types, but disease may recur in the graft; risk diminishes with time. In anti-GBM antibody disease, the anti-GBM titers should be undetectable for at least 12 months before transplantation [34]. For patients with pauci-immune RPGN, disease activity should be quiescent for at least 6 months before transplantation; ANCA titers do not need to be suppressed. Continuous advancement in the understanding of the pathogenesis of various forms of GN has led to the discovery of novel therapeutic targets.

Clinical Pearls

- Consider rapidly progressive glomerulonephritis if patients have acute kidney injury with hematuria and dysmorphic RBCs or RBC casts, particularly with subacute constitutional or non-specific symptoms (e.g., fatigue, fever, anorexia, arthralgia, abdominal pain).
- Perform serologic tests and early renal biopsy. Early diagnosis (biopsy with immunofluorescence and serology) and therapy are essential to minimize the degree of irreversible renal injury.
- Initiate treatment early with corticosteroids, cyclophosphamide, rituximab, and often plasma exchange.

REFERENCES

[1] Naqvi R, Mubarak M, Ahmed E, Akhtar F, Bhatti S, Naqvi A, et al. Spectrum of glomerular diseases causing acute kidney injury; 25 years experience from a single center. *J Renal Inj Prev.* 2015;4(4):113-6.

[2] Hebert L A, Parikh S, Prosek J, Nadasdy T, Rovin BH. Differential diagnosis of glomerular disease: a systematic and inclusive approach. *Am J Nephrol.* 2013;38(3):253-66.

[3] Lv J, Yang Y, Zhang H, Chen W, Pan X, Guo Z, et al. Prediction of outcomes in crescentic IgA nephropathy in a multicenter cohort study. *J Am Soc Nephrol.* 2013;24(12):2118-25.

[4] Magistroni R, D'Agati VD, Appel GB, Kiryluk K. New developments in the genetics, pathogenesis, and therapy of IgA nephropathy. *Kidney Int.* 2015;88(5):974-89.

[5] Segelmark M, Butkowski R, Wieslander J. Antigen restriction and IgG subclasses among anti-GBM autoantibodies. *Nephrol Dial Transplant.* 1990;5(12):991-6.

[6] Chapter 9: Infection-related glomerulonephritis. *Kidney Int. Suppl.* (2011). 2012;2(2):200-8.

[7] Trimarchi H, Barratt J, Cattran D C, Cook H T, Coppo R, Haas M, et al. Oxford Classification of IgA nephropathy 2016: an update from the IgA Nephropathy Classification Working Group. *Kidney Int.* 2017;91(5):1014-21.

[8] Barbour S J, Reich H N. Risk stratification of patients with IgA nephropathy. *Am J Kidney Dis*. 2012;59(6):865-73.

[9] Turner N, Mason P J, Brown R, Fox M, Povey S, Rees A, et al. Molecular cloning of the human Goodpasture antigen demonstrates it to be the alpha 3 chain of type IV collagen. *J Clin Invest.* 1992;89(2):592-601.

[10] Nadasdy T, Hebert LA. Infection-related glomerulonephritis: understanding mechanisms. *Semin Nephrol.* 2011;31(4):369-75.

[11] Falk R J, Hogan S, Carey T S, Jennette J C. Clinical course of anti-neutrophil cytoplasmic autoantibody-associated glomerulonephritis and systemic vasculitis. The Glomerular Disease Collaborative Network. *Ann Intern Med.* 1990;113(9):656-63.

[12] Brouet J C, Clauvel J P, Danon F, Klein M, Seligmann M. Biologic and clinical significance of cryoglobulins. A report of 86 cases. *Am J Med.* 1974;57(5):775-88.

[13] Bengtsson U, Larsson O, Lindstedt G, Svalander C. Monoclonal IgG cryoglobulinemia with secondary development of glomerulonephritis and nephrotic syndrome. *Q . Med.* 1975;44(175):491-503.

[14] Trejo O, Ramos-Casals M, Garcia-Carrasco M, Yague J, Jimenez S, de la Red G, et al. Cryoglobulinemia: study of etiologic factors and clinical and immunologic features in 443 patients from a single center. *Medicine (Baltimore).* 2001;80(4):252-62.

[15] Leung N, Bridoux F, Hutchison C A, Nasr S H, Cockwell P, Fermand J P, et al. Monoclonal gammopathy of renal significance: when MGUS is no longer undetermined or insignificant. *Blood.* 2012;120(22):4292-5.

[16] Vastni P S, Erickson D G, Williams R C, Jr., Tung K. S. Benign monoclonal gammaglobulinemia and glomerulonephritis. *Am J Med.* 1977;62(3):324-9.

[17] Bomback AS, Smith RJ, Barile GR, Zhang Y, Heher EC, Herlitz L, et al. Eculizumab for dense deposit disease and C3 glomerulonephritis. *Clin J Am Soc Nephro. l*2012;7(5):748-56.

[18] Bajema I M, Wilhelmus S, Alpers C E, Bruijn J A, Colvin R B, Cook H T, et al. Revision of the International Society of Nephrology/Renal Pathology Society classification for lupus nephritis: clarification of definitions, and modified National Institutes of Health activity and chronicity indices. *Kidney Int.* 2018;93(4):789-96.

[19] Weening J J, D'Agati V D, Schwartz M M, Seshan S V, Alpers C E, Appel G B, et al. The classification of glomerulonephritis in systemic lupus erythematosus revisited. *Kidney Int.* 2004;65(2):521-30.

[20] Hutchison C A, Plant T, Drayson M, Cockwell P, Kountouri M, Basnayake K, et al. Serum free light chain measurement aids the diagnosis of myeloma in patients with severe renal failure. *BMC Nephrol.* 2008;9:11.

[21] Nowrousian M R, Brandhorst D, Sammet C, Kellert M, Daniels R, Schuett P, et al. Serum free light chain analysis and urine immunofixation electrophoresis in patients with multiple *myeloma. Clin Cancer Res.* 2005;11(24 Pt 1):8706-14.

[22] Maixnerova D, Reily C, Bian Q, Neprasova M, Novak J, Tesar V. Markers for the progression of IgA nephropathy. *J Nephrol.* 2016;29(4):535-41.

[23] Crowson AN, Mihm MC, Jr., Magro CM. Cutaneous vasculitis: a review. *J Cutan. Pathol.* 2003;30(3):161-73.

[24] McAdoo S P, Pusey C D. Anti-Glomerular Basement Membrane Disease. *Clin J Am Soc Nephrol.* 2017;12(7):1162-72.

[25] Damoiseaux J, Csernok E, Rasmussen N, Moosig F, van Paassen P, Baslund B, et al. Detection of antineutrophil cytoplasmic antibodies (ANCAs): a multicentre European Vasculitis Study Group (EUVAS) evaluation of the value of indirect immunofluorescence (IIF) versus antigen-specific immunoassays. *Ann Rheum Dis.* 2017;76(4):647-53.

[26] Baldwin D S, Neugarten J, Feiner H D, Gluck M, Spinowitz B. The existence of a protracted course in crescentic glomerulonephritis. *Kidney Int.* 1987;31(3):790-4.

[27] Krmar R T, Holtback U, Linne T, Berg U B, Celsi G, Soderberg M P, et al. Acute renal failure in dense deposit disease: complete recovery after combination therapy with immunosuppressant and plasma exchange. *Clin Nephrol.* 2011;75 Suppl 1:4-10.

[28] Roccatello D, Baldovino S, Rossi D, Giachino O, Mansouri M, Naretto C, et al. Rituximab as a therapeutic tool in severe mixed cryoglobulinemia. *Clin Rev. Allergy Immunol.* 2008;34(1):111-7.

[29] Evans T W, Nicholls A J, Shortland J R, Ward A M, Brown C B. Acute renal failure in essential mixed cryoglobulinemia: precipitation and reversal by plasma exchange. *Clin Nephrol.* 1984;21(5):287-93.

[30] Furie R, Rovin B H, Houssiau F, Malvar A, Teng Y K O, Contreras G, et al. Two-Year, Randomized, Controlled Trial of Belimumab in Lupus Nephritis. *N Engl J Med.* 2020;383(12):1117-28.

[31] Rovin B H, Solomons N, Pendergraft W F, 3rd, Dooley M A, Tumlin J, Romero-Diaz J, et al. A randomized, controlled double-blind study comparing the efficacy and safety of dose-ranging voclosporin with placebo in achieving remission in patients with active lupus nephritis. *Kidney Int.* 2019;95(1):219-31.

[32] Goldberg R, Dennen P. Long-term outcomes of acute kidney injury. *Adv Chronic Kidney Dis.* 2008;15(3):297-307.

[33] Little M A, Nightingale P, Verburgh C A, Hauser T, De Groot K, Savage C, et al. Early mortality in systemic vasculitis: relative contribution of adverse events and active vasculitis. *Ann Rheum Dis.* 2010;69(6):1036-43.

[34] Levy J B, Turner A N, Rees A J, Pusey C D. Long-term outcome of anti-glomerular basement membrane antibody disease treated with plasma exchange and immunosuppression. *Ann Intern Med.* 2001;134(11):1033-42.

In: Issues in Kidney Disease – Acute Kidney Injury
Editors: S. Z. Fadem and A. Arslan Yousuf Awan

ISBN: 978-1-68507-002-1

Chapter 11

ACUTE KIDNEY INJURY SECONDARY TO DYSPROTEINEMIAS

Sohail Riaz, MD and Pascale Khairallah*, MD
Selzman Institute for Kidney Health, Section of Nephrology, Department of Medicine, Baylor College of Medicine, Houston, TX, USA

ABSTRACT

Dysproteinemias encompass a group of diseases which are characterized by the overproduction of immunoglobulins. Some immunoglobulins are present in high concentrations that classify them as a hematologic malignancy. In some cases, the immunoglobulin is present in low quantities that do not classify it as a hematological malignancy; however, they can cause kidney injury via various mechanisms. This entity is referred to as monoclonal gammopathy of renal significance (MGRS). MGRS results in acute kidney injury which can result in progressive chronic kidney disease and eventual end-stage kidney disease if untreated. Diagnosis, workup, and management will be discussed in detail.

Keywords: monoclonal gammopathy, electrophoresis, kappa, gamma, light chains, heavy chains

INTRODUCTION

Dysproteinemias encompass a group of diseases which are characterized by the overproduction of immunoglobulins. These monoclonal immunoglobulins (MIg) are a result of clonal proliferation of immunoglobulin-producing cells (plasma cells or B cells). Dysproteinemias can cause acute kidney injury (AKI) secondary to various forms of injury in different locations in the kidney. Nephrologists should be actively involved in the management

* Corresponding Author's E-mail: Pascale.khairallah@bcm.edu.

of paraprotein-mediated disorders and not defer completely to oncologists. Usually there is only one type of paraprotein-associated kidney disorder present at one time. In this chapter, different types of dysproteinemias, their clinical presentation, diagnosis and treatment, as well as their presentation in the kidney biopsy will be highlighted.

Multiple myeloma (MM) is caused by the presence of ≥10% plasma cell clonal proliferation, the detection of an M protein >3g/dl in the serum and the presence of defining features (Table 1).

Monoclonal gammopathy of undetermined significance (MGUS) is diagnosed when there is <10% plasma cell clonal proliferation, <3g/dl of an M protein in the serum and no defining MM features. In some cases, the MIg is present in low quantities that do not classify it as a hematological malignancy, however, they can cause kidney injury via various mechanisms. This entity is referred to as monoclonal gammopathy of renal significance (MGRS). MGRS results in AKI which can result in progressive chronic kidney disease (CKD) and eventual end-stage kidney disease (ESKD) if untreated (Table 1).

DIAGNOSIS

Monoclonal protein testing can be done to screen for the disease, confirm the disease, and as a tool to follow up response to treatment (Table 2).

MIg is usually screened for or diagnosed by serum protein electrophoresis (SPEP). Adding immunofixation and serum free light chain assay increases the sensitivity even further to >97%. Therefore, most experts will recommend performing all 3 tests for screening and/or diagnosis.

24-hour urine collection for protein electrophoresis and immunofixation will increase the sensitivity of the other tests even further, therefore it is reserved in cases when SPEP/immunofixation/serum free light chain assays are negative (Table 2 and 3).

The serum free light chain assay is a ratio of κ to λ light chains which is significantly increased in the case of a κ light chain–producing clone and significantly decreased in the case of a λ light chain–producing clone. Thus, the normal free κ-to-λ ratio is 0.26 – 1.65. Importantly, in the setting of impaired renal function, the ratio rises to 0.34 – 3.1 owing to reduced renal clearance. The presence of a κ-clone or λ-clone is inferred from an abnormal ratio (Table 2 and 3).

For definitive diagnosis, however, a bone marrow or lymph node biopsy is required. If a kidney biopsy is performed before the above tests are conducted, then immunofluorescence performed on the kidney tissue using different antibodies targeting different immunoglobulins (heavy chains of IgG, IgM, and IgA, Ig light chains (κ and λ), and IgG subclasses (IgG1–IgG4)) will specify which immunoglobulin is causing the kidney disease.

Clinical Pearls
• Dysproteinemias can cause acute kidney injury (AKI) secondary to various forms of injury in different locations in the kidney.
• Usually there is only one type of paraprotein associated kidney disorder present at one time.

Table 1. Hematologic conditions associated with kidney diseases

	Monoclonal Gammopathy of Unknown Significance (MGUS)	**Monoclonal Gammopathy of Clinical Significance (MGCS)**	**Monoclonal Gammopathy of Renal Significance (MGRS)**	**Smoldering Multiple Myeloma**	**Multiple Myeloma**
Diagnosis	<10% Clonal bone marrow plasma cells without myeloma-defining events or amyloidosis	<10% Clonal bone marrow plasma cells with organ involvement (skin, nervous system, kidney, etc.)	<10% Clonal bone marrow plasma cells with one or more kidney lesions that are related to the immunoglobulin	10% – 60% Clonal bone marrow plasma cells without myeloma-defining events or amyloidosis	Clonal plasma cell disorder with ≥10% clonal bone marrow plasma cells AND myeloma-defining events which include: hypercalcemia, renal insufficiency, anemia or bone disease.
Lab Abnormality	<3 g/dl M protein	<3 g/dl M protein	<3 g/dl M protein	≥3g/dl Serum M protein (IgG or IgA) or ≥500mg/24h urinary M protein	M protein in serum and/or urine

Table 2. Tests used to screen monoclonal gammopathies

Test	How It Is Performed	What It Is Measuring	Sensitivity
SPEP	separates proteins by electrophoresis on agarose gel or using light absorbance techniques by capillary zone followed by quantification of the M protein using densitometer tracing of the gel	Quantifies the monoclonal protein in the serum	64%
UPEP	separates proteins by electrophoresis on agarose gel or using light absorbance techniques by capillary zone followed by quantification of the M protein using densitometer tracing of the gel	Quantifies the monoclonal protein in the urine	75%
IFE	applies antibodies to the specific Ig heavy- and light-chain components	Classifies the immunoglobulin	93%
Serum Free light chain assay		quantitation of total serum free (unbound) κ-light chain and λ-light chain	88%

Table 3. Serum, urine and bone marrow findings of different monoclonal gammopathies

	Monoclonal Protein	SPEP or UPEP	SIFE or UIFE	Bone Marrow
Multiple Myeloma	Kappa>Lambda	Positive	Positive	High % PC
AL Amyloidosis	Lambda>Kappa	Often negative	Usually positive	Low % PC
LCDD	Kappa>Lambda	Often positive	Usually positive	Low % PC
LHCDD	Kappa>Lambda	Often positive	Usually positive	Low % PC
Immunotactoid GN	Usually none	Negative	Usually negative	Usually normal
PGNMID	Kappa>Lambda	Often negative	May be negative	Low % PC
C3 glomerulopathy	Kappa>Lambda	Often negative	May be negative	Low % PC
Cast Nephropathy	Kappa>Lambda	Often positive	Often positive	High % PC
Fibrillary GN	Lambda>Kappa	Often negative	Often negative	Low % PC

Clinical Pearls

- MIg is usually screened or diagnosed by serum protein electrophoresis (SPEP). Adding immunofixation and serum free light chain assay increases the sensitivity even further to >97%
- Multiple myeloma (MM) is caused by the presence of ≥10% plasma cell clonal proliferation, the detection of an M protein >3 g/dl in the serum and the presence of defining features

Clinical Presentation

The physicochemical properties and size of the MIg are important as they determine where in the kidney the MIg will deposit, and as such dictate the clinical presentation. MIg can deposit in the glomeruli, in the tubulointerstitium, or in the blood vessels.

Glomerular Deposition

Ig Light Chain Amyloidosis/Ig Heavy Chain Amyloidosis

Amyloidosis is caused by protein misfolding, which leads to protein aggregation and fibril formation. Amyloidosis (light or heavy chain) usually presents with nephrotic-range proteinuria owing to the deposition of amyloid in the glomerulus. Amyloid can also deposit in the tubulointerstitial space and in the blood vessels. When no glomerular deposition is involved, patients will present with progressive CKD and with autonomic dysfunction with orthostatic hypotension as a major feature. Patients usually have cardiac involvement, as well; and the extent of cardiac involvement is the primary determinant of survival [1].

A monoclonal protein can be detected in 95% of cases using a combination of SPEP with IFE and urine IFE. However, the most sensitive test is serum free light chain assay which will be abnormal in >98% of patients. The latter can be used for diagnosis and to monitor treatment response.

On light microscopy, kidney biopsy will show amyloid pale pink deposits in the mesangium and spikes in the glomerular basement membranes. The amyloid deposits can also involve the blood vessels. When the Congo red staining method is utilized, an apple-green birefringence will present under polarized light. Immunofluorescence will show predominant stain for either lambda (the most common form of amyloid) or kappa light chain or for heavy chain (the rarest form of amyloid). On electron microscopy, amyloid fibrils with a diameter of 7 - 12nm are randomly arranged in the mesangium and glomerular basement membrane. Foot process effacement is also seen (AJKD atlas of pathology figures).

Treatment of Ig Amyloidosis has improved through the years. Bortezomib, dexamethasone, and cyclophosphamide or bortezomib, dexamethasone, and melphalan remain the most commonly used first-line treatments for patients with AL amyloidosis. Daratumumab-based regimens are increasingly being used. Stem cell transplant (SCT) is the preferred treatment, but only 20% of patients are eligible. Requirements for safe SCT include systolic blood pressure >90 mmHg, troponin T < 0.06 ng/mL and serum creatinine ≤1.7mg/dL [2].

Clinical Pearls

- Amyloidosis is caused by protein misfolding which leads to protein aggregation and fibril formation.
- Bortezomib, dexamethasone, and cyclophosphamide or bortezomib, dexamethasone, and melphalan remain the most commonly used first-line treatments for patients with AL amyloidosis. Daratumumab-based regimens are increasingly being used.

Monoclonal Immunoglobulin Deposition Disease (MIDD)

MIDD is classified into three types [3]:

- light chain deposition disease (LCDD) where deposits are composed of light chains only (in most cases the deposits are composed of κ-light chains),
- heavy chain deposition disease (HCDD) where deposits are composed of truncated γ-chains,
- light heavy chain deposition (LHCD) disease where deposits are composed of both light and heavy chains.

These chains deposit in the mesangium, glomerular, and tubular basement membranes; therefore, patients present with proteinuria and AKI, which can progress to CKD. The chains can also deposit in other organs. The extra-renal deposition and presence of concomitant multiple myeloma are the main determinants of patient survival.

In LCDD, a monoclonal protein can be detected in 65% of cases using SPEP with IFE. However, the most sensitive test is serum free light chain assay which will be abnormal in almost all patients with LCDD.

Light microscopy on kidney biopsy will show mesangial expansion in early stages of the disease and nodular sclerosis in later stages of the disease. Immunofluorescence will show monoclonal light chain staining in the mesangium, glomerular, and tubular basement membranes. On electron microscopy, ground-pepper-like deposits in the mesangium, glomerular, and tubular basement membranes and foot process effacement are seen.

Treatment of LCDD consists of regimens that target the hematologic clone such as bortezomib-based regimens. Stem cell transplantation can also be done in select cases.

In HCDD, 80% of cases can be detected by SPEP with IFE. However, the most sensitive test is serum free light chain assay which will be abnormal in almost all patients with HCDD.

Upon examination of a kidney biopsy, utilization of light microscopy (LM) shows glomerular, tubular basement membrane and arterial wall deposits; and in more advanced cases, nodular sclerosis. Immunofluorescence (IF) will show staining for monoclonal heavy chain, and electron microscopy (EM) will show deposits along the glomerulus, tubular basement membrane and arterial wall. With utilization of electron microscopy, ground-pepper-like deposits and double contours may be seen.

As with light chain deposition disease (LCDD), treatment of HCDD consists of regimens that target the hematologic clone with mainly bortezomib-based regimens. Stem cell transplantation can also be done in select cases.

MIDD is classified into three types: LCDD where deposits are composed of light chains only (in most cases the deposits are composed of κ-light chains), HCDD where deposits are composed of truncated γ-chains, and LHCD disease where deposits are composed of both light and heavy chains.

Monoclonal Gammopathy-Associated Proliferative Glomerulonephritis

This includes 2 main diseases:

- Proliferative glomerulonephritis with monoclonal immunoglobulin deposits (PGNMID),
- C3 glomerulopathy with monoclonal gammopathy

PGNMID

PGNMID is the result of glomerular MIg deposition in mesangial and glomerular capillary wall distribution. The most common monoclonal immunoglobulin found in PGNMID biopsies is IgG3κ (50%) followed by IgG3λ (15%). Patients present with proteinuria, hematuria, and AKI. Serum complement levels are low in a significant number of patients [4].

With PGNMID, most patients will NOT have positive SPEP or abnormal free light chain assays.

Kidney biopsy will show membranoproliferative pattern and glomerular basement membrane double contours on light microscopy. Immunofluorescence will stain for monoclonal immunoglobulins which most commonly is IgG3κ (50%) followed by IgG3λ (15%). C3 deposits are seen in certain cases. Electron microscopy is positive for mesangial and subendothelial deposits.

In patients with PGNMID in whom a clone is detected, treatment includes clone-directed therapy. If the clone is a plasma-cell clone, then bortezomib-based regimens are preferred. If the clone is a B-cell clone, then rituximab-based regimens as most B cell clones are CD20 positive. In patients who have no detectable clone but have a detectable immunoglobulin in the serum or urine, then chemotherapy is advised to treat the monoclonal immunoglobulin. In patients without a detectable clone and without a detectable immunoglobulin in the serum or urine, chemotherapy is typically reserved for patients with worsening kidney function or >1g of proteinuria [5].

C3 Glomerulopathy with Monoclonal Gammopathy

C3 glomerulopathy with monoclonal gammopathy refers to a group of patients who have a detectable monoclonal gammopathy as well as staining for C3 on the kidney biopsy. It is hypothesized that the MIg activates the alternate complement pathway resulting in C3 deposition [6].

In one study, 38% of patients had positive serum or urine IFE.

Kidney biopsy is notable for mesangial proliferative lesions on light microscopy and C3 mesangial staining on immunofluorescence. Electron microscopy shows mesangial and capillary wall deposits [7].

Treatment is similar to other MIg diseases where clone-directed therapy is used.

- PGNMID is the result of glomerular MIg deposition in mesangial and glomerular capillary wall distribution and in C3 glomerulopathy with monoclonal gammopathy. It is hypothesized that the MIg activates the alternate complement pathway resulting in C3 deposition. Treatment for both includes clone-directed therapy.
- If the clone is a plasma-cell clone, then bortezomib-based regimens are preferred. If the clone is a B-cell clone, then rituximab-based regimens as most B cell clones are CD20 positive.

IMMUNOTACTOID GLOMERULOPATHY

Immunotactoid glomerulopathy is due to IgG deposits in the glomerulus, and capillary walls. Therefore, patients present with proteinuria, hematuria, and nephrotic syndrome. They can also present with hypertension (HTN) and AKI.

Hematologic disorders are present in 66% of patients, including lymphoma in 41% (mainly chronic lymphocytic leukemia/small lymphocytic lymphoma), monoclonal gammopathy in 20%, and multiple myeloma in 6% [8].

The most common pattern in immunotactoid GN is membranoproliferative with mesangial expansion, hypercellularity, and double contouring. Large subendothelial deposits can be seen in some cases.

Table 4. Biopsy Findings of different monoclonal gammopathies

	Glomerular Nodularity	Mesangial PAS	Proliferative Changes	Congo Red	Fibrils
Multiple Myeloma	Yes	Strong	No	No	No
AL Amyloidosis	Yes	Weak	No	Yes	Yes
LCDD	Yes	Strong	No	No	No
LHCDD	Yes	Strong	No	No	No
Immunotactoid GN	No	No	No	No	Yes
PGNMID	No	Weak	Yes	No	No
C3 glomerulopathy	Yes	Weak	Yes	No	No
Cast Nephropathy	No	No	No	No	No
Fibrillary GN	No	Strong	Yes	No	Yes

It could also present with thickening basement membranes and spikes either globally or segmentally. With immunofluorescence, nearly 90% have IgG staining. C3 staining follows the same pattern as the IgG [9].

Fibrillary GN

Fibrillary GN is a rare form of glomerulonephritis that is characterized by the ultrastructural finding of organized, randomly oriented, nonbranching fibrils with a mean diameter of 20nm (range 15 – 25nm).

The diagnosis of FGN can only be established by renal biopsy, and the incidence of FGN in native renal biopsies is less than 1%. Fibrillary GN presents with 5 different types of glomerular involvement. Mesangial proliferative GN is the most common pattern in FGN seen in approximately 70% of patients [10].

4 - 43% of patients have a monoclonal gammopathy. Other conditions associated with fibrillary GN include malignancies, autoimmune diseases, and diabetes [11].

TUBULAR DEPOSITION

Light Chain Cast Nephropathy

Multiple myeloma (MM) is one of the most common hematologic malignancies. Up to 30% of patients with MM will present with AKI and in most patients with AKI, the underlying case is myeloma cast nephropathy. In myeloma cast nephropathy, casts bind to the Tamm-Horsfall protein in the distal tubules resulting in obstruction and inflammatory reaction. Medications that precipitate cast nephropathy include NSAIDs and ACEIs/ARBs.

AKI is the most common presentation. Proteinuria but not albuminuria will be detected in the urine. If the diagnosis of cast nephropathy precedes the diagnosis of MIg, then a detailed evaluation for the underlying type of hematological malignancy should be performed.

A kidney biopsy is the gold standard for diagnosis of cast nephropathy. Serum free light chain is abnormal in almost all cases and when >500mg/dL are pathognomonic for cast nephropathy obviating the need for a kidney biopsy [12]

Treatment should be initiated as soon as possible following diagnosis in order to reduce the concentration of free light chains in an attempt to reverse the kidney injury. A 60% reduction of in serum free light chains within 2 - 3 weeks is usually associated with improvement in kidney function [13]. Patients are typically treated with a 3-drug regimen including high dose steroids and bortezomib. There is currently no role for plasmapheresis in aiding with the removal of serum free light chains [14].

Clinical Pearls

- In myeloma cast nephropathy, casts bind to the Tamm-Horsfall protein in distal tubules resulting in obstruction and inflammatory reaction.
- Patients with cast nephropathy are typically treated with a 3-drug regimen including high dose steroids and bortezomib. There is currently no role for plasmapheresis in aiding with the removal of serum free light chains.

Light Chain Proximal Tubulopathy (LCPT)

LCPT is characterized by cytoplasmic inclusions of monoclonal light chains (more commonly κ than λ) within proximal tubular cells. Patients present with proteinuria and AKI and classically Fanconi syndrome with hypophosphatemia, hypokalemia, hypouricemia, glucosuria and aminoaciduria.

Crystalline LCPTs are κ-restricted and display acute tubular injury. One-third of noncrystalline LCPT patients display λ-restriction or acute tubular injury [12].

Achievement of remission of the underlying hematologic malignancy is the cornerstone of therapy. Treatment of Fanconi syndrome resultant electrolyte abnormalities should occur as well.

REFERENCES

[1] Leung N, Bridoux F, Batuman V, Chaidos A, Cockwell P, D'Agati VD, et al. The evaluation of monoclonal gammopathy of renal significance: a consensus report of the International Kidney and Monoclonal Gammopathy Research Group. *Nat Rev Nephrol.* 2019;15(1):45–59.

[2] Varga C, Titus SE, Toskic D, Comenzo RL. Use of novel therapies in the treatment of light chain amyloidosis. *Blood Rev.* 2019;37:100581.

[3] Nasr SH, Valeri AM, Cornell LD, Fidler ME, Sethi S, D'Agati VD, et al. Renal monoclonal immunoglobulin deposition disease: a report of 64 patients from a single institution. *Clin J Am Soc Nephrol.* 2012;7(2):231–9.

[4] Nasr SH, Satoskar A, Markowitz GS, Valeri AM, Appel GB, Stokes MB, et al. Proliferative glomerulonephritis with monoclonal IgG deposits. *J Am Soc Nephrol.* 2009;20(9):2055–64.

[5] Gumber R, Cohen JB, Palmer MB, Kobrin SM, Vogl DT, Wasserstein AG, et al. A clone-directed approach may improve diagnosis and treatment of proliferative glomerulonephritis with monoclonal immunoglobulin deposits. *Kidney Int.* 2018;94(1):199–205.

[6] Chauvet S, Frémeaux-Bacchi V, Petitprez F, Karras A, Daniel L, Burtey S, et al. Treatment of B-cell disorder improves renal outcome of patients with monoclonal gammopathy-associated C3 glomerulopathy. *Blood.* 2017;129(11):1437–47.

[7] Ravindran A, Fervenza FC, Smith RJ, Sethi S. C3 glomerulopathy associated with monoclonal Ig is a distinct subtype. *Kidney Int.,* 2018;94:178 - 186. Kidney Int. 2018;94(5):1025.

[8] Nasr SH, Kudose SS, Said SM, Santoriello D, Fidler ME, Williamson SR, et al. Immunotactoid glomerulopathy is a rare entity with monoclonal and polyclonal variants. *Kidney Int.* 2021;99(2):410-420

[9] Rosenstock JL, Markowitz GS, Valeri AM, Sacchi G, Appel GB, D'Agati VD. Fibrillary and immunotactoid glomerulonephritis: distinct entities with different clinical and pathologic features. *Kidney Int.* 2003 Apr;63(4):1450–61.

[10] Fogo A, Qureshi N, Horn RG. Morphologic and clinical features of fibrillary glomerulonephritis versus immunotactoid glomerulopathy. *Am J Kidney Dis.* 1993 Sep;22(3):367–77.

[11] Rosenstock JL, Markowitz GS. Fibrillary Glomerulonephritis: an Update. *Kidney Int* Rep. 2019 Apr;4(7):917–22.

[12] Hutchison CA, Plant T, Drayson M, Cockwell P, Kountouri M, Basnayake K, et al. Serum free light chain measurement aids the diagnosis of myeloma in patients with severe renal failure. *BMC Nephrol.* 2008;9:11.

[13] Hutchison CA, Cockwell P, Stringer S, Bradwell A, Cook M, Gertz MA, et al. Early reduction of serum-free light chains associates with renal recovery in myeloma kidney. *J Am Soc Nephrol*. 2011;22(6):1129–36.

[14] Clark WF, Stewart AK, Rock GA, Sternbach M, Sutton DM, Barrett BJ, et al.; Canadian Apheresis Group. Plasma exchange when myeloma presents as acute renal failure: a randomized, controlled trial. *Ann Intern Med*. 2005;143(11):777–84.

In: Issues in Kidney Disease – Acute Kidney Injury
Editors: S. Z. Fadem and A. Arslan Yousuf Awan
ISBN: 978-1-68507-002-1

Chapter 12

ACUTE KIDNEY INJURY AND COVID-19

Stephen Z. Fadem**, MD, FACP, FASN
Selzman Institute for Kidney Health, Section of Nephrology, Department of Medicine,
Baylor College of Medicine, Houston, TX, USA
Michael E. DeBakey VA Medical Center, Houston, TX, USA
Kidney Associates, Houston, TX, USA

ABSTRACT

The SARS-CoV-2 virus has disrupted an entire planet creating a pandemic that has led to 1.3 million global deaths in a 10-month period. It is a spiked virus that attaches to an ACE2 receptor on lung and respiratory cells. In addition to damage caused by the virus, ACE2 receptor binding causes an increase in angiotensin 2, which also can damage cells. Targeting respiratory cells can result in acute respiratory distress syndrome, requiring assisted ventilation. This population of critically ill patients frequently develops acute kidney injury. Patients with chronic kidney disease are more susceptible to having bad outcomes from COVID-19. African Americans with two APOL1 gene variants are at risk to develop collapsing glomerulopathy as the consequence of increased interferon production by viral infected cells. Transplant patients are also more likely to have poor outcomes from COVID-19. Although transplantation was halted for a brief time early in the pandemic, the number of kidney transplants performed in 2020 is similar to 2019. Vaccines were developed and implemented against the SARS-CoV-2 virus. However, mutations threaten at least blunted resistance to the vaccines unless boosters can be developed. It is not clear whether effective neutralizing antibody responses to the currently available SARS-CoV-2 vaccines will fully develop and protect patients with advanced kidney disease and transplant populations, and until this question is answered, CKD and transplant patients should remain vigilant with respect to wearing masks and social distancing.

Keywords: COVID-19, AKI, acute kidney injury, SARS-CoV-2, coronavirus, pandemic

---

* Corresponding Author's E-mail: fadem@bcm.edu.

INTRODUCTION

In mid-November 2019, a shopper at the Huanan Seafood Wholesale Market in Wuhan, China became ill with an unusual type of pneumonia. Others were soon determined to have a similar pneumonia presentation associated with fever and cough. By December 15, there were 27 cases. Within two additional weeks, the number of cases had reached 44, and the World Health Organization (WHO) was notified. It was determined that this was a novel virus and, by January 7, its genetic code was determined and shared internationally. The virus was thought to originate in bats and possibly spread to a secondary animal. It was found to be a coronavirus, highly similar to the SARS virus of 2003. By January 31, the viral disease was declared a global health emergency by WHO. By March 11, it was declared a pandemic. By November 14, there were 53,747,027 global cases with 1,308,122 deaths. 245,453 of these deaths were in the United States (SOURCE: http://coronavirus.jhu.edu - accessed November 14, 2020).

The knowledge and literature surrounding COVID-19 is rapidly evolving. To date, there is no definitive cure for COVID-19. Most people will have a mild course, but the elderly and those with underlying medical conditions such as diabetes, chronic kidney disease, or kidney transplants are highly vulnerable to have bad outcomes. Efforts to mitigate the spread of the disease are limited to social distancing and the avoidance of crowd gathering. Such efforts also include wearing a face mask in public, frequent sanitizing of one's hands and touch-point surfaces, as well as the act of self-quarantine when one begins to feel sick. Vaccines and monoclonal antibodies show great promise for the general population. But it is not clear whether they will sufficiently protect the immunocompromised host, such as the patient who has received an organ transplant.

SARS-CoV-2

The SARS-CoV-2 virus consists of a nucleocapsid of RNA that is surrounded by a membrane that includes envelope proteins and spike proteins, S1 and S2. The crown-like spikes on the outer edge of the virus particle gives the virus its name, coronavirus. The S2 proteins connect with the membrane and terminate at the other end with a fusion protein that is bound to the S1 protein that contains the receptor binding domain (RBD). Through an evolutionary process that refined the coronavirus from SARS-CoV to SARS-CoV-2, the binding protein developed the ability to successfully attach to the ACE2 receptor. The ACE2 receptor is ubiquitous but found in the lungs in type II alveolar cells and the upper respiratory tract, heart, blood vessels, ileum, esophagus, and kidneys. Its binding promotes the activation of transmembrane serine protease 2 (TMPRSS2) that in turn cleaves S1 from S1, leaving the fusion protein exposed. It meanwhile liberates the ACE2 receptor from the membrane so that either fusion or endocytosis can allow the virus to enter the cell. Once inside the cell, the RNA can break out of its membrane shell and transcribe new RNA as well as assemble a new envelope-membrane-spike package that produces new viral particles ready for exocytosis.

The ACE2 receptor is anti-inflammatory by breaking down angiotensin 2 from a 9 amino acid to a 7 amino acid peptide, and by releasing the endogenous peptide, apelin, which also blocks the angiotensin 2 (AII) AT1R receptor. As the ACE2 receptor is internalized with the virus, its anti-inflammatory properties are diminished and no longer counterbalance

Angiotensin 2, leading to an increased AII effect. Angiotensin 2 plays a key role in the pathogenesis of kidney disease and is proinflammatory. It may play a key role in increasing vascular permeability and acute respiratory distress syndrome (ARDS), as well as play a role in the endothelial damage observed in patients with COVID-19 [1]. It may be that angiotensin receptor blockers such as losartan and valsartan, as well as converting enzyme inhibitors such as captopril and lisinopril, may be protective against the decrease in ACE2 receptor activity and consequent increase in angiotensin 2.

The activation of the innate immune system results in a series of inflammatory cytokines being released. These cytokines attack and destroy the virus and help set up an adaptive immune response – the development of antibodies. Unfortunately, the overstimulation of inflammatory cytokines can result in tissue damage known as the cytokine storm. The immune reaction is induced by toll-like receptors (TLR), a class of proteins that detect microbial signals. While there are several TLR pathways, all TLR activity culminates in the activation of NFκB, a protein complex that controls transcription [2]. It is both ubiquitous across the animal kingdom and involved in adverse stimuli including bacteria, viral particles, chemical agents, and ionizing radiation. Its activity is increased in aging and obesity and is upregulated by activation of the ATR1 receptor. ADAM17 is also upregulated by the ATR1 receptor and is responsible for increasing IL6 and tumor necrosis factor α(TNFα) responsiveness. TNFα, IL6 and interferons are released from the cell in response to viral stimuli. IL6 in turn amplifies NFκB activation.

It is not entirely clear whether the hypercoagulability, micro-thromboses, and vasculopathy are worsened by ACE2 receptor depletion, or consequent target organ damage is the direct result of endothelial infection by the virus, or the result of an inflammatory cytokine reaction to TNFα with triggering of the coagulation pathway. The coagulation cascade occurs when a series of serine proteases activate a chain of factors that result in thrombin, and the conversion of fibrinogen to a clot. The clot is then broken by plasmin activation. Tissue factors that initiate coagulation can be activated by inflammatory responses through G protein-coupled receptors, and procoagulant activation occurs on monocytes, macrophages and endothelial cells [3]. Tissue factors are exposed with endothelial damage and complex with factors VII to initiate the cascade that culminates in a clot. It is thus likely that endothelial cell vulnerability plays a role in initiating the coagulation response common in COVID-19.

Type 1 interferons (1-IFN) consist of a group of molecules that have potent antiviral activity. They are activated when toll-like receptors recognize viral particles early in the course of the disease, and their production is essential for an effective antiviral response. The interferons stimulate the receptors on inflammatory cells that turn on Janus-Kinase (JAK) signal transduction that in turn activates transcription through a mechanism known as the STAT pathway to turn on the responses each will play in fighting the virus. Interferons act on dendritic cells and macrophages. Dendritic cells have several functions, including the triggering of an adaptive immune response, the triggering of antigen presentation to T and B lymphocytes to differentiate and produce anti-viral antibodies. They also produce additional interferons and cytokines. In COVID-19, it is presently thought that macrophages are the major producers of inflammatory cytokines such as IL-6, TNFα, and other cytokines, and play a role in defense against the virus. They also play a role in promoting the cytokine storm associated with COVID-19. Lymphocyte depletion has been seen with COVID-19 and may also be the paradoxical consequence of a cytokine storm. Increased neutrophils are also part of the complex that results in the cytokine storm.

A balanced immune response may be the difference between a mild and a severely complicated course of COVID-19. This requires ample CD4 T cells that can activate a cytotoxic CD8 T cell response and promote neutralizing antibody formation. The aging patient is at high risk for severe complications from COVID-19, and this could relate to a lower density of ACE2 receptor, the availability of T cells, the functionality of T cells, and the ability to make antibodies. TLR response to the virus may be dampened in the elderly, who may have a lower proportion of interferon secreting cells [4]. Regardless of age, it appears viral load is a determinant of outcome [5].

COVID-19 and Chronic Kidney Disease

The association between COVID-19 and chronic kidney disease has been clear from the outset and is indeed universal. In a review of 336 consecutive patients in Istanbul, 61 had a baseline eGFR of less than <60 mL/min/1.73m^2. There was an independent association between eGFR on admission and mortality (Odds Ratio - OR 0.94 CI .956-.992 $p = 0.005$). Predictors of mortality in this study were age, eGFR, diabetes, hypertension, chronic obstructive pulmonary disease, and heart failure. Among the 336 patients admitted with an eGFR < 60 ml/min/1.73m^2 vs. those with a GFR $\geq$ 60 ml/min/1.73m^2 resulted in a significantly higher incidence of AKI ($p < 0.001$), ICU admissions 34.4 v 13.8% ($p < 0.001$) and mortality – 34.4 v 8% ($p < 0.001$) [6].

When a phenome-wide association study was performed at the Geisinger Health System, kidney disorders emerged as the strongest factor associated with hospitalization. End-stage renal disease or stage 5 CKD had odds ratios of 11.07, $p = 1.96X10^{-8}$ [7].

OpenSAFELY is a secure health analytics platform based in the United Kingdom. It was used to analyze 10,926 COVID-19 related deaths between February 1 and May 6, 2020. This population-based database analysis showed that CKD was a risk factor for COVID-19 mortality by comparing those with Stage 3 CKD (GFR 30-60 ml/min/1.73m^2) to those with Stage 4 & 5 CKD (GFR < 30 ml/min/1.73m^2) and those who had a kidney transplant. The hazard ratios (HR) in the CKD 3 group was 1.33 (CI 1.28-1.40) but with advanced CKD and transplantation jumped to 2.52 (CI 2.33-2.72) and 3.53 (CI 2.77-4.49) respectively. Reduced kidney function hazard ratios were higher than that of uncontrolled diabetes (1.95 CI 1.83-2.08). The database also revealed higher hazard ratios with BMI > 40 (1.92 CI 1.72-2.13). Ethnicity also played a role with Blacks having a HR of 1.48 (CI 1.29-1.69) [8].

A study from Wuhan included 49 hospitalized patients receiving maintenance hemodialysis and 52 patients who served as controls. All had COVID-19 and were evaluated between January 30 and March 10, 2020. Fever was a less common presentation in the dialysis population than controls (47 vs. 90%). CT scans of the lungs were more likely abnormal in the dialysis population (82 vs. 69% $p = 0.15$) but not significant. Shock, ARDS, and acute cardiac injury were significantly higher in patients undergoing dialysis; 25 vs. 6% required assisted ventilation ($P = 0.008$). The death rate was also higher in the dialysis population with a mortality rate of 14% in contrast to 4% in the non-dialysis group [9].

Although social distancing is an important practice that may help decrease the spread of the COVID-19 virus, it is impossible in the dialysis setting. The impact of COVID-19 on a dialysis patient was studied as management evolved. In a review of 1530 patients, 300 (19.6%)

developed COVID-19. Older age was a risk factor for infection. Clustering of cases around nursing staff, shifts and units was also observed. As management evolved, screening of symptoms and temperature were implemented and flattened the epidemic course to R = 2.2. The authors also found that transportation was not a factor. Although the most spacious units had the least number of infections, the infection rate was not linear [10].

ACUTE KIDNEY INJURY (AKI)

AKI and Critical Illness

Several studies have now confirmed an association between acute kidney injury (AKI) and COVID-19. Comorbidities are generally diabetes, hypertension, and chronic kidney disease. The AKI rate varied and was not reported in some series. But in the majority of studies, it occurred at between 3 to 5 percent in 4 studies to 8 percent and above in 13 studies, as published in the 25th Acute Disease Quality Initiative Workgroup report. In a New York series of 1,000 patients up to 34% had AKI, of which 78% were in the ICU. In a multicenter study of 2,215 patients, 43% had AKI and 20% required renal replacement therapy. Risk factors for AKI in COVID-19 patients include older age, diabetes, hypertension cardiovascular disease, obesity, immunosuppression, smoking history and APOL1 or ACE2 polymorphisms. The degree of viremia and respiratory status plays a role, as does hypovolemia, the use of vasopressors, the administration of nephrotoxins, and the requirement for assisted ventilation [11].

A study by Ochsner Medical Center looked at 575 COVID-19 admissions in the New Orleans area. 70% were of African American origin and 34% were obese. 35% had preexisting chronic kidney disease. Most of the cases (70%) were ischemic acute tubular necrosis. 30% were admitted to the intensive care unit. The mortality rate of patients who developed AKI during admission was 50% [12].

A large study of 5,449 patients admitted to 13 New York hospitals between March 1 to April 5 with COVID-19 demonstrated an AKI rate of 36.6%. This was strongly associated with respiratory failure, as 87.7% of patients developed AKI as opposed to the development of AKI in 21.7% of patients not on assisted ventilation. 52.2% developed AKI within 24 hours of intubation. There were 694 deaths among the AKI patients, 35% of the subpopulation of AKI [13].

AKI is a major complication of COVID-19, leading to the emergence of several possible explanations for its pathogenesis. In a review by Batlle et al. [14], the authors comment on autopsy findings from deceased COVID-19 patients. Although proximal tubular injury is present, so is evidence of microvascular injury - peritubular erythrocyte aggregation, fibrin thrombi and ischemic collapse, endothelial damage, and hemosiderin deposition. The report also includes other autopsy reports that confirm increased clotting and disseminated intravascular coagulation, microthrombi and elevated d-dimer levels. Early biopsies were felt to demonstrate viral particles, suggesting trophism [15-17]. Although it is a source of controversy, more recent studies have found no evidence of SARS-CoV-2 viral particles by either electron microscopy, immunochemistry or in situ hybridization. Viral particles have not been demonstrated in pathology samples reviewed in more recent articles. Acute tubular necrosis was a common finding in a series of 10 kidney biopsies performed in patients with

COVID-19. In this series, five of the patients were Black, two were White, and three were Hispanic. All the patients had proteinuria, and 8 had severe AKI requiring renal replacement therapy. Two of the patients had microangiopathy; one of the Black patients had collapsing glomerulonephritis; and the other had pauci-immune crescentic glomerulonephritis. No viral particles were found [18].

In a renal biopsy study of a population of patients who developed kidney disease during admission for COVID-19, 15 of 17 had AKI and 9 had the nephrotic syndrome. 16 of the 17 patients were either hypertensive, obese, diabetic, or had either cancer, kidney, or heart transplants. In 9 of the biopsied patients, pneumonia was present. The biopsies revealed 4 instances of acute tubular necrosis, 5 cases of collapsing glomerulonephritis, and 2 of membranous glomerulonephritis. There was 1 each of crescentic lupus nephritis, anti-glomerular basement membrane (GBM) disease or minimal change disease. This series suggested that patients with preexisting glomerular disease had a high likelihood of developing COVID-19 disease, but also demonstrated the relationship between collapsing glomerulonephritis and COVID-19. The patient with minimal change glomerulonephritis and three of the patients with collapsing nephropathy had the high risk APOL1 gene variants. There were no viral particles seen in the biopsy specimens [19].

Collapsing Glomerulonephritis and the APOL1 Story

The tsetse fly in Africa is similar to the house fly but, with one exception, it is a vampire. It has a long proboscis and can bite mammals. In the process it can transfect humans with protozoans such as the trypanosome. These unicellular motile parasites develop in the gut of the fly and move to the salivary ducts. In humans who have been bitten, the trypanosomes easily cross the blood-brain barrier and cause disease resulting in seizures, ataxia, and mental deterioration. The disease has been termed African sleeping sickness.

APOL1 is an apolipoprotein that is involved in autophagy. It kills invading trypanosomes by inducing chloride channels in their lysosomes, causing them to swell. But over centuries the trypanosomes developed resistance. That resistance was overcome with genetic variants referred to as G1 and G2 that produced minor variations in APOL1 and enabled a successful attack and defeat of the trypanosome. African Americans with two copies of the gene variant are at higher risk for chronic kidney disease, lupus and HIV associated nephritis, preeclampsia, end-stage renal disease, and focal sclerosing glomerulosclerosis – particularly collapsing glomerulonephritis. Collapsing GN has been associated with receiving therapeutic interferon in patients who have had two variants of the APOL1 gene. Viruses such as HIV and COVID-10 also stimulate interferons, and receptors for interferon are found at the APOL1 transcription start site. When interferons stimulate these APOL1 receptors, they turn on Janus-Kinase (JAK) signal transduction, activating the STAT pathway. In turn, interferons are stimulated [20]. Interferons can also stimulate APOL1 expression 200 fold [21].

In one series, 6 African American patients with a mean serum creatinine of 6.5 mg/dL/1.73m^2 underwent kidney biopsies. They were all diagnosed with COVID-19, and all had high risk APOL1 gene variations. The kidney biopsy showed collapsing glomerulonephritis, foot process effacement and acute tubular injury. No viral particles were seen [22]. This has also been demonstrated in other kidney biopsies of COVID-19 patients [19].

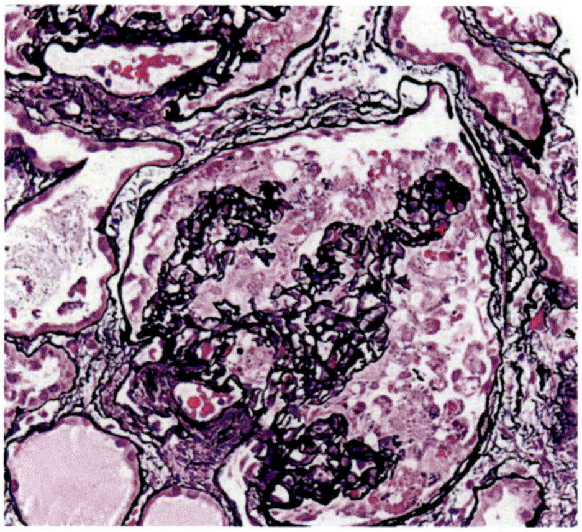

Figure 1. Silver stain showing a collapsed glomerular tuft in a patient with COVID-19 collapsing glomerulonephritis (Picture courtesy of Luong Truong, Houston Methodist Hospital).

It appears that COVID-19 induces interferon which increases APOL1 transcription. It has been suggested that high levels of APOL1 underlie podocyte injury. Just how APOL1 is related to the podocyte damage resulting in collapsing glomerulonephritis is being elucidated. It has been shown that when APOL1 localizes to the podocyte surface, the pore-forming domain is exposed. The endoplasmic reticulum is a tubular organelle that is lined with ribosomes. A main function of the ER is to synthesize and fold proteins. It has been shown that APOL1 is found and causes damage in the plasma membrane, mitochondrion, and endoplasmic reticulum and plasma membrane [23-29].

COVID-19 AND KIDNEY TRANSPLANTATION

Kidney transplant patients who develop COVID-19 have worse outcomes. A study in Paris looked at 66 transplant patients with COVID-19. In this group the mean age was 56.4 ± 12.5. Obesity was a risk factor with an odds ratio (OR) of 2.19 (95%CI 1.19-4.05; P = 0.01). Patients with lung disease such as asthma or COPD had a high OR of 3.09 (CI 1.49-6.41; P = 0.0002), as did diabetics (OR 3.33 CI 1.92-5.77; p < 0.001) The mortality rate in the transplant subset with COVID-19 patients was 24% in contrast to 1% for non-transplanted COVID-19 patients [30].

In a study of 36 transplant patients at Montefiore Medical Center with COVID-19, 34 (94%) had hypertension, 25 (69%) had diabetes mellitus, 13 (36%) were either present or former smokers, and 6 (17%) had cardiac disease. 14 patients were Black (39%), and 15 were Hispanic (42%). Major symptoms were fever (21;58%) and diarrhea (8;22%). Laboratory markers demonstrated lymphopenia in 22 (79%) of patients, thrombocytopenia in 12 (43%) of patients, a C-reactive protein greater than 5 mg/dL in 12 (43%) of patients, D-dimer greater than 0.5 μg/dL in 12 (43%) patients, a low CD3 in 19 (68%), low CD4 in 20 (71%), and a low CD8 in 8 (29%) patients. 78% of patients required hospitalization and 8 (22%) were treated at home. 21% (6 patients) required renal replacement therapy. 11 (39%) patients required intubation, of whom 7 died. The death rate in the transplanted patients with COVID-19 was

28% (10 patients). The transplant patients with COVID-19 had a rapid deterioration compared with the general population, and a higher mortality rate [31].

A review of data from over 50 transplant centers demonstrated that solid organ transplants have a mortality rate of 20.5%. 66% of the patients were either kidney or kidney/pancreas recipients [32].

The COVID-19 pandemic had an impact on the number of kidney transplants performed during the initial days of the epidemic. In a survey of 63 transplant centers, complete suspension of live donor transplantation occurred in 71.8% of centers. 98.4% of centers limited visits, and 96.8% adopted telemedicine [33]. This was associated with a general lockdown and suspension of elective surgery nationwide during March and April. Several patients had transplants cancelled as a result of the pandemic creating stress, confusion, and feelings of despair among patients [34]. During the month of April, transplantation in the USA started to increase as hospitals adopted strategies to minimize risks to patients and staff. Deceased donor transplants have surpassed 2019, while living related donor transplants have lagged. Year-to-date donor transplants for 2020 are nearly equal to those of 2019.

Table 1. UNOS data comparing the number of kidney transplants with year to date from 2020 with 2019

	11/12/2019	11/12/2020
Living donor	5,898	4,547
Deceased donor	14,294	15,268
All transplants	20,241	19,815

Source: https://unos.org/covid accessed 11/14/2020.

Vaccines and Variants

There are currently three vaccines available in the USA; two are messenger RNA (mRNA) varieties; the third is a viral vector vaccine. None of these vaccines are live viruses. mRNA vaccines induce the immune system to make antibodies that will attack a future virus. The Pfizer BNT162b2 vaccine is administered in the deltoid over two injections three weeks apart. In a large clinical trial, 43,548 participants were randomized to receive either the placebo-control or vaccination. 8 cases of COVID-19 occurred 7 days after receiving the second vaccine dose in contrast to 162 cases among those who received the placebo; it was considered 95% effective. Side effects included headache, fatigue and injection site pain,; symptoms were short-lived. The occurrence of serious adverse events between the control and placebo group was similar [35].

The Moderna mRNA1273 vaccine is administered in two injections four weeks apart and has no concerning safety issues. 30,420 volunteers randomized to either placebo-control or vaccination group demonstrated an incidence of symptomatic COVID-19 cases after the second dose of the vaccine 94.1% lower than placebo. Of the 185 cases of symptomatic COVID-19 in the placebo group, 30 were severe. In the 11 cases of post vaccine COVID-19, none were severe. Local reactions included mild arm pain, headache, fatigue, and muscle aches [36].

The Johnson & Johnson (Janssen) vaccine Janssen's product, JNJ-78436735, is a viral vector vaccine that can be administered in either one or two doses. The single dose trial enrolled over 44,000 participants and was conducted in areas where variants were emerging. Its reported side effects included local arm pain, redness and swelling, as well as generalized fatigue, headache, muscle pain, fever, nausea and chills. It was 66.3% effective at preventing illness, and protection was noted two weeks post vaccine. It was 85% effective against preventing severe disease and completely protective against COVID-19 related hospitalizations and death.

As the virus infects more and more patients, it mutates, particularly in the spike protein area in response to neutralizing antibodies. This creates the potential for resistant strains. The two major variants are the B1.351 and the P.1 variant, both of which evolved during neutralizing antibody selection pressure. The B.1.351 variant is partially resistant to the Moderna, Pfizer and Novavax vaccinations. In South Africa, the JNJ vaccine was 95% effective against the B.1.351 variant. It is 69% effective against the P.2. variant in Brazil. In the USA it was 96% effective against the dominant D614G variant. It is not clear whether the vaccine is effective against the B.1.1.7 variant from the UK. All leading vaccine companies are in the process of redesigning their vaccines to counter the new variants [37].

There are currently two additional vaccines awaiting approval from use in the USA: the Astra Zeneca and the Novavax inoculations - both expected to be released this year. Astra Zeneca claims 79% effectiveness with a two-dose viral vector vaccine, AZD1222. Novavax's NVXCoV2373 is a protein inoculation that is dispensed in 2 doses three weeks apart.

So far there have been nearly 500 million persons worldwide who have been inoculated against COVID-19. In the USA there have been 128 million persons vaccinated. Presently, dialysis facilities are vaccinating patients as well as staff. Given the odds of dialysis patients having poor outcomes when contracting COVID-19, this is wise.

However, the immunogenicity of the mRNA SARS-CoV-2 vaccine against recipients of solid organ transplants has been called into question as the majority did not develop any appreciable neutralizing antibodies. This was demonstrated in a study of 436 transplant patients. Only 17% (CI, 14% to 21%) had an antibody response. An antibody response was less likely in patients on anti-metabolite maintenance. The Moderna mRNA-1273 was more effective than the Pfizer BNT162b2 (69% vs 31%, respectively; adjusted IRR, 2.15; CI 1.29 to 3.57; p=.003). The weakness of the study was that only one injection of two had been administered, and follow-up data will be essential to review [38].

CONCLUSION

The COVID-19 pandemic has disrupted life on this planet since its emergence in December 2019. However, it has had a particularly drastic impact on patients with kidney disease who have had outcomes worse even than diabetic patients. Patients who contract COVID-19 generally do well, but a fraction develops severe respiratory disease. This fraction is more likely to develop acute kidney injury. Patients with APOL1 gene variants are at risk to develop collapsing glomerulopathy. The pathogenesis related to kidney disease appears to be indirect and may be the consequence of interferons and other cytokines, microvascular disease, and the acute tubular necrosis associated with multisystem failure and critical illness.

Transplant patients are especially vulnerable to have severe consequences of COVID-19. Despite a lockdown period where elective surgery and transplantation stopped in March, the number of kidney transplants performed in the USA has not significantly decreased. Although it is recommended that transplant recipients receive the COVID-19 vaccine, preliminary studies suggest they will have a relatively poor response.

REFERENCES

[1] Iwasaki M, Saito J, Zhao H, Sakamoto A, Hirota K, Ma D, et al. Inflammation Triggered by SARS-CoV-2 and ACE2 Augment Drives Multiple Organ Failure of Severe COVID-19: Molecular Mechanisms and Implications. *Inflammation*. 2020:1-22.

[2] Kawai T, Akira S. Signaling to NF-kappaB by Toll-like receptors. *Trends Mol Med*. 2007;13(11):460-9.

[3] Zelaya H, Rothmeier AS, Ruf W. Tissue factor at the crossroad of coagulation and cell signaling. *J Thromb Haemost*. 2018;16(10):1941-52.

[4] Sattler A, Angermair S, Stockmann H, Heim KM, Khadzhynov D, Treskatsch S, et al. SARS–CoV-2–specific T cell responses and correlations with COVID-19 patient predisposition. *J Clin Investig*. 2020;130(12).

[5] Lega S, Naviglio S, Volpi S, Tommasini A. Recent Insight into SARS-CoV2 Immunopathology and Rationale for Potential Treatment and Preventive Strategies in COVID-19. *Vaccines* (Basel). 2020;8(2).

[6] Trabulus S, Karaca C, Balkan II, Dincer MT, Murt A, Ozcan SG, et al. *Kidney function on admission predicts in-hospital mortality in COVID-19. medRxiv*. 2020:2020.06.18. 20134627.

[7] Oetjens MT, Luo JZ, Chang A, Leader JB, Hartzel DN, Moore BS, et al. Electronic health record analysis identifies kidney disease as the leading risk factor for hospitalization in confirmed COVID-19 patients. *PloS One*. 2020;15(11):e0242182.

[8] Gansevoort RT, Hilbrands LB. CKD is a key risk factor for COVID-19 mortality. *Nat Rev Nephrol* 2020.

[9] Wu J, Li J, Zhu G, Zhang Y, Bi Z, Yu Y, et al. Clinical Features of Maintenance Hemodialysis Patients with 2019 Novel Coronavirus-Infected Pneumonia in Wuhan, China. *Clin J Am Soc Nephrol*. 2020;15(8):1139.

[10] Corbett RW, Blakey S, Nitsch D, Loucaidou M, McLean A, Duncan N, et al. Epidemiology of COVID-19 in an Urban Dialysis Center. *J Am Soc Nephrol*. 2020;31(8):1815.

[11] Nadim MK, Forni LG, Mehta RL, Connor MJ, Liu KD, Ostermann M, et al. COVID-19-associated acute kidney injury: consensus report of the 25th Acute Disease Quality Initiative (ADQI) Workgroup. *Nat Rev Nephrol*. 2020.

[12] Mohamed MMB, Lukitsch I, Torres-Ortiz AE, Walker JB, Varghese V, Hernandez-Arroyo CF, et al. Acute Kidney Injury Associated with Coronavirus Disease 2019 in Urban New Orleans. *Kidney 360*. 2020;1(7):614.

[13] Hirsch JS, Ng JH, Ross DW, Sharma P, Shah HH, Barnett RL, et al. Acute kidney injury in patients hospitalized with COVID-19. *Kidney Intl*. 2020;98(1):209-18.

[14] Batlle D, Soler MJ, Sparks MA, Hiremath S, South AM, Welling PA, et al. Acute Kidney Injury in COVID-19: Emerging Evidence of a Distinct Pathophysiology. *J Am Soc Nephrol*. 2020;31(7):1380.

[15] Farkash EA, Wilson AM, Jentzen JM. Ultrastructural Evidence for Direct Renal Infection with SARS-CoV-2. *J Am Soc Nephrol*. 2020:ASN.2020040432.

[16] Braun F, Lütgehetmann M, Pfefferle S, Wong MN, Carsten A, Lindenmeyer MT, et al. SARS-CoV-2 renal tropism associates with acute kidney injury. *Lancet* (London, England). 2020;396(10251):597-8.

[17] Puelles VG, Lütgehetmann M, Lindenmeyer MT, Sperhake JP, Wong MN, Allweiss L, et al. Multiorgan and Renal Tropism of SARS-CoV-2. *N Engl J Med*. 2020;383(6):590-2.

[18] Sharma P, Uppal NN, Wanchoo R, Shah HH, Yang Y, Parikh R, et al. COVID-19–Associated Kidney Injury: A Case Series of Kidney Biopsy Findings. *J Am Soc Nephrol ology*. 2020;31(9):1948-58.

[19] Kudose S, Batal I, Santoriello D, Xu K, Barasch J, Peleg Y, et al. Kidney Biopsy Findings in Patients with COVID-19. *J Am Soc Nephrol*. 2020;31(9):1959.

[20] Limou S, Dummer PD, Nelson GW, Kopp JB, Winkler CA. APOL1 toxin, innate immunity, and kidney injury. *Kidney Intl*. 2015;88(1):28-34.

[21] Nichols B, Jog P, Lee JH, Blackler D, Wilmot M, D'Agati V, et al. Innate immunity pathways regulate the nephropathy gene Apolipoprotein L1. *Kidney Intl*. 2015;87(2):332-42.

[22] Wu H, Larsen CP, Hernandez-Arroyo CF, Mohamed MMB, Caza T, Sharshir Md, et al. AKI and Collapsing Glomerulopathy Associated with COVID-19 and APOL1 High-Risk Genotype. *J Am Soc Nephrol*. 2020;31(8):1688.

[23] Gupta N, Wang X, Wen X, Moran P, Paluch M, Hass PE, et al. Domain-Specific Antibodies Reveal Differences in the Membrane Topologies of Apolipoprotein L1 in Serum and Podocytes. *J Am Soc Nephrol*. 2020;31(9):2065-82.

[24] Scales SJ, Gupta N, De Mazière AM, Posthuma G, Chiu CP, Pierce AA, et al. Apolipoprotein L1-Specific Antibodies Detect Endogenous APOL1 inside the Endoplasmic Reticulum and on the Plasma Membrane of Podocytes. *J Am Soc Nephrol*. 2020;31(9):2044-64.

[25] Datta S, Kataria R, Zhang JY, Moore S, Petitpas K, Mohamed A, et al. Kidney Disease-Associated APOL1 Variants Have Dose-Dependent, Dominant Toxic Gain-of-Function. *J Am Soc Nephrol*. 2020;31(9):2083-96.

[26] Kopp JB, Rosenberg AZ. One Actor, Many Roles: Histopathologies Associated With APOL1 Genetic Variants. *Adv Anat Pathol*. 2019;26(3):215-9.

[27] Ma L, Ainsworth HC, Snipes JA, Murea M, Choi YA, Langefeld CD, et al. APOL1 Kidney-Risk Variants Induce Mitochondrial Fission. *Kidney Intl Rep*. 2020;5(6):891-904.

[28] Carney EF. APOL1 risk variants induce opening of the mitochondrial permeability transition pore. *Nat Rev Nephrol*. 2019;15(12):730-.

[29] Friedman DJ, Pollak MR. APOL1 Nephropathy: From Genetics to Clinical Applications. *Clin J Am Soc Nephrol*. 2020:CJN.1516 1219.

[30] Elias M, Pievani D, Randoux C, Louis K, Denis B, Delion A, et al. COVID-19 Infection in Kidney Transplant Recipients: Disease Incidence and Clinical Outcomes. *J Am Soc Nephrol*. 2020;31(10):2413.

[31] Akalin E, Azzi Y, Bartash R, Seethamraju H, Parides M, Hemmige V, et al. Covid-19 and Kidney Transplantation. *N Engl J Med*. 2020;382(25):2475-7.

[32] Kates OS, Haydel BM, Florman SS, Rana MM, Chaudhry ZS, Ramesh MS, et al. Coronavirus Disease 2019 in Solid Organ Transplant: A Multicenter Cohort Study. *Clin Infect Dis*. 2020.

[33] Boyarsky BJ, Po-Yu Chiang T, Werbel WA, Durand CM, Avery RK, Getsin SN, et al. Early impact of COVID-19 on transplant center practices and policies in the United States. *Am J Transplant*. 2020;20(7):1809-18.

[34] Guha C, Tong A, Baumgart A, Scholes-Robertson N, Isbel N, Kanellis J, et al. Suspension and resumption of kidney transplant programmes during the COVID-19 pandemic: perspectives from patients, caregivers and potential living donors – a qualitative study. *Transplant Intl*. 2020;33(11):1481-90.

[35] Polack FP, Thomas SJ, Kitchin N, Absalon J, Gurtman A, Lockhart S, et al. Safety and Efficacy of the BNT162b2 mRNA Covid-19 Vaccine. *N Engl J Med.* 2020;383(27):2603-15.

[36] Baden LR, El Sahly HM, Essink B, Kotloff K, Frey S, Novak R, et al. Efficacy and Safety of the mRNA-1273 SARS-CoV-2 Vaccine. *N Engl J Med.* 2021;384(5):403-16.

[37] Moore JP. Approaches for Optimal Use of Different COVID-19 Vaccines: Issues of Viral Variants and Vaccine Efficacy. *JAMA*. 2021.

[38] Boyarsky BJ, Werbel WA, Avery RK, Tobian AAR, Massie AB, Segev DL, et al. Immunogenicity of a Single Dose of SARS-CoV-2 Messenger RNA Vaccine in Solid Organ Transplant Recipients. *JAMA*. 2021.

In: Issues in Kidney Disease – Acute Kidney Injury
Editors: S. Z. Fadem and A. Arslan Yousuf Awan

ISBN: 978-1-68507-002-1

Chapter 13

KIDNEY INJURY ASSOCIATED WITH PRESCRIPTION AND NON-PRESCRIPTION DRUGS

Kavitha Ramaswamy[1,*], MD, Samuel Y. Suen[2], PharmD, Vidhi A. Gandhi[2], PharmD, Hector Madariaga[3], MD, Beje Thomas[4], MD, Annelise Nolan[2], PharmD, and Edgar V. Lerma[5], MD

[1]Wellspan Chambersburg Hospital, Department of Medicine, Chambersburg, PA, USA
[2]Medstar Georgetown University Hospital, Department of Pharmacy, Washington DC, USA
[3]Good Samaritan Medical Center-Brockton, Department of Medicine, Brockton, MA, USA
[4]MedStar Georgetown University Hospital, MedStar Georgetown Transplant Institute, Washington DC, USA
[5]University of Illinois at Chicago College of Medicine/Advocate Christ Medical Center, Section of Nephrology, Chicago, IL, USA

ABSTRACT

Kidney injury due to prescription and non-prescription medications is periodically encountered. There are multiple factors that potentiate the side effects of drugs and contribute to injury. These include direct toxic effects, drug interactions, metabolism, and the effects of poor kidney clearance. Whenever acute kidney injury or chronic kidney disease is identified, medications are always on the differential list. Medications can affect the kidney in multiple areas of the glomerulus and collecting system and are associated with specific abnormalities. A kidney biopsy might be indicated to prove that drug induced kidney injury has occurred. The healthcare provider must always be aware of the potential toxicity of both prescription and non-prescription medications. This chapter summarizes preventative measures and interventions that can resolve drug-induced kidney injury.

* Corresponding Author's E-mail: drkavitha@gmail.com.

Proper dosing of medications in the hospital, especially with altered renal function and altered volume of distribution, is an important responsibility shared by nephrologists, pharmacists, and hospitalists/intensivists [1].

Keywords: acute kidney injury, chronic kidney disease (CKD), clearance, drugs, drug-induced, drug interactions, function, interstitial nephritis, medications, nephrolithiasis, nephrotoxic, non-prescription, pharmacology, prescription, risk factors, thrombotic microangiopathy, toxins, tubular injury

INTRODUCTION

Kidney injury due to prescription and non-prescription medications is periodically encountered. There are multiple factors that contribute to this, including direct toxic effects, drug interactions, metabolism, and the effects of poor kidney clearance of drugs potentiating their side effects. When acute kidney injury (AKI) or chronic kidney disease (CKD) is identified, medications are always on the differential list. Medications can affect the kidney in multiple areas of the glomerulus and collecting system and are associated with specific abnormalities. In the case of kidney injury where drug-induced kidney injury is suspected but not certain, a kidney biopsy may be indicated. The healthcare provider must always be aware of the potential toxicity of both prescription and non-prescription medication.

DEFINITION

Medications are a common cause of kidney injury especially in hospitalized patients and, in particular, ICU [2].

EPIDEMIOLOGY

Drug-induced nephrotoxicity is approximately 14-26% in the adult population. Newer chemotherapeutic agents are increasingly used, which have been associated with toxicity. However, challenges in diagnosing and reporting exist, especially if the drug is used short term [3]. Drugs that contribute to nephrotoxicity include 20% of AKI related hospital admissions, 8-60% of hospitalized AKI, and 19-25% ICU-related AKI [2].

The factors that contribute to nephrotoxicity can be divided into the following categories:

1. Nephrotoxic medication
2. Patient characteristic
3. Kidney handling of the ingested substance

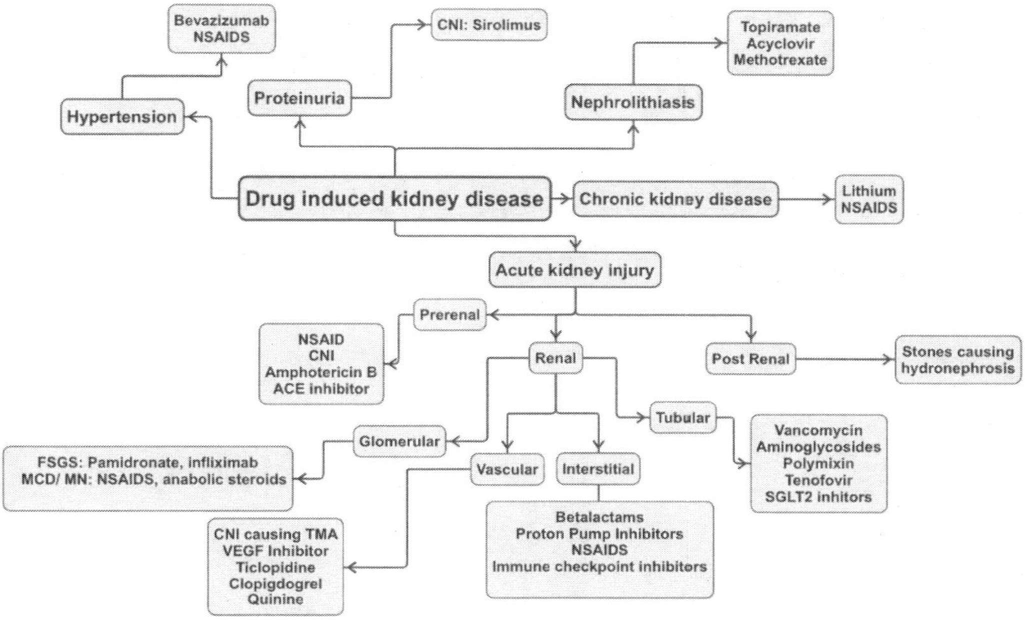

Figure 1. Mechanisms of drug-induced nephrotoxicity traced to the cause.

Nephrotoxic Medication

The first step in kidney injury involves use of nephrotoxic medications such as antimicrobials, anticancer agents, and non-steroidal anti-inflammatory drugs (NSAIDs). In addition, the innate nephrotoxicity of certain agents like aminoglycosides, especially with higher and longer courses, leads to kidney injury, even in patients with no underlying risk [4]. Figure 1 shows the various mechanisms of how a drug can cause kidney disease.

Drug Characteristics

It is of utmost importance to tailor drug dosing to kidney function. High doses, as well as long treatment durations of certain drugs, can lead to increased nephrotoxicity. Certain drugs (e.g., methotrexate, acyclovir, indinavir/atazanavir) are insoluble in urine, leading to crystalline nephropathy. Drug combination (e.g., vancomycin and Zosyn, NSAIDs and ACE inhibitors, tacrolimus and fluconazole, tacrolimus and phenytoin) can potentiate nephrotoxicity. Commonly used drugs, mechanism of action, and their nephrotoxicity are discussed in Table 1.

Table 1. Medications and specific nephrotoxicities

Nephrotoxic Medication	**Injury Mechanism leading to AKI/CKD**	**Additional Information**
Non-Steroidal Anti-Inflammatory Drugs (NSAIDs) [5]	Vasoconstriction AA/AIN/ATN/MCD/MN	• Known to cause acute kidney injury (AKI) via reducing renal blood flow through a decrease in prostaglandins (controls vasodilation at the glomerular level). • Cause vasoconstriction of the afferent renal arteriole and reduces the kidney's ability to regulate glomerular blood flow. • Disrupt compensatory vasodilation by renal prostaglandins resulting in acute renal function decline. • Also cause AKI via acute interstitial nephritis (AIN), commonly occurring after taking NSAIDs for ~1 week. AIN constitutes ~15% patients presenting with unexplained AKI.
Calcineurin Inhibitors (CNIs)	Vasoconstriction AA/TMA/IFTA	• Causes both acute and chronic nephrotoxicity • Acute nephrotoxicity o Reversible vasoconstriction of intrarenal vessels causing decreased blood flow to kidneys and clinically presenting as an increase in serum creatinine • Chronic nephrotoxicity o Associated with long-term CNI use regardless of appropriate tacrolimus/cyclosporine concentrations o Severe tubular atrophy, interstitial fibrosis, and focal hyalinosis with occasional glomerular scarring seen on kidney biopsy
Aminoglycosides	Tubular injury	• Preferentially target S1 and S2 segments of the proximal tubular epithelial cells after initially interacting with phospholipids on brush border membranes. • This ultimately causes renal vasoconstriction, manifesting as a gradual increase in serum creatinine and hypoosmolar urinary output after several days of aminoglycoside exposure.
Polymyxins [6]	Tubular injury	• Accumulate extensively within proximal tubular cells of the kidneys, the primary site at which megalin and PEPT2 are expressed in the kidney, leading to AKI in up to 50-60% of patients (23) [7].
Amphotericin B [8]	Vasoconstriction AA	• Tubular injury is a well-known documented problem with amphotericin-B, specifically binding to sterols in cell membranes and cholesterol in human cell membranes. • Liposomal-based amphotericin B is associated with less nephrotoxicity.
Tenofovir [9]	Tubular injury/CIN	• Tenofovir causes proximal tubulopathy, possibly in part due to decreasing mitochondrial DNA replication through inhibition of mitochondrial DNA polymerase γ.

Nephrotoxic Medication	Injury Mechanism leading to AKI/CKD	Additional Information
Beta-Lactams [10]	AIN	• Mechanisms of injury include: (1) transport into the tubular cell, mainly through the antiluminal organic anion secretory carrier; (2) acylation of target proteins, causing respiratory toxicity by inactivation of mitochondrial anionic substrate carriers; and (3) lipid peroxidation.
Vancomycin [11, 12][1]	Tubulopathy	• Exact mechanism of nephrotoxicity remains unclear, but current data suggests vancomycin exerts an oxidative effect on the proximal renal tubule causing renal tubular ischemia. • Vancomycin associated nephrotoxicity (VANT) is defined as an increase in serum creatinine (SCr) by 0.5 mg/dL or 50% above baseline SCr after several days of vancomycin therapy without an alternative cause. • Potential risk factors with VANT include: loading dose, total daily dose, duration, continuous versus intermittent infusion, obesity, critically ill patients, ICU exposure, CKD, concurrent nephrotoxins (i.e., aminoglycosides, piperacillin-tazobactam).
VEGF Inhibitors [13]	Podocyte injury/TMA	• *In vitro*, VEGF induces the formation of fenestrations in endothelium which are necessary for the unique permeability characteristics of the glomerular filtration barrier. • Loss of VEGF from the glomerulus leads to a loss of the healthy fenestrated phenotype and promotes the development of microvascular injury and thrombotic microangiopathy.
PPIs [14]	AIN	• One of the most widely used medications in both OTC and prescription sales. • Shown to be attributed to increasing AKI risk; however, various studies have demonstrated conflicting data. • Proposed mechanism with how PPIs cause AKI may be explained via interstitial nephritis. Most studies documenting relationship between PPIs and AKI specifically referred to acute interstitial nephritis (AIN) as the primary association with an elevated risk in younger patients (<60 years old). • Healthcare providers are encouraged to monitor patients taking PPIs and potential renal injury via monitoring urinalysis and renal function tests.
Topiramate [15]	Nephrolithiasis	• Inhibition of carbonic anhydrase in renal tubules causes mixed renal tubular acidosis ultimately leads to systemic metabolic acidosis • These metabolic changes present with low plasma bicarbonate concentration, alkaline urine pH with low urine citrate concentration calcium phosphate stone formation.

Table 1. (Continued)

Nephrotoxic Medication	Injury Mechanism leading to AKI/CKD	Additional Information
Acyclovir [16]	Nephrolithiasis	• Excreted rapidly in the urine via glomerular filtration and tubular secretion resulting in reaching elevated concentrations in the tubular lumen. • SCr and crystalluria is seen to increase within 24-48 hours of acyclovir initiation.
Methotrexate [17]	Nephrolithiasis	• Methotrexate is excreted renally, meaning rapid MTX elimination can largely cause MTX-induced AKI.
Pamidronate	Collapsing FSGS	• Within the clinicopathologic spectrum of FSGS, collapsing FSGS has been defined as a distinct morphologic variant characterized by marked wrinkling and "collapse" of the glomerular basement membranes and hypertrophy and hyperplasia of overlying podocytes. • Dose-related toxicity; seen in patients with doses that exceed recommended levels >90 mg/month for prolonged period (15-48 months).
Infliximab	Collapsing FSGS	• Given the frequent induction of autoantibodies following anti-TNFα therapy, it is hypothesized that this phenomenon may give rise to either lupus-like immune complex glomerulonephritis or ANCA-related necrotizing and crescentic glomerulonephritis in susceptible individuals.
ACE Inhibitors	Decrease in intraglomerular pressure	• Inhibits efferent renal arterioles resulting in lower glomerular filtration pressure and increased vasoconstriction.
SGLT2 Inhibitors [6]	Tubular injury	• SGLT2 inhibitors-induced uricosuria is associated with renal toxicity due to uric acid crystal deposition within the renal tubules as well as to crystal-independent mechanisms related to pro-inflammatory effects and oxidative stress. • Increased glucose reabsorption in the S_3 segment of the proximal renal tubules is associated with elevated fructose production and metabolism through fructokinase leading to oxidative stress and increased chemokine production, local tubular injury and inflammation.

(AA) Afferent arteriole; (AIN) Acute interstitial nephritis; (ACE) angiotensin-converting enzyme; (ATN) Acute tubular necrosis; (CIN) Chronic interstitial nephritis; (FSGS) Focal segmental glomerulosclerosis; (IFTA) Interstitial fibrosis and tubular atrophy; (MCD) Minimal change disease; (MN) Membranous nephropathy; (NSAIDs) Non-steroidal anti-inflammatory drugs; (PEPT2) Oligopeptide transporter 2; (TMA) Thrombotic microangiopathy; (PPIx) Proton pump inhibitors; (SGLT2) Sodium glucose transporter-2; (VEGF) Vascular endothelial growth factor.

Table 2. Dietary supplements and associated nephrotoxicity

Common names	Indications	Nephrotoxicity
Licorice	Anti-inflammatory	Renal tubular injury due to prolonged Hypokalemia
Vitamin C	Antioxidant and wound healing	Nephrolithiasis from oxaluria
Willow bark	Analgesic and Anti-inflammatory	Analgesic Nephropathy
Yohimbine	Erectile Dysfunction	SLE with renal dysfunction
Creatine	Muscle performance	Acute interstitial nephritis and tubular dysfunction with rhabdomyolysis

CHARACTERISTICS OF DRUG TOXICITY

Important risk factors for drug-induced nephrotoxicity [4] include older age, female sex due to lean body mass and decreased body water, genetic make-up, volume depletion, as well as comorbidities such as chronic kidney disease, cardiac disease, and liver disease. Increased drug delivery to the kidney is 25 percent of the cardiac output, exposing the kidney to drug toxicity. The tubular cells in the loop of Henle reside in a hypoxic environment and have metabolic requirements generated by sodium potassium ATPase active transport. Failure to meet this metabolic demand can potentiate nephrotoxicity. In addition to hepatic metabolism, many drugs undergo biotransformation by enzymatic processes in the kidney, including CYP450. This can result in toxic metabolites as seen with aminoglycosides, platinums, and several other medications.

Alternative medicine is a multibillion industry; half of the American population uses some form of herbs or supplements in addition to prescription medications. Dietary supplements are a cause of renal dysfunction, accounting for 7% of all medication-related toxicities [18]. Aristolochic acid (AA) is a naturally occurring substance found in birthwort plants. It is the most documented adulterant with nephrotoxic adverse events, leading to interstitial fibrosis. It is also a carcinogen, and has been associated with urothelial malignancies [19]. Other common contaminants are heavy metals such as arsenic, lead, and mercury. A few common herbs are listed in Table 2.

THE 6R APPROACH

The 6R approach to drug nephrotoxicity was developed by Linda Awdishu and Ravindra Mehta. The approach is based on Risk assessment, early Recognition, a targeted Response, timely Renal support, and Rehabilitation coupled with Research [20].

Risk

Drug reactions can be either idiosyncratic or dose-related. Dose-related nephrotoxicity is predictable and can be individualized to specific patients. Factors to consider when assessing risk include age, level of kidney function, cumulative dose, and concurrent nephrotoxin exposure.

Recognition

This refers to the recognition of a change in kidney function, including certainty that the change is related to the attributable drug. This depends on timing and the measurement in kidney function.

Response

Therapy may include simply adjusting or stopping the attributable medication, but also requires determining substitute management. Management to resolve the toxicity depends on the adverse event. Causation might not be straightforward and may require a kidney biopsy.

Renal Support

Renal replacement therapy may be beneficial to remove the offending toxin, or may be required to support the patient until renal recover can occur.

Rehabilitation

Although most cases of nephrotoxicity resolve quickly, some may be complicated by a prolonged recovery period. This may depend upon the underlying medical condition. During the period of recovery management, therapeutic monitoring is necessary.

Research

The dynamics that contribute to a varied incidence of drug-induced kidney disease need to be more carefully studied. Research offers opportunities to determine factors that predict patient vulnerability and goes beyond post marketing surveillance, which is voluntary and unable to determine causality. The benefits of well-designed research are valid predictive modeling tools, practical biomarkers, a better understanding of drug metabolism, and more effective therapies that avoid or minimize drug toxicity while achieving optimal results. Clinical trials and the updating of clinical practice guidelines can help reduce the incidence of drug toxicity.

DIAGNOSIS

There are multiple tests ordered in the differentiation of AKI in the search for a cause. Medication-induced AKI must be appropriately evaluated so that a patient is correctly diagnosed and managed. Laboratory assessments include a complete blood count, kidney function indices such as serum creatinine, liver function tests, urine tests, and other specialized testing. Urine tests include urinalysis for pyuria, hematuria, proteinuria, and cellular casts (i.e., white blood or red blood cell casts). Pyuria is found in almost 60-80% of patients affected by drug-induced interstitial nephritis, but there are almost a third of patients who do not have pyuria. Proteinuria related to drug toxicity can in certain cases can reach nephrotic range (>3.5 g of proteinuria/24 hours). Nephrotic range proteinuria is particularly associated with NSAID use. Urine chemistries are not traditionally helpful in the workup of AKI from drug causes. Serum eosinophilia is present in only about a third of cases and urine eosinophils are unreliable with a sensitivity and specificity of only about 30% and 70%, respectively [21].

Crystal nephropathy is another finding on manual microscopy and can be seen with drugs including sulfadiazine, acyclovir, indinavir, triamterene, methotrexate, orlistat, and ciprofloxacin [22]. Some of these drugs such as indinavir or topiramate can cause kidney stones seen on imaging with CT and kidney ultrasound. As with tenofovir toxicity (reported to cause Fanconi syndrome) [23], other drugs have very specific urinary findings, such as phosphaturia and glucosuria.

ROLE OF KIDNEY BIOPSY

Kidney biopsy is an invasive procedure with potential risks, especially bleeding. Contraindications to kidney biopsy are uncontrolled hypertension, anticoagulation, small echogenic kidneys, horseshoe kidneys or kidneys with large cysts and solitary kidney. Two absolute contraindications are with patients with active kidney infection or skin infection.

Uremia, thrombocytopenia, and coagulopathies increase the risk of bleeding. Risk vs. benefit assessment is necessary. In general, renal biopsies should not be performed if they will not change the management of the patient. If it is obvious that a suspected drug has resulted in a reaction, the majority of clinicians would first discontinue a drug rather than subjecting the patient to a renal biopsy. If the persistent injury persists despite stopping the drug altogether or mitigating the reaction to the suspected culprit medication, a renal biopsy may be warranted. The renal function should be trending back to baseline within 7 to 14 days past the injury, and if that is not the case, an evaluation of the histology might be necessary [24].

PREVENTION STRATEGIES

To target safety of the drug, precautionary steps include monitoring its toxicity, and controlling or reducing effects of its risk factors. Before starting any medication, it is prudent to know the patient risk factors and home medications. While therapy is ongoing, one must ensure adequate hydration, and avoid other potentially nephrotoxic agents.

Clinicians should use the lowest effective dose possible, maintain drug concentrations during drug therapy, and monitor renal function. It is necessary to use the lowest dose of iodinated contrast agents in patients with existing renal disease, heart failure, or diabetes. It is prudent to use the lowest effective dose of medications such as aspirin and acetaminophen [25].

Clinical Pearls

- NSAIDs cause AIN, CIN, acute and chronic papillary necrosis, CKD, Nephrotic syndrome (MCD, MGN)
- Phenytoin, as well as Rifampin, induces Tacrolimus metabolism, hence its dose should be increased while using combination
- Fluconazole, Macrolides, Quinolones can inhibit metabolism of Tacrolimus and hence its dose should be monitored and decreased
- Gemcitabine can cause Thrombotic Microangiopathy.
- Pamidronate, Interferon Alpha can cause collapsing FSGS
- SLE like nephritis; Quinidine, Methyldopa, Hydralazine, Procainamide
- Aminoglycosides can cause ATN but sometimes an acquired Bartter syndrome with hypokalemia and metabolic alkalosis [26]
- Most common agents to cause AIN: Antibiotics, NSAIDS, PPIs

Patient Information

Patients should be advised to consult with their family physician before taking any over the counter medications due to the ease of access to drugs like NSAIDS, PPI, or herbal supplements. They can lead to nephrotoxicity.

CONCLUSION

Nephrotoxicity with prescription and nonprescription drugs is very common in both community and hospital settings. Increased awareness and heightened screening, especially on older individuals with comorbidities, are required. Dietary supplements are a significant component of over-the-counter market, which is viewed as safe by the consumers. Further lack of regulations complicates the use. Dietary supplement use should be monitored closely on patients who have or are at risk for renal dysfunction. Educating patients in general to avoid taking any medications and supplements without consulting with their family physician should be encouraged.

REFERENCES

[1] Matzke GR, Aronoff GR, Atkinson AJ, Bennett WM, Decker BS, Eckardt K-U, et al. Drug dosing consideration in patients with acute and chronic kidney disease-a clinical update from Kidney Disease: Improving Global Outcomes (KDIGO). *Kidney Int.* 2011 Dec;80(11):1122–37.

[2] Perazella MA. Drug use and nephrotoxicity in the intensive care unit. *Kidney Int.* 2012 Jun;81(12):1172–8.

[3] Nolin TD, Perazella MA. Introduction to Nephropharmacology for the Clinician: A New CJASN Series. *Clin J Am Soc Nephrol.* 2018;13(7):1083–4.

[4] Perazella MA. Pharmacology behind Common Drug Nephrotoxicities. *Clin J Am Soc Nephrol.* 2018;13(12):1897–908.

[5] Dixit M, Doan T, Kirschner R, Dixit N. Significant Acute Kidney Injury Due to Non-steroidal Anti-inflammatory Drugs: Inpatient Setting. *Pharmaceuticals* (Basel). 2010;3(4):1279–85.

[6] Tsimihodimos V, Filippatos TD, Elisaf MS. SGLT2 inhibitors and the kidney: Effects and mechanisms. *Diabetes Metab Syndr.* 2018;12(6):1117–23.

[7] Zavascki AP, Nation RL. Nephrotoxicity of Polymyxins: Is There Any Difference between Colistimethate and Polymyxin B? *Antimicrob Agents Chemother.* 2017;61(3):02319-16

[8] Fanos V, Cataldi L. Amphotericin B-induced nephrotoxicity: a review. *J Chemother.* 2000;12(6):463–70.

[9] Fernandez-Fernandez B, Montoya-Ferrer A, Sanz AB, Sanchez-Niño MD, Izquierdo MC, Poveda J, et al. Tenofovir nephrotoxicity: 2011 update. *AIDS Res Treat.* 2011;2011:354908.

[10] Tune BM. Nephrotoxicity of beta-lactam antibiotics: mechanisms and strategies for prevention. *Pediatr Nephrol.* 1997;11(6):768–72

[11] Filippone EJ, Kraft WK, Farber JL. The Nephrotoxicity of Vancomycin. *Clin Pharmacol Ther.* 2017;102(3):459–69.

[12] Vora S. Acute renal failure due to vancomycin toxicity in the setting of unmonitored vancomycin infusion. *Proc (Bayl Univ Med Cent).* 2016;29(4):412–3

[13] Eremina V, Jefferson JA, Kowalewska J, Hochster H, Haas M, Weisstuch J, et al. VEGF inhibition and renal thrombotic microangiopathy. *N Engl J Med.* 2008;358(11):1129–36.

[14] Yang Y, George KC, Shang W-F, Zeng R, Ge S-W, Xu G. Proton-pump inhibitors use, and risk of acute kidney injury: a meta-analysis of observational studies. *Drug Des Devel Ther.* 2017;11:1291–9

[15] Fariba K, Saadabadi A. Topiramate. In: *StatPearls* [Internet]. Treasure Island (FL): StatPearls Publishing; 2021 [cited 2021 Aug 8]. Available from: http://www.ncbi.nlm.nih.gov/books/NBK554530/

[16] Yildiz C, Ozsurekci Y, Gucer S, Cengiz AB, Topaloglu R. Acute kidney injury due to acyclovir. *CEN Case Rep.* 2013;2(1):38–40.

[17] Widemann BC, Adamson PC. Understanding and managing methotrexate nephrotoxicity. *Oncologist.* 2006;11(6):694–703.

[18] Gabardi S, Munz K, Ulbricht C. A review of dietary supplement-induced renal dysfunction. *Clin J Am Soc Nephrol.* 2007;2(4):757–65

[19] Debelle FD, Vanherweghem J-L, Nortier JL. Aristolochic acid nephropathy: a worldwide problem. *Kidney Int.* 2008;74(2):158–69.

[20] Awdishu L, Mehta RL. The 6R's of drug induced nephrotoxicity. *BMC Nephrol.* 2017;18(1):124.

[21] Lusica M, Rondon-Berrios H, Feldman L. Urine Eosinophils for Acute Interstitial Nephritis. *J Hosp Med.* 2017;12(5):343–5.

[22] Yarlagadda SG, Perazella MA. Drug-induced crystal nephropathy: an update. *Expert Opin Drug Saf.* 2008;7(2):147–58.

[23] Matlaga BR, Shah OD, Assimos DG. Drug-induced urinary calculi. *Rev Urol.* 2003;5(4):227–31.

[24] Luciano RL, Moeckel GW. Update on the Native Kidney Biopsy: Core Curriculum 2019. *Am J Kidney Dis*. 2019;73(3):404–15.

[25] Ghane Shahrbaf F, Assadi F. Drug-induced renal disorders. *J Renal Inj Prev.* 2015;4(3):57–60.

[26] Singh J, Patel ML, Gupta KK, Pandey S, Dinkar A. Acquired Bartter syndrome following gentamicin therapy. *Indian J Nephrol.* 2016;26(6):461–3.

In: Issues in Kidney Disease – Acute Kidney Injury
Editors: S. Z. Fadem and A. Arslan Yousuf Awan
ISBN: 978-1-68507-002-1

Chapter 14

ACUTE KIDNEY INJURY ASSOCIATED WITH CARDIORENAL DISEASE

Carl P. Walther**, MD

Selzman Institute for Kidney Health, Section of Nephrology, Department of Medicine, Baylor College of Medicine, Houston, TX, USA

ABSTRACT

The health and function of the heart and kidney are tightly and inextricably linked. Crosstalk between the organs drives diverse cardiorenal disease processes, whose tenuous pathophysiological state predisposes to AKI from diverse superimposed insults. In recent years, improved mechanistic understanding and diagnostics in the cardiorenal setting have markedly changed the understanding of AKI in many cardiorenal disease states in recent years and have also begun to influence management. Understanding of the roles in cardiorenal disease of flow-mediated derangements (both macro- and microcirculatory), local and systemic inflammatory processes, and local and systemic neurohormonal activation have all advanced in recent years, opening the doors for therapeutic and other management advances. One of the most salient advances is in the situation of AKI complicating acute decompensated heart failure (HF), where new kidney biomarkers directly reflecting parenchymal kidney damage have demonstrated that all substantial creatinine elevations are not necessarily reflective of AKI. Another crucial advance is the validation in a randomized trial that an approved urine biomarker tool enables decreased AKI complicating cardiac surgery, through early identification of AKI enabling adaptive management. Therapeutic advances have also yielded promising results. Background, pathophysiology, diagnosis, and therapy of AKI associated with frequently encountered cardiorenal disease states are discussed in this chapter.

Keywords: AKI, cardiorenal syndrome, heart failure, cardiac surgery, kidney biomarkers

---

* Corresponding Author's E-mail: Carl.Walther@bcm.edu.

INTRODUCTION

The health and function of the heart and kidney are inextricably linked through numerous pathways, and dysfunction of either organ can set the stage for development of acute kidney injury (AKI). In the most basic physiologic conception, the heart is a pump and the kidney is a filter, and dysfunction of either the pumping or the filtering process results in dysfunction of the other. From a clinical standpoint, cardiorenal interactions are often discussed in terms of the cardiorenal syndromes Types 1-5, which are determined by the primary organ driving the deleterious cardiorenal interaction, and the acuity of the effect [1]. These simplified models and categories have undoubted value and applicability. For example, the pump/filter model may explain parts of what is initially observed in oliguric acute kidney injury complicating acute cardiogenic shock. Moreover, the cardiorenal syndrome Types 1-5 have clear prototypical examples that are regularly encountered in clinical practice. However, to further improve care of the growing number of people with both heart and kidney dysfunction, the complexity of the organ crosstalk must be accounted for, and in many patients the organ crosstalk does not appear to be driven obviously by one organ or the other, but by a cyclic continuum of a multiplicity of harmful processes [2]. An ever-expanding understanding of the numerous mechanisms for the subtle interdependencies between heart and kidney health/function, mechanisms beyond the more obvious macrocirculatory parameters such as arterial blood pressure and cardiac output, mechanisms operant in the acute, subacute, and chronic settings, is driving this field forward. This increased understanding of the mechanisms of heart-kidney crosstalk will be covered in this chapter in terms of clinically relevant diagnostic, prognostic, and therapeutic implications. Additionally, beyond the diverse mechanistic interdependencies for heart and kidney dysfunction underlying increased susceptibility to AKI, there are numerous specific clinical scenarios where heart-kidney interactions are important for clinical management of AKI. This chapter is divided into some of the most important of these different clinical scenarios of AKI in cardiorenal disease that clinicians encounter commonly, with discussion of the background and underlying pathophysiology, followed by discussion of diagnostic, management and prognostic considerations.

CARDIORENAL DISEASE AND PREDISPOSITION TO AKI

Pathophysiological Concepts Underlying a Tenuous State

Diverse cardiorenal stresses may set the stage for predisposition to AKI. In this section, these underlying cardiorenal stresses and mechanisms are summarized.

Macrocirculation

As discussed in the introduction, arterial blood pressure and cardiac output are important macrocirculatory parameters, and derangements in these parameters certainly can degrade kidney (and cardiac) health/function over the short or long term [1]. Other macrocirculatory parameters are also important to both heart and kidney function, and may be more important in many common situations, particularly central venous pressure [3]. Driven by many factors, including volume status and cardiac filling pressures, elevations in central venous pressure can decrease glomerular filtration rate (GFR) by causing renal venous hypertension which then causes increased renal resistance and finally leads to disordered intrarenal blood flow [1, 4]. While this is most commonly seen in left heart failure, primary right ventricular dysfunction can also cause GFR decline by elevating central venous pressure directly, in addition to impairing left ventricular filling.

Neurohormonal Activation

Neurohormonal activation is a characteristic of many cardiorenal disease states, including acute and chronic HF with preserved or reduced ejection fraction, acute myocardial infarction, and arrhythmias [5-8]. Neurohormonal activation may be local and organ specific, or systemic [9]. This activation, with increased sympathetic nervous system, renin-angiotensin-aldosterone system (RAAS), arginine vasopressin (AVP), and endothelin activity, often occurs in the body's attempts to maintain cardiovascular homeostasis in the setting of a disease or stressor [6, 7]. This activation can occur acutely or chronically and can cause afferent renal arterioles to constrict, reducing kidney perfusion and function [10]. Over the short term, this vasoconstriction may cause a reversible decrement in GFR; over the long term, this may result in hypoxic damage and irreversible injury [11]. The acute and chronic neurohormonal activation characteristic of disordered cardiorenal physiology may play a predisposing or directly causative role in many cases of AKI complicating cardiorenal syndrome, as discussed in the clinical section. Both neurohormonal activation and endothelial dysfunction play important roles in the disordered kidney microcirculation that occurs in cardiorenal syndromes [12].

Inflammation

In many acute and chronic heart disease phenotypes, with HF and atherosclerotic disease being the most studied, systemic and local inflammation are concomitant processes [13, 14]. Inflammation, local and systemic, is nearly ubiquitous in AKI and CKD as well, as alluded to earlier in the chapter [15]. Inflammatory crosstalk between the two organs, and the contribution of both to an overall systemic inflammatory milieu, is a likely contributor to a tenuous cardiorenal state sensitive to relatively mild insults, and these inflammatory effects have been directly observed in experimental animal studies [16]. This immune dysregulation in cardiorenal disease seems to include both the innate and adaptive immune responses [7]. The innate response is characterized by myeloid cell activation, including neutrophils, lymphocytes, dendritic cells, and others, along with release of chemokines and cytokines [7]. The adaptive response targets specific antigens, with humoral and cellular pathways. Decreased kidney function contributes to inflammation through reduced cytokine clearance, oxidative stress, among numerous other experimentally determined drivers [17]. Cardiac dysfunction and injury—through numerous processes—can activate the innate and adaptive immune responses, both within the heart and systemically [18]. Reversal of inflammation with a monoclonal antibody has been shown to improve outcomes in people with atherosclerotic disease [19]. Also in the therapeutic realm, reduction in inflammation in kidney disease is posited as a mechanism of action for medications which have been demonstrated to be effective in reducing adverse kidney outcomes [20]. Combined improvement of heart and kidney outcomes observed with some medications may be due, at least in part, to anti-inflammatory effects [21]. This is one explanation for the striking improvement in cardiac and kidney outcomes with Sodium Glucose Cotransporter 2 Inhibitors (SGLT2 inhibitors), which have been found to reduce activity of the nucleotide-binding oligomerization domain-like receptor P3 (NLRP3) inflammasome, a protein complex important to interleukin-1β and interleukin-18 production [22]. In summary, cardiorenal disease can be characterized as a highly proinflammatory state, which sets the stage for AKI, and this inflammatory milieu may be one of the contributors to a sensitivity to any additional insult, lowering the threshold for insults to precipitate AKI [23, 24].

Endothelial Dysfunction

Endothelial dysfunction is a characteristic of both cardiac and kidney dysfunction. The most obvious clinical implication of this is the markedly heightened risk of both kidney and heart disease among patients with albuminuria, the most frequently measured marker of endothelial dysfunction [25]. Endothelial dysfunction is characterized by arterial stiffness (affecting both the heart and kidney), and characterized by reduced nitric oxide (NO) bioavailability, increased oxidative stress, and pro-inflammatory and pro-thrombotic effects [26]. A continuum of endothelial dysfunction plays a role in cardiorenal interactions and disease, ranging from (reversible) activation of endothelial cells, to (irreversible) endothelial apoptosis and necrosis [26]. Endothelial dysfunction is likely present across the range of cardiorenal disease states. The specific drivers and feedback loops may differ by cardiorenal phenotype, but likely involve, to varying degrees, shear stress, neurohormonal activation (impairing the L-arginine-nitric oxide pathway) [27], oxidative stress, and inflammation [26]. Existing endothelial dysfunction may then reduce the ability of the kidneys to deal with additional stresses, making them susceptible to induction of AKI by a second hit [28].

Oxidative Stress

Oxidative stress is due to excess cellular production of reactive oxygen species (ROS), and reduced endogenous antioxidant defenses. Derangements in the mitochondrial electron transport chain, NADPH oxidases, nitric oxide synthases, and xanthine oxidase all can contribute to oxidative stress in the heart and kidney [29, 30]. Increased oxidative stress can occur acutely or chronically in the heart and kidney [31, 32]. Therapeutics to counteract oxidative stress have been an area of active research in cardiology and nephrology [33, 34].

DIAGNOSIS OF ACUTE KIDNEY INJURY IN CARDIORENAL SYNDROMES

Conventional Markers of AKI

Conventional AKI diagnostic criteria use urine output or serum creatinine-based definitions [35]. Both of these factors, however, have limitations, limitations that are especially pertinent to cardiorenal disease. Serum creatinine is used in AKI diagnosis (and kidney function estimation) as an endogenous marker of glomerular filtration. However, it takes time to increase following a decrement in GFR, as serum creatinine must accumulate over time, and thus may not identify an AKI event until 24-48 hours after the event. Additionally, it may be altered acutely by factors other than GFR. Particularly relevant in cardiorenal disease is the effect that fluid balance has on creatinine concentration, independent of GFR changes (examples: worsening fluid accumulation can dilute serum creatinine concentration, resulting in a decrease in serum creatinine with unchanged GFR; diuresis can cause a decrease in total body volume, thus increasing serum creatinine concentration). Similar issues arise with the other commonly used endogenous filtration markers, serum cystatin C, and blood urea nitrogen (BUN). While serum cystatin C has demonstrated advantages in estimating chronic kidney function, it has not been used for AKI determination. BUN, while it has been investigated for use particularly in acute heart failure exacerbations and may be relevant in some cases, has the added disadvantage (over serum creatinine and cystatin C) of being sensitive to protein intake. In many cases of injury to the kidney, a change in GFR may not be detected at all, because of compensatory hyperfiltration from undamaged nephrons, or because the injury affected other aspects of kidney function than glomerular filtration (for example, exclusive tubular injury). Finally, serum creatinine elevations may reflect processes other than AKI, such as decreased eGFR due to RAASi use. Urine output is an insensitive marker for AKI, and many cases of AKI, even of severe AKI, in a variety of settings, are non-oliguric.

Serum creatinine's limitations in cardiorenal disease outside of the AKI realm are relevant here, as well. In many settings, reliance on serum creatinine results in underestimation of the severity of cardiorenal dysfunction as, for example, in the setting of severe HF, where sarcopenia commonly develops, reducing the generation of creatinine and thus driving down serum concentrations. In this state, severe kidney dysfunction can go undetected [36, 37]. (This sarcopenic situation is analogous to what occurs in advanced cirrhosis.) Detailed studies using exogenous filtration markers have shown that serum creatinine (and derived estimating equations) do not accurately reflect the one aspect of kidney health/function they are supposed to measure in heart failure [36, 37].

Newer Markers of AKI

Given the limitations of serum creatinine- and urine-based definitions of AKI, many investigations have been performed looking for other diagnostic markers. Numerous biomarkers of AKI have been identified, most of which are measured in the urine. Several new markers of kidney damage have been identified that, unlike endogenous filtration markers, may directly reflect kidney parenchymal injury, particularly tubulointerstitial injury [38, 39]. The tubulointerstitial component of the kidney is responsible for much of kidney functionality, and damage to this compartment is the principal process in progression of kidney disease and overt kidney failure [40, 41]. As just one example of investigations into use of these markers in cardiorenal disease, tubular damage, assessed by urine biomarkers, is common in chronic HF and is associated with reduced survival (independently of glomerular filtration rate) in HF with reduced ejection fraction [42-44]. This observed tubulointerstitial damage in HF may be due to altered local renal perfusion with hypoxic injury, venous congestion with elevated interstitial pressures, and intrarenal RAAS activation [45-48].

While these newer biomarkers have not made it into routine clinical practice, specific novel biomarker applications are discussed when relevant in some of the case scenarios.

Common Clinical Cardiorenal Scenarios Complicated by AKI

Acute Decompensated Heart Failure

Background

AKI in acute decompensated HF is a common and vexing cardiorenal scenario. It may be particularly challenging because a mainstay of treatment in most patients, relief of congestion from volume overload, often causes a rise in serum creatinine, a rise that commonly reaches the thresholds defining AKI. However, it appears that this rise in serum creatinine is due to hemodynamic effects rather than to parenchymal kidney injury [49]. Moreover, rising serum creatinine during treatment of acute decompensated HF has been shown to be associated with lower risk for readmissions, perhaps suggesting that rather than an indication of AKI, a rising serum creatinine with diuresis in acute decompensated HF indicates more adequate decongestion [49]. The cardiology literature thus refers to these increases in creatinine as worsening renal function (WRF), rather than AKI. Use of novel biomarkers reflecting parenchymal kidney injury have shown that tubulointerstitial kidney damage does not usually accompany diuresis. A minority of patients with acute decompensated HF will have hypotension, and even fewer will have cardiogenic shock, necessitating inotropic medications and potential support devices such as aortic balloon pump counterpulsation or a ventricular assist device. This subgroup of patients, especially prior to hemodynamic resuscitation, may sustain parenchymal kidney injury.

Diagnosis, Management, and Prognosis

The most important aspect of management of kidney dysfunction in this setting is recognition of the acute decompensated HF state, and optimization of the deranged hemodynamics. This is done at the same time as the cause of the acute decompensation is determined. This entails a detailed investigation to determine the HF phenotype and cause of HF, and identifying and treating congestion and, less commonly, to identify and treat hypoperfusion [50]. Given that congestion is the "predominant clinical profile" in most patients with acute HF, relief of congestion is the mainstay of therapy and of improving organ function for most patients [50]. Thus, intravenous loop diuretics are recommended for all patients with acute HF admitted with signs and symptoms of volume overload [51]. Kidney dysfunction, acute or chronic, may require increased loop diuretic doses to achieve adequate diuretic response. Goal-directed titration protocols, with adjustment of diuretic doses in response to urine output, have been used successfully in trials, although no specific regimen has been demonstrated to be superior [52, 53]. As discussed earlier, often serum creatinine rises during diuresis, which may reach the threshold defining AKI, and clinicians may wonder whether harm is occurring and may be tempted to decrease or hold the diuretic dose. However, it does not appear that these observed serum creatinine increases are associated with damage to the kidneys and increasing serum creatinine has been found to be associated with better outcomes [54, 55]. Thus, the goal of decongestion is paramount, and rising serum creatinine or BUN levels should not dissuade the clinician from continued (or increased) diuresis if the patient remains volume overloaded [49]. Different strategies of adjusting diuretic-induced decongestion based on changes in kidney function have not been studied. Continuous and intermittent IV diuretics have demonstrated similar effectiveness [52]. Consensus recommendations highlight the need for early monitoring for effectiveness of diuretic dosing, and algorithmically intensifying diuretics to achieve goals [49].

Less commonly, a patient with acute HF will be (or will become) diuretic resistant in the face of continued volume overload and congestion, and will not respond to even aggressive stepped therapy with increased loop diuretic doses and adjunctive distal tubule diuretics. In these cases, mechanical ultrafiltration is often needed, at least on a temporary basis [49]. Once euvolemia achieved, the patient may be able to be transitioned back to diuretic therapy, or may require long-term mechanical ultrafiltration. These challenging cases require close collaboration between nephrologists and cardiologists.

As biomarkers directly reflecting parenchymal kidney injury move into broader clinical use, these may assist with differentiating benign creatinine increases from true parenchymal kidney injury in cases where there may be uncertainty, or disagreement among clinicians.

In the minority of acute HF patients with hypoperfusion (which commonly manifests with cold extremities, confusion, dizziness, hypotension, narrow pulse pressure, and oliguria), improving systemic perfusion (which often involves finding and treating an inciting cause) is central. This often entails supportive care with use of inotropic agents such as milrinone or dobutamine to bridge until more definitive therapy (reversal of the inciting factor with, for example, coronary revascularization; mechanical device therapy) can be implemented [56].

Coronary Angiography and Revascularization

Background

Coronary angiography and revascularization is a common diagnostic and treatment strategy for atherosclerotic cardiovascular disease. It is used in both acute clinical situations (such as ST elevation myocardial infarction [STEMI]) and non-acute situations (such as chronic ischemic heart disease). People undergoing these procedures commonly have underlying kidney dysfunction and thus fit into the cardiorenal phenotypes (perhaps most commonly due to underlying diabetes driving both heart and kidney disease, or due to the heart disease itself). Because iodinated radiocontrast media is used in the vast majority of these procedures, practitioners are often concerned about AKI, and nephrologists are often consulted for risk assessment prior to the procedure, or in response to an apparent AKI following the procedure.

The importance and severity of contrast-induced AKI in modern practice are unclear. Animal studies have shown that contrast media can cause acute tubular necrosis (ATN) through inducing medullary hypoxia (through viscosity alterations and changes in nitric oxide, endothelin, and adenosine pathways), and through direct cytotoxicity to tubular cells [57, 58]. Previous reports suggest that substantial serum creatinine increases occur in more than 5 percent of patients undergoing cardiac catheterization [59]. However, in modern practice, non-ionic, low- or iso-osmolal contrast agents are used almost exclusively, which may substantially reduce the risk.

A major difficulty in understanding contrast-induced AKI in general, and particularly in the setting of coronary angiography, are the other factors that are often present (other than the contrast media) that may cause AKI. These include diminished kidney perfusion (from hypotension), atheroembolic injury, hypoxia, and inflammation [58]. Disentangling the effects of these complicated factors from the effects of contrast media is exceptionally challenging.

Prevention, Diagnosis, and Management

There have been extensive investigations into prevention of contrast-induced AKI. However, the only strategy supported by consistent evidence is volume expansion, typically with intravenous isotonic crystalloid [60]. Another strategy that has been studied extensively is treatment with oral acetylcysteine. This molecule, a precursor to glutathione, has not been consistently shown to be of benefit, and is not generally recommended [60]. Numerous other strategies have been used, yet none have supporting evidence for general use [61]. Mechanistic, experimental, and epidemiological evidence supports the use of low-osmolal, or preferably even iso-osmolal contrast agents to minimize damage to the kidneys through ischemic and cytotoxic mechanisms [62]. Discontinuation of non-steroidal anti-inflammatory drugs (NSAIDS) prior to angiography is reasonable, to prevent additive vasoconstriction that could potentiate hypoxic medullary injury.

An important conundrum that commonly arises in clinical practice is often whether to proceed with coronary angiography among those with pre-existing cardiorenal disease. Expert consensus is to not allow concern about AKI to deter the use of coronary angiography and revascularization if it is needed, given the centrality of cardiac health and function to overall health in cardiorenal settings.

Monitoring of serum creatinine following coronary angiography often shows an increase, although the importance of this is often unclear. More widespread use of urinary biomarkers will likely provide more and better information. There are no effective treatments for AKI if it develops, so monitoring is primarily relevant from a prognostic perspective, or in those with severe preexisting kidney dysfunction for whom a modest kidney insult could precipitate failure needing kidney replacement therapy. General kidney preserving strategies such as holding NSAIDs, ensuring euvolemia, and avoiding or minimizing any additional contrast procedures are appropriate.

Cardiac Surgery

Background

AKI is the most frequent major complication of cardiac surgery, impacting up to 42% of surgeries [63]. Additionally, AKI in this setting is associated with substantially higher mortality and longer length of stay. Cardiac surgery can damage the kidneys through numerous pathways. These include mechanisms initiated by use of cardiopulmonary bypass, with hemolysis and production of free radicals, inflammatory and oxidative stress and activation of complement, reduced kidney perfusion with low, non-pulsatile flow, and neurohormonal activation, among others [63]. AKI commonly complicates cardiac surgery even in the absence of overt hypotension. Patients who are undergoing cardiac surgery commonly have metabolic syndrome and/or diabetes, in addition to atherosclerosis. These factors lead to high rates of pre-existing, known kidney disease, in addition to likely high rates of undetected CKD where serum creatinine has not risen, despite substantial underlying chronic kidney damage. This pre-existing kidney dysfunction or disease leads to low tolerance for the additional, multipronged insults from cardiac surgery.

Prevention, Diagnosis, and Management

Most studies aiming to identify factors that can prevent AKI are observational, and have demonstrated an association of possible beneficial effect of statins in prevention of cardiac surgery associated AKI [63]. Given the strong indications for statins in the majority of patients undergoing cardiac surgery, most patients will be on these agents. Remote ischemic preconditioning, with short occlusions of blood flow to the extremities, has been studied as a means of preventing AKI. However, meta-analysis has found no conclusive prevention benefit from remote ischemic preconditioning [64]. Preventive management is primarily built on optimal supportive care, with avoidance of nephrotoxic medications, optimization of hemodynamics, and usual surgical strategies to minimize surgical insults such as blood loss, surgical time, aortic clamp time, and cardiopulmonary bypass time [64].

There is recent evidence of the importance of early detection diagnosis of cardiac surgery associated AKI in improving outcomes. Previously, detection was either by oliguria (in the case of severe dysfunction) or, in non-oliguric bases, by increasing levels of serum creatinine (or cystatin C and/or BUN) as these endogenous filtration markers accumulated over days. However, recent biomarker advancements allow for earlier detection and focused management, with diagnosis of AKI as early as 1 hour after cardiopulmonary bypass [65]. Use of a US Food and Drug Administration (FDA) approved urine biomarker score, obtained by multiplying the urine concentrations of tissue inhibitor of metalloproteinase 2 (TIMP-2) and insulin-like growth factor binding protein 7 (IGFBP7), has been shown to be effective for early detection of AKI allowing for altered management [66, 67]. A randomized trial using an AKI score derived from two cell-cycle arrest markers has demonstrated reductions in subsequent development of AKI based on the Kidney Disease Improving Global Outcomes (KDIGO) guidelines [68], resulting in a recommendation for use in cardiac surgery by the Enhanced Recovery After Surgery Society [65]. This demonstrates the importance of moving beyond sole reliance on serum creatinine and urine assessments in the diagnosis and management of AKI.

Additionally, pharmacologic therapy may soon play a role in prevention of cardiac surgery induced AKI. Detailed mechanistic animal studies and a phase 1 human trial suggest that nicotinamide administered prior to surgery may prevent AKI [69]. Larger trials are ongoing, and results are needed before this treatment could be considered in clinical practice.

Neurohormonal Blockade and Blood Pressure Control

Background

Blood pressure control and neurohormonal blockade are paramount management goals in coronary heart disease and in heart failure. While discussion of specific indications for various agents is beyond the scope of this chapter, adequate treatment of HTN is essential in the general population, and even more so in persons with cardiorenal dysfunction. Beta-blockers are essential therapy in coronary heart disease and in HF with reduced ejection fraction (HFrEF), while ACEi/ARBs are important in coronary heart disease, HFrEF, diabetes, and CKD. Generally, these medications are titrated to achieve appropriate blood pressure control, or in the setting of heart disease, are often titrated to the maximal tolerated doses that do not result in excessively low blood pressure or heart rate. This is done because of the mortality and morbidity benefits shown in many circumstances with these agents. A concern faced by some clinicians is increasing serum creatinine in these circumstances of tight blood pressure control or ACEi/ARB maximization. The rising serum creatinine in these situations appears to be driven largely by macro- and microcirculatory hemodynamic alterations diminishing the GFR, which may at times cause serum creatinine increases that meet threshold definitions for AKI. However, no clear harm has been shown to occur from this and, given the strong evidence of benefits with maximization of these agents in many scenarios, it is reasonable to continue these agents unless there is evidence of incipient kidney failure or severe decreases in kidney function suggesting underlying tenuous kidney circulatory status, such as in renal artery stenosis.

The Future of AKI in Cardiorenal Syndromes

Management of the cardiorenal syndrome, and of AKI in the cardiorenal syndrome in particular, has been stymied in the past by limited diagnostic tools, uncertain prognostic implications, and absent therapies. However, all these roadblocks are rapidly diminishing. Improved biomarkers, with lessened reliance on endogenous filtration markers, is one crucially important facet of this. While not yet widely clinically used, biomarkers reflecting damage to the kidneys more directly—during the relatively short period of their availability—have already altered understandings of several acute kidney processes within the domain of cardiorenal syndromes and have enabled improved care. Ultimately, directed therapeutics to protect the kidneys from acute harms, and to reverse harms that have occurred before they progress to irreversible chronic damage, are what are most essential, and it is likely that these will be available in the near future, revolutionizing nephrology care of the cardiorenal syndromes.

Clinical Pearls

- Cardiorenal disease sets up a tenuous state where relatively mild insults may cause important kidney dysfunction.
- Underlying chronic kidney disease (CKD) may be present in many states of heart disease, without any elevation in serum creatinine being apparent.
- In acute decompensated HF with volume overload, adequate decongestion (usually with diuretics) is a paramount goal, and serum creatinine elevations in this setting are to be expected and accepted, and do not usually reflect parenchymal kidney injury.
- Urine biomarkers that directly reflect parenchymal kidney injury are now available, and are recommended for clinical use to reduce cardiac surgery-associated AKI.

References

[1] Rangaswami EAJ, Bhalla IV, Blair LJ, Chang VT, Costa WS, Lentine AK, et al. Cardiorenal syndrome: classification, pathophysiology, diagnosis, and treatment strategies: a scientific statement from the American Heart Association. *Circulation.* 2019;139(16):e840-e78.

[2] Zannad F, Rossignol P. Cardiorenal syndrome revisited. *Circulation.* 2018;138(9):929-44.

[3] Bock JS, Gottlieb SS. Cardiorenal syndrome: new perspectives. *Circulation.* 2010;121(23):2592-600.

[4] Damman K, van Deursen VM, Navis G, Voors AA, van Veldhuisen DJ, Hillege HL. Increased central venous pressure is associated with impaired renal function and mortality in a broad spectrum of patients with cardiovascular disease. *J Am Coll Cardiol.* 2009;53(7):582-8.

[5] Obokata M, Kane GC, Reddy YN, Melenovsky V, Olson TP, Jarolim P, et al. The neurohormonal basis of pulmonary hypertension in heart failure with preserved ejection fraction. *Eur Heart J.* 2019;40(45):3707-17.

[6] Hartupee J, Mann DL. Neurohormonal activation in heart failure with reduced ejection fraction. *Nat Rev Cardiol.* 2017;14(1):30-8.

[7] Clementi A, Virzì GM, Battaglia GG, Ronco C. Neurohormonal, endocrine, and immune dysregulation and inflammation in cardiorenal syndrome. *Cardiorenal Med.* 2019;9(5):265-73.

[8] Carnagarin R, Kiuchi MG, Ho JK, Matthews VB, Schlaich MP. Sympathetic nervous system activation and its modulation: role in atrial fibrillation. *Front Neurosci.* 2019;12:1058.

[9] Hartupee J, Mann DL. Neurohormonal activation in heart failure with reduced ejection fraction. *Nat Rev Cardiol.* 2017;14(1):30-8.

[10] Dube P, Weber KT. Congestive heart failure: pathophysiologic consequences of neurohormonal activation and the potential for recovery: part I. *Am J Med Sci.* 2011;342(5):348-51.

[11] Evans RG, Ince C, Joles JA, Smith DW, May CN, O'Connor PM, et al. Haemodynamic influences on kidney oxygenation: clinical implications of integrative physiology. *Clin Exp Pharmacol Physiol.* 2013;40(2):106-22.

[12] Ronco C, Cicoira M, McCullough PA. Cardiorenal syndrome type 1: pathophysiological crosstalk leading to combined heart and kidney dysfunction in the setting of acutely decompensated heart failure. *J Am Coll Cardiol.* 2012;60(12):1031-42.

[13] Libby P, Nahrendorf M, Swirski FK. Leukocytes link local and systemic inflammation in ischemic cardiovascular disease: an expanded "cardiovascular continuum." *J Am Coll Cardiol.* 2016;67(9):1091-103.

[14] Swirski FK, Nahrendorf M. Leukocyte behavior in atherosclerosis, myocardial infarction, and heart failure. *Science.* 2013;339(6116):161-6.

[15] Sato Y, Yanagita M. Immune cells and inflammation in AKI to CKD progression. *Am J Physiol Renal Physiol.* 2018;315(6):F1501-F12.

[16] Matsushita K, Saritas T, Eiwaz MB, McClellan N, Coe I, Zhu W, et al. The acute kidney injury to chronic kidney disease transition in a mouse model of acute cardiorenal syndrome emphasizes the role of inflammation. *Kidney Int.* 2020;97(1):95-105.

[17] Zoccali C, Vanholder R, Massy ZA, Ortiz A, Sarafidis P, Dekker FW, et al. The systemic nature of CKD. *Nat Rev Nephrol.* 2017;13(6):344-58.

[18] Adamo L, Rocha-Resende C, Prabhu SD, Mann DL. Reappraising the role of inflammation in heart failure. *Nat Rev Cardiol.* 2020:17(5):269-85.

[19] Ridker PM, Everett BM, Thuren T, MacFadyen JG, Chang WH, Ballantyne C, et al. Antiinflammatory therapy with canakinumab for atherosclerotic disease. *New Engl J Med.* 2017;377(12):1119-31.

[20] Bakris GL, Agarwal R, Anker SD, Pitt B, Ruilope LM, Rossing P, et al. Effect of finerenone on chronic kidney disease outcomes in type 2 diabetes. *New Engl J Med.* 2020;383(23):2219-29.

[21] Zelniker TA, Braunwald E. Mechanisms of cardiorenal effects of sodium-glucose cotransporter 2 inhibitors: JACC state-of-the-art review. *J Am Coll Cardiol.* 2020;75(4):422-34.

[22] Birnbaum Y, Bajaj M, Yang H-C, Ye Y. Combined SGLT2 and DPP4 inhibition reduces the activation of the Nlrp3/ASC inflammasome and attenuates the development of diabetic nephropathy in mice with type 2 diabetes. *Cardiovasc Drugs Ther.* 2018;32(2):135-45.

[23] Yuan Y, Qiu H, Hu X, Luo T, Gao X, Zhao X, et al. Predictive value of inflammatory factors on contrast-induced acute kidney injury in patients who underwent an emergency percutaneous coronary intervention. *Clin Cardiol.* 2017;40(9):719-25.

[24] Bonavia A, Singbartl K. A review of the role of immune cells in acute kidney injury. *Pediatr Nephrol.* 2018;33(10):1629-39.

[25] Van Dijk CG, Oosterhuis NR, Xu YJ, Brandt M, Paulus WJ, Van Heerebeek L, et al. Distinct endothelial cell responses in the heart and kidney microvasculature characterize the progression of heart failure with preserved ejection fraction in the obese ZSF1 rat with cardiorenal metabolic syndrome. *Circ Heart Fail.* 2016;9(4):e002760.

[26] Zhang J, Bottiglieri T, McCullough PA. The central role of endothelial dysfunction in cardiorenal syndrome. *Cardiorenal Med.* 2017;7(2):104-17.

[27] Rajapakse NW, Nanayakkara S, Kaye DM. Pathogenesis and treatment of the cardiorenal syndrome: implications of L-arginine-nitric oxide pathway impairment. *Pharmacol Ther.* 2015;154:1-12.

[28] Marrazzo F, Spina S, Zadek F, Lama T, Xu C, Larson G, et al. Protocol of a randomised controlled trial in cardiac surgical patients with endothelial dysfunction aimed to prevent postoperative acute kidney injury by administering nitric oxide gas. *BMJ Open.* 2019;9(7):e026848.

[29] Burgoyne JR, Mongue-Din H, Eaton P, Shah AM. Redox signaling in cardiac physiology and pathology. *Circ Res.* 2012;111(8):1091-106.

[30] Small DM, Coombes JS, Bennett N, Johnson DW, Gobe GC. Oxidative stress, anti-oxidant therapies and chronic kidney disease. *Nephrology.* 2012;17(4):311-21.

[31] Liguori I, Russo G, Curcio F, Bulli G, Aran L, Della-Morte D, et al. Oxidative stress, aging, and diseases. *Clin Interv Aging.* 2018;13:757.

[32] Virzì GM, Clementi A, de Cal M, Brocca A, Day S, Pastori S, et al. Oxidative stress: dual pathway induction in cardiorenal syndrome type 1 pathogenesis. *Oxid Med Cell Longev.* 2015, 391790–391799.

[33] Nasri H. Antioxidant therapy to ameliorate chronic kidney disease induced by oxidative stress; an updated mini-review. *J Prev Epidemiol.* 2017;2(1):e04-e.

[34] Sorriento D, De Luca N, Trimarco B, Iaccarino G. The antioxidant therapy: new insights in the treatment of hypertension. *Front Physiol.* 2018;21:9:258.

[35] Acosta-Ochoa I, Bustamante-Munguira J, Mendiluce-Herrero A, Bustamante-Bustamante J, Coca-Rojo A. Impact on outcomes across KDIGO-2012 AKI criteria according to baseline renal function. *J Clin Med.* 2019;8(9):1323.

[36] Kervella D, Lemoine S, Sens F, Dubourg L, Sebbag L, Guebre-Egziabher F, et al. Cystatin c versus creatinine for GFR estimation in CKD due to heart failure. *Am J Kidney Dis.* 2017;69(2):321-3.

[37] Brisco M, Hale A, Zile M, Heyward D, Cook J, Uber W, et al. Patients undergoing LVAD placement demonstrate marked sarcopenia leading to overestimation of pre-implant glomerular filtration rate. *J Heart Lung Transplant.* 2015;34(4):S165.

[38] Srisawat N, Kellum JA. The role of biomarkers in acute kidney injury. *Crit Care Clin.* 2020;36(1):125-40.

[39] Chawla LS, Bellomo R, Bihorac A, Goldstein SL, Siew ED, Bagshaw SM, et al. Acute kidney disease and renal recovery: consensus report of the Acute Disease Quality Initiative (ADQI) 16 Workgroup. *Nat Rev Nephrol.* 2017;13(4):241-57.

[40] Youhua L. Cellular and molecular mechanisms of renal fibrosis. *Nat Rev Nephrol.* 2011;7(12):684.

[41] Takaori K, Nakamura J, Yamamoto S, Nakata H, Sato Y, Takase M, et al. Severity and frequency of proximal tubule injury determines renal prognosis. *J Am Soc Nephrol.* 2016;27(8):2393-406.

[42] Damman K, van Veldhuisen DJ, Navis G, Voors AA, Hillege HL. Urinary neutrophil gelatinase associated lipocalin (NGAL), a marker of tubular damage, is increased in patients with chronic heart failure. *Eur J Heart Fail.* 2008;10(10):997-1000.

[43] Damman K, Van Veldhuisen DJ, Navis G, Vaidya VS, Smilde TDJ, Westenbrink BD, et al. Tubular damage in chronic systolic heart failure is associated with reduced survival independent of glomerular filtration rate. *Heart.* 2010;96(16):1297.

[44] Damman K, Masson S, Hillege HL, Voors AA, van Veldhuisen DJ, Rossignol P, et al. Tubular damage and worsening renal function in chronic heart failure. *JACC Heart Fail.* 2013;1(5):417-24.

[45] Damman K, Voors AA, Navis G, van Veldhuisen DJ, Hillege HL. The cardiorenal syndrome in heart failure. *Prog Cardiovasc Dis.* 2011;54(2):144-53.

[46] Jin WC, Hu WC, Polichnowski WA, Mori WT, Skelton WM, Ito WS, et al. Effects of renal perfusion pressure on renal medullary hydrogen peroxide and nitric oxide production. *Hypertension.* 2009;53(6):1048-53.

[47] Wysocki J, Batlle D. Urinary angiotensinogen: a promising biomarker of AKI progression in acute decompensated heart failure: what does it mean? *Clin J Am Soc Nephrol;* 2016; 11(9):1515-7.

[48] Maki U, Hiroyuki K. Intrarenal renin-angiotensin system activation in end-stage renal disease. *Hypertens Res.* 2017;40(4):351-2.

[49] Mullens W, Damman K, Harjola VP, Mebazaa A, Brunner-La Rocca HP, Martens P, et al. The use of diuretics in heart failure with congestion—a position statement from the Heart Failure Association of the European Society of Cardiology. *Eur J Heart Fail.* 2019;21(2):137-55.

[50] Harjola VP, Mullens W, Banaszewski M, Bauersachs J, Brunner-La Rocca HP, Chioncel O, et al. Organ dysfunction, injury and failure in acute heart failure: from pathophysiology to diagnosis and management. A review on behalf of the Acute Heart Failure Committee of the Heart Failure Association (HFA) of the European Society of Cardiology (ESC). *Eur J Heart Fail.* 2017;19(7):821-36.

[51] Ponikowski P, Voors AA, Anker SD, Bueno H, Cleland JGF, Coats AJS, et al. 2016 ESC Guidelines for the diagnosis and treatment of acute and chronic heart failure: The Task

Force for the diagnosis and treatment of acute and chronic heart failure of the European Society of Cardiology (ESC) Developed with the special contribution of the Heart Failure Association (HFA) of the ESC. *Eur Heart J.* 2016;37(27):2129-200.

[52] Felker GM, Lee KL, Bull DA, Redfield MM, Stevenson LW, Goldsmith SR, et al. Diuretic strategies in patients with acute decompensated heart failure. *New Engl J Med.* 2011;364(9):797-805.

[53] Lala A, McNulty SE, Mentz RJ, Dunlay SM, Vader JM, AbouEzzeddine OF, et al. Relief and recurrence of congestion during and after hospitalization for acute heart failure: insights from Diuretic Optimization Strategy Evaluation in Acute Decompensated Heart Failure (DOSE-AHF) and Cardiorenal Rescue Study in Acute Decompensated Heart Failure (CARESS-HF). *Circ Heart Fail.* 2015;8(4):741-8.

[54] Ahmad T, Jackson K, Rao VS, Tang WW, Brisco-Bacik MA, Chen HH, et al. Worsening renal function in patients with acute heart failure undergoing aggressive diuresis is not associated with tubular injury. *Circulation.* 2018;137(19):2016-28.

[55] Brisco MA, Zile MR, Hanberg JS, Wilson FP, Parikh CR, Coca SG, et al. Relevance of changes in serum creatinine during a heart failure trial of decongestive strategies: insights from the DOSE trial. *J Cardiac Fail.* 2016;22(10):753-60.

[56] Yancy CW, Jessup M, Bozkurt B, Butler J, Casey DE, Drazner MH, et al. 2013 ACCF/AHA guideline for the management of heart failure: a report of the American College of Cardiology Foundation/American Heart Association Task Force on Practice Guidelines. *J Am Coll Cardiol.* 2013;62(16):e147-e239.

[57] Persson PB, Hansell P, Liss P. Pathophysiology of contrast medium–induced nephropathy. *Kidney Intl.* 2005;68(1):14-22.

[58] Fähling M, Seeliger E, Patzak A, Persson PB. Understanding and preventing contrast-induced acute kidney injury. *Nat Rev Nephrol.* 2017;13(3):169-180.

[59] Tommaso CL. Contrast-induced nephrotoxicity in patients undergoing cardiac catheterization. *Cathet Cardiovasc Diagn.* 1994;31(4):316-21.

[60] Kellum JA, Lameire N, Aspelin P, Barsoum RS, Burdmann EA, Goldstein SL, et al. KDIGO clinical practice guideline for acute kidney injury. *Kidney Int Suppl.* 2012;2(1):1-138.

[61] Chalikias G, Drosos I, Tziakas DN. Prevention of contrast-induced acute kidney injury: an update. *Cardiovasc Drugs Ther.* 2016;30(5):515-24.

[62] Seeliger E, Sendeski M, Rihal CS, Persson PB. Contrast-induced kidney injury: mechanisms, risk factors, and prevention. *Eur Heart Jl.* 2012;33(16):2007-15.

[63] Wang Y, Bellomo R. Cardiac surgery-associated acute kidney injury: risk factors, pathophysiology and treatment. *Nat Rev Nephrol.* 2017;13(11):697-711.

[64] Pierce B, Bole I, Patel V, Brown DL. Clinical outcomes of remote ischemic preconditioning prior to cardiac surgery: a meta-analysis of randomized controlled trials. *J Am Heart Assoc.* 2017;6(2):e004666.

[65] Engelman DT, Ali WB, Williams JB, Perrault LP, Reddy VS, Arora RC, et al. Guidelines for perioperative care in cardiac surgery: enhanced recovery after surgery society recommendations. *JAMA Surgery.* 2019;154(8):755-66.

[66] Gunnerson KJ, Shaw AD, Chawla LS, Bihorac A, Al-Khafaji A, Kashani K, et al. TIMP2*IGFBP7 biomarker panel accurately predicts acute kidney injury in high-risk surgical patients. *J Trauma Acute Care Surg.* 2016;80(2):243-9.

[67] Kashani K, Al-Khafaji A, Ardiles T, Artigas A, Bagshaw SM, Bell M, et al. Discovery and validation of cell cycle arrest biomarkers in human acute kidney injury. *Crit Care.* 2013;17(1):1-12.

[68] Mayer T, Bolliger D, Scholz M, Reuthebuch O, Gregor M, Meier P, et al. Urine biomarkers of tubular renal cell damage for the prediction of acute kidney injury after cardiac surgery—a pilot study. *J Cardiothorac Vasc Anesth.* 2017;31(6):2072-9.

[69] Mehr AP, Tran MT, Ralto KM, Leaf DE, Washco V, Messmer J, et al. De novo NAD+ biosynthetic impairment in acute kidney injury in humans. *Nat Med.* 2018;24(9):1351-9.

In: Issues in Kidney Disease – Acute Kidney Injury
Editors: S. Z. Fadem and A. Arslan Yousuf Awan
ISBN: 978-1-68507-002-1

Chapter 15

HEPATORENAL SYNDROME

Juan Carlos Q. Velez*[1,*]*, MD and Luis A. Juncos*[2]*, MD

[1]Department of Nephrology, Ochsner Clinic Foundation, New Orleans, LA, USA;
Ochsner Clinical School, The University of Queensland, Brisbane, Australia
[2]Division of Nephrology, Department of Medicine,
University of Arkansas for Medical Sciences, Little Rock, AR, USA;
Renal Section, Department of Medicine, Central Arkansas Veterans Affairs Medical Center, Little Rock, AR, USA

ABSTRACT

Acute kidney injury (AKI) in patients with end-stage liver disease constitutes one of the most challenging clinical scenarios in in-hospital and critical care medicine. Hepatorenal syndrome type 1 (HRS-1), which is a specific type of AKI that occurs in the context of advanced cirrhosis and portal hypertension, is associated with particularly high mortality. The pathogenesis of HRS-1 is largely viewed as a functional derangement that ultimately affects kidney perfusion. Non-hemodynamic tubulo-toxic factors, such as endotoxins and bile acids, might also mediate parenchymal kidney injury and contribute to the development of AKI. The diagnosis of HRS-1 is clinical. Exclusion of other causes of AKI is required because patients with cirrhosis are at risk of AKI due to a wide range of factors. The cornerstone of pharmacological treatment is goal-directed hemodynamically targeted vasoconstrictor therapy. Renal replacement therapy in this patient population must be considered with close attention to the severity of the acute illness and the estimated life expectancy and/or impact on quality of life. Ultimately, liver transplantation is the most effective treatment for HRS-1.

Keywords: hepatorenal, acute kidney injury, cirrhosis, bilirubin, renal dysfunction, end-stage liver disease, vasoconstrictor

[*] Corresponding Author's E-mail: juancarlos.velez@ochsner.org.

Introduction

Cirrhosis is an advanced form of chronic liver disease characterized by fibrosis of the hepatic parenchyma. Individuals with cirrhosis are at high risk of developing acute kidney injury (AKI), with a reported incidence of AKI of 20% among hospitalized patients with cirrhosis [1]. In addition to the vulnerability of their effective arterial blood volume, patients with cirrhosis are frequently exposed to medications that promote gastrointestinal or urinary losses, such as lactulose or diuretics, respectively. In addition, these patients are exposed to potentially nephrotoxic antibiotics to treat infections such as spontaneous bacterial peritonitis (SBP) of ascitic fluid, undergo large volume paracentesis (LVP), which has potential to cause hemodynamic instability, and are at risk of gastrointestinal bleeding with a resultant reduction in serum hemoglobin and oxygen carrying capacity. Beyond these inherent risk factors for AKI, advanced cirrhosis with portal hypertension can lead to the development of a specific form of AKI: hepatorenal syndrome type 1 (HRS-1).

Historical Overview of HRS-1

The coexistence of liver and kidney disease was described as early as 1863 [2], leading to recognition, in the early twentieth century, that individuals with advanced cirrhosis could succumb to acute kidney failure and die shortly after [3-5]. A report describing near-normal renal histology on autopsy despite the presence of severe renal impairment before death in patients with cirrhosis [6] led to the hypothesis that acute kidney failure in patients with cirrhosis is a functional disorder, rather than a disease characterized by specific morphological changes in kidney parenchyma. A subsequent seminal study used postmortem angiography to demonstrate remarkable restoration of renal blood flow immediately following resection of the kidneys, solidifying the notion that the renal dysfunction of patients with HRS-1 is associated with near complete cessation of renal blood flow and suggesting that circulating humoral factors are responsible for this effect [7]. These findings were supported by a later study of 70 individuals, which used invasive measurement of renal blood flow to demonstrate that patients with cirrhosis, azotemia, and oliguria had markedly reduced renal blood flow compared to that of patients with cirrhosis and ascites without azotemia and oliguria, patients with compensated cirrhosis and individuals without cirrhosis (Figure 1) [8]. However, perhaps the most convincing evidence that HRS-1 is primarily a functional disorder comes from experience in transplantation medicine, whereby kidneys from patients with cirrhosis and HRS-1 exhibited excellent allograft function following transplantation into patients with end-stage renal disease (ESRD) [9]. Conversely, liver transplantation in patients with HRS-1 led to normalization of kidney function within 2 weeks [10]. Together, this evidence pointed to the existence of a reversible form of AKI of humoral nature.

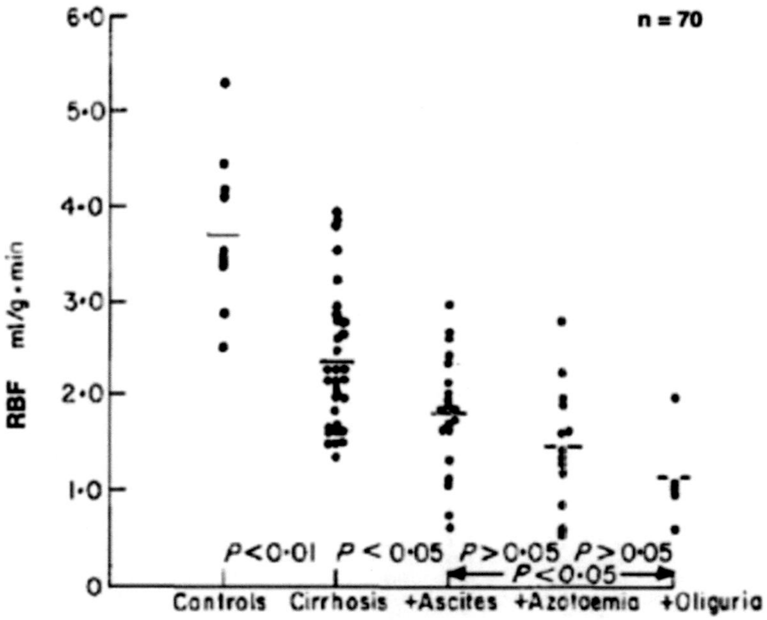

Figure 1. Marked reduction in kidney perfusion in hepatorenal syndrome type 1 (HRS-1). *In vivo* assessment of renal blood flow (RBF) by direct puncture of femoral artery and cannulation of renal artery in a cohort of control individuals as well as in subjects with cirrhosis without ascites, cirrhosis with ascites, cirrhosis with ascites and azotemia, and cirrhosis with ascites, azotemia and oliguria. Measurements illustrate progressive decline in RBF as the disease progresses.
Adapted with permission from Ring-Larsen H, Scand J Clin Lab Invest 37: 635-42, 1977.

EPIDEMIOLOGY

Patients with cirrhosis and ascites have up to a 40% probability of developing HRS-1 within a 5 year period [11]. It is well established that HRS-1 is a severe form of AKI that is associated with considerable mortality [12-14]. As liver disease progresses, the circulatory and renal abnormalities advance to the point that they not only predispose the kidney to injury, but also directly incite it — a phenomenon known as hepatorenal physiology. In parallel, patients with cirrhosis can be exposed to numerous potentially nephrotoxic elements, such as hypovolemia, infections, bile acids, and nephrotoxic medications. Thus, standard etiologies of AKI such as prerenal azotemia and acute tubular injury (ATI) can also occur in cirrhosis. The relative incidence of prerenal azotemia, ATI, HRS-1, or other causes of AKI among patients with cirrhosis varies between studies depending on their design and origin. Overall, ATI (which affects ~15 – 60% of patients) and prerenal azotemia (affecting ~15 – 45% of patients) seem to be more common than HRS-1 (which affects ~10 – 40% of patients) [1, 15-18]. However, we now recognize that in many instances, AKI in patients with cirrhosis may be caused by overlap of more than one etiology (Figure 2) [19]. Although the prognosis of HRS-1 is often ominous, the condition can potentially be reversed by implementation of vasoconstrictor therapy or liver transplantation at an appropriate juncture. Liver transplantation is the treatment modality most likely to lead to complete resolution of HRS-1, but it is not widely available.

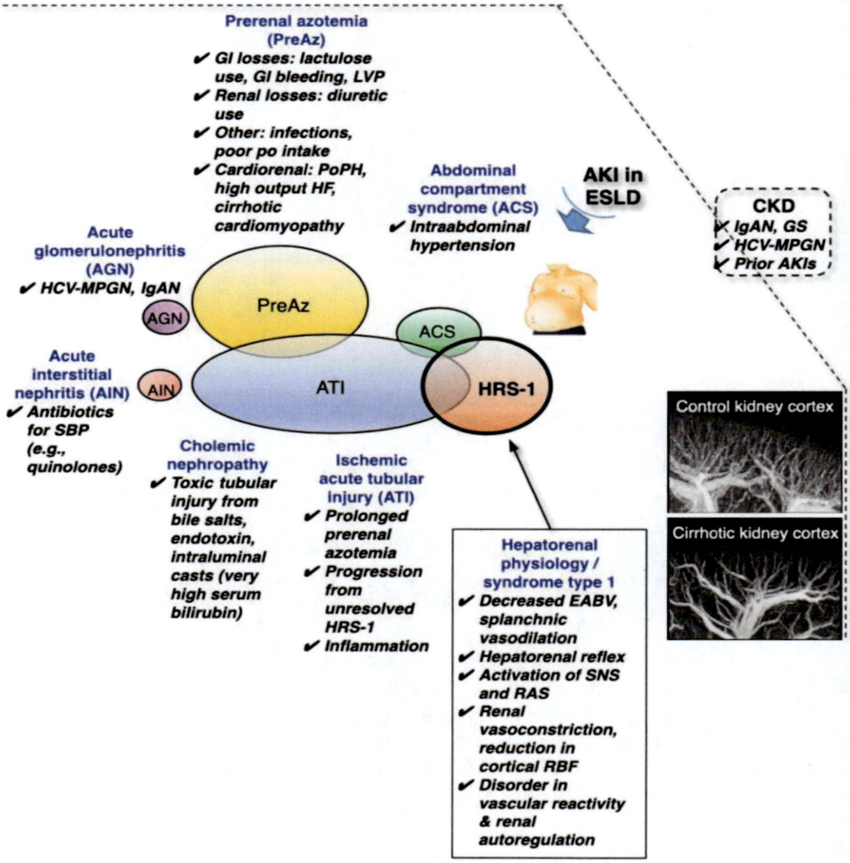

Figure 2. Differential diagnosis for acute kidney injury (AKI) in cirrhosis and hepatorenal syndrome type 1 (HRS-1). Different pathogenic mechanisms might contribute to AKI in patients with cirrhosis. Notably, considerable potential exists for overlap in the mechanisms, suggesting that the various disease processes might not always represent distinct entities. Prerenal azotemia (PreAz), acute tubular injury (ATI) or necrosis (ATN), HRS-1 and abdominal compartment syndrome (ACS) constitute the prevailing forms of AKI in cirrhosis. The size of the individual ovals corresponds to the observed frequency of each diagnosis based on the published literature [1, 15-18] and our own perspective. A key mechanism involved in the development of HRS-1 is a reduction in cortical blood flow within the kidney, as evidenced by micro-computed tomography image reconstruction of a control and cirrhotic rat kidney cortex (induced by common bile duct ligation). A reduction in renal blood flow (RBF) is at the center of HRS-1 pathogenesis. Portal hypertension and maladaptive splanchnic arterial vasodilation lead to overactivation of sympathetic nervous system (SNS) and the renin-angiotensin system (RAS) resulting in renal vasoconstriction. In addition, enhanced vascular reactivity, loss of renal autoregulation, the hepatorenal reflex and hepatocardiorenal physiology can also reduce RBF and glomerular filtration rate (GFR). Ischemia resulting from sustained reduction of RBF or prolonged PreAz can lead to ATI. In addition, inflammatory (endotoxin) and toxic (cholemic) triggers can further contribute to ATI. Acute glomerulonephritis (AGN) and acute interstitial nephritis (AIN) can be a cause of AKI in cirrhosis. Exposure to antibiotics to treat spontaneous bacterial peritonitis or other infections can cause AIN and certain forms of AGN are prevalent in cirrhosis, such as hepatitis C virus-associated membranoproliferative glomerulonephritis (HCV-MPGN). Obstructive uropathy is rare in this setting. CKD resulting from cirrhosis-associated IgA nephropathy (IgAN) or HRS-2 can also coexist with AKI. GI: gastrointestinal; LVP: large volume paracentesis; PoPH: Portopulmonary hypertension; HF: heart failure; ESLD: end-stage liver disease; SBP: spontaneous bacterial peritonitis; EABV: effective arterial blood volume.

PATHOGENESIS

The overarching mechanism of renal dysfunction in HRS-1 relates to a circulatory derangement that ultimately leads to impairment in renal blood flow and resulting fall in glomerular filtration rate (GFR). In this section, different hemodynamically mediated pathophysiological processes will be reviewed that are thought to contribute to the development of HRS-1, as well as some non-hemodynamic factors that may play a role in the pathogenesis.

Hemodynamic Mechanisms

Cirrhosis-Induced Circulatory Dysfunction

In patients with cirrhosis, damage to the hepatic parenchyma leads to an increase in intrahepatic vascular resistance, portal vein pressure, portosystemic shunting, and shear stress that in turn lead to local production of various vasodilators that act on the splanchnic vascular bed. Of these mediators, nitric oxide is of particular interest for a number of reasons. First, it is a key regulator of systemic and regional hemodynamics in the mesenteric and renal vascular beds [20]. Second, it is generated by the portal endothelium in response to increased shear stress [20]. Third, it is sufficiently potent to generate the hemodynamic derangements observed in cirrhosis. Finally, nitric oxide levels are increased in human and experimental cirrhosis, and blocking nitric oxide production blunts cirrhosis-induced circulatory and renal impairment in animals [21].

Renal Vasoconstriction

The hyperdynamic circulation, decrease in systemic vascular resistance, nitric oxide-mediated splanchnic arterial vasodilation, and resulting pooling of blood volume leads to a reduction in the effective circulatory volume [20-22]. This arterial underfilling triggers activation of the sympathetic nervous system (SNS) and renin-angiotensin system (RAS) in an attempt to restore effective circulatory volume [23-26]. The release of norepinephrine and angiotensin II as a result of SNS and RAS activation induces profound renal vasoconstriction and reductions in renal blood flow, which leads to an acute loss of glomerular filtration rate (GFR) [27, 28]. Elevated plasma levels of norepinephrine, angiotensin II and plasma renin activity in patients with HRS-1 support the notion that these hormonal systems have a fundamental role in its pathogenesis [28]. Release of nitric oxide and prostaglandins counterbalance the action of vasoconstrictors and transiently maintain GFR. However, as the severity of the underlying liver disease manifests, splanchnic and systemic arterial vasodilation reach levels that overwhelm the compensatory capacity, leading to a reduction in mean arterial pressure (MAP) [28], further activation of the RAS and SNS and fall in kidney perfusion. This cascade of events has been termed the underfilling hypothesis. Experimental evidence also supports a role for other vasoconstrictors, including endothelin-1, thromboxane A_2 and adenosine in the pathogenesis of cirrhosis-induced renal vasoconstriction; however, the contribution of these factors to human HRS-1 remains unclear.

Derangements in Renal Microcirculation

Unlike other ischemic forms of AKI that are characterized by a preferential reduction in medullary blood flow, the reduction in renal blood flow that occurs in HRS-1 primarily affects cortical blood flow [29-31] (Figure 2). It has been proposed that this shunting of renal blood flow to the salt-avid juxtamedullary nephrons, which occurs in tandem with cirrhosis-induced hypertrophy of the thick ascending limbs, might impair renal sodium excretory capacity, thus further augmenting salt retention [32]. However, this proposal arose from observations in animal studies, and the relevance of these processes to humans remains speculative. Use of microcomputed tomography has demonstrated that chronic bile duct ligation to induce liver fibrosis in rats induces a decrease in renal perfusion characterized by decreased vascular filling of the renal cortex [31]. This decrease in vascular volume was most likely caused by profound, refractory regional vasoconstriction. However vascular rarefaction may also have a role, particularly in the more advanced stages of disease [29]. Thus, prolonged activation of neurohumoral systems such as the SNS and RAS in cirrhosis and the resulting protracted hypoperfusion may incite an ischemic insult, thereby triggering renal microvascular endothelial injury, vascular rarefaction and other irreversible defects in the kidney cortex [33, 34, 35].

Vascular Reactivity

Vascular reactivity refers to the responsiveness of a blood vessel to a specific stimulus or compound. Enhanced renal vascular reactivity, for instance, an augmented response to a stimulus compared to that of a physiological state, has been recognized in animal models of cirrhosis. For example, renal arterioles of rats models of hepatobiliary disease exhibit a diminished vasodilatory response to bradykinin [36] and an augmented contractile response to norepinephrine [37], endothelin-1 [38], and angiotensin II. Endotoxemia and reactive oxygen species have been implicated in those mechanisms [39-41]. As seen clinically, the renal hemodynamic alterations characteristic of HRS-1 eventually become more difficult to treat with therapeutic measures, suggesting the existence of mechanisms that perpetuate renal dysfunction. A logical explanation for the development of treatment resistance is that the sustained renal cortical hypoperfusion and rarefaction together with renal vascular hyperresponsiveness, promote the progression of renal functional impairment akin to that of an ischemic insult and intrinsic tubular injury, eventually leading to irreversible kidney damage and dysfunction.

The Hepatorenal Reflex

Experimental evidence supports the existence of a hepatorenal baroreflex that originates in the liver and leads to changes in renal sympathetic nerve activity [42]. Changes in hepatic sinusoidal pressure stimulate local release of adenosine, which in turn activates the hepatic afferent SNS, which signals to the brain and subsequently to the kidneys via the efferent renal SNS, to induce renal vasoconstriction [43-46]. The monoamine neurotransmitter serotonin has also been implicated in the activation of the hepatic afferent SNS [47]. An elegant study in individuals in whom portal pressure and renal blood flow was measured demonstrated a connection between portal hypertension and renal circulation [48]. Occluding the portal vein to increase portal pressure induced an immediate reduction in renal blood flow, which was rapidly restored when the catheter was deflated, and portal pressure normalized. This phenomenon occurred in the absence of a decrease in MAP or effective circulatory volume, suggesting that this liver-kidney crosstalk is independent of the systemic neuro-humoral activation observed in HRS-1. Further supporting this hypothesis, hepatic denervation led to a reduction in renal sympathetic nerve activity in rat model of cirrhosis [49], whereas lumbar sympathetic block led to improvement in kidney function in 5 cirrhotic patients with estimated GFR < 25 ml/min [50]. Thus, the hepatorenal reflex remains an enigmatic mechanism that may play an important role in the pathogenesis of HRS-1 independently of the underfilling hypothesis.

Cirrhotic Cardiomyopathy

Circulatory homeostasis in cirrhosis in response to a decreased peripheral vascular resistance is maintained by a hyperdynamic circulation, which is characterized by increased cardiac output, heart rate, and plasma volume. With disease progression, however, patients evolve from a state of high cardiac output to one of cardiac dysfunction, characterized by blunted cardiac responsiveness, impaired diastolic relaxation, electrophysiological conductance abnormalities with chronotropic incompetence, and decreased cardiac output — a disorder called cirrhotic cardiomyopathy [51]. The contribution of cirrhotic cardiomyopathy to circulatory dysfunction is supported by the association of low cardiac output with decreased renal blood flow, decreased GFR, and a higher probability of developing HRS-1 among patients with cirrhosis and refractory ascites [52, 53]. Studies have reported decreased cardiac output in the setting of HRS-1 [54]. Systolic dysfunction might manifest under conditions of hemodynamic stress such as in the presence of beta-blockers; indeed, the use of nonselective beta-blockers in patients with decompensated cirrhosis might predispose to HRS-1 [55]. Autonomic dysfunction and reduced baroreflex sensitivity might also contribute to altered hemodynamics and the reduction in cardiac output that occurs with advanced cirrhosis [56-58]. Further evidence to support a mechanistic link between cardiac dysfunction and kidney dysfunction in the context of liver cirrhosis was provided by a detailed study, which showed that placement of a transjugular intrahepatic portosystemic shunt (TIPS) results in considerable displacement of blood to the central vascular compartment, causing a marked increase in preload, stroke volume, and kidney function [59]. Thus, the term “hepatocardiorenal” syndrome has been recently proposed to describe the interaction between the kidney, liver, and heart in the context of cirrhosis [60].

Porto-Pulmonary Hypertension

Individuals with cirrhosis and portal hypertension are at increased risk of pulmonary hypertension, with some studies reporting an incidence of 5 - 10% [61-63, 64]. This entity, termed porto-pulmonary hypertension (PoPH), is often identified during evaluation for liver transplantation eligibility. The pathogenesis of PoPH involves lung vascular smooth muscle cell hypertrophy, *in situ* thrombosis, vasoconstriction and the development of venovenous shunts, triggered by factors such as serotonin, interleukin 1, endothelin-1 and thromboxanes [65, 66]. Of note, altered systemic hemodynamics and venous congestion are well-described features of acute decompensated pulmonary hypertension regardless of its aetiology [67]. Thus, although PoPH further compromises the circulatory derangements of HRS-1, the extent to which PoPH itself contributes to renal impairment in HRS-1 remains unclear.

Intra-Abdominal Hypertension

Paracentesis-induced circulatory dysfunction (PICD) is a well-described phenomenon characterized by a transient rise in plasma renin activity following large volume paracentesis

(LVP) [68]. Initial reports of patients with HRS-1 identified LVP as an event that preceded the development of renal dysfunction [6]; however, causality has not been established as LVP is a common procedure in patients with advanced cirrhosis. Of note, studies of PICD have been primarily conducted in patients with normal kidney function or stable chronic kidney disease, not in patients with AKI [69-71]. In addition, the incidence of PICD among patients with cirrhosis has decreased by approximately half with increasing prophylactic use of intravenous albumin as means to optimize the arterial blood volume during the ascitic fluid removal [72]. However, it is increasingly recognized that increased intra-abdominal pressure (IAP) associated with tense ascites can lead to abdominal compartment syndrome, an increase in renal vein pressure and impaired kidney function [73-75]. Accordingly, use of LVP to relieve abdominal pressure has been shown to induce a transient rise in GFR and urinary output in patients with cirrhosis [76-78]. One study showed that only 5% of patients with cirrhosis undergoing LVP developed AKI afterwards, whereas 10% improved kidney function following LVP [79]. Moreover, cases of AKI resolution following therapeutic LVP have emerged [80, 81]. Nonetheless, whether systematic surveillance of IAP and reactive LVP could favorably impact the clinical course of patients with HRS-1 remains to be determined.

Non-Hemodynamic Mechanisms

Progression to Acute Tubular Injury

Some lines of evidence suggest that persistence of HRS-1 can eventually evolve into an established tubular insult. Electron microscopy studies of kidneys obtained from patients with HRS-1 soon after death demonstrated tubulorrhexis and the presence of dark bodies in mitochondria, indicative of acute tubular necrosis (ATN) [82]. Furthermore, a distinctive lesion involving reflux of proximal convoluted tubule epithelium into the Bowman space has also been described in autopsy specimens from patients with HRS-1 [82, 83]. Studies from the transplantation literature also support the existence of progressive kidney injury in patients with HRS-1. Standard protocols across most transplant centers recommend liver transplantation alone in situations where a donor liver becomes available within 4–6 weeks of a patient with HRS-1 initiating dialysis and combined liver-kidney transplantation for patients who have been dialysis-dependent for ≥ 6 weeks [84]. This approach originates from data showing that the likelihood of achieving resolution of HRS-1 and dialysis independence after liver transplantation is inversely proportional to the duration of time on dialysis prior to transplantation [84, 85]. Perhaps a logical explanation for this observation is that sustained AKI and renal vasoconstriction in the context of cirrhosis can eventually transform into an ischemic insult and intrinsic tubular injury. Furthermore, the observation that the response of HRS-1 to treatment with vasoconstrictor therapy decreases with increasing serum bilirubin level [86] suggests that higher levels of serum bilirubin may promote AKI through mechanisms similar to those involved in the development of cholemic nephropathy (discussed below). This contention is supported by findings from a study reporting an association between the severity of hyperbilirubinemia and the likelihood of detecting renal tubular epithelial cell casts, which are markers or ATN [87]. Studies in animal models of cirrhosis have also shown time-dependent development of intrinsic tubular injury [88]. Together, these observations indicate that the pathogenesis of HRS-1 might be best viewed as a spectrum that evolves from purely functional renal impairment into overt tubular damage, which becomes superimposed on the functional derangements. However, conclusive evidence that temporal progression of HRS-1 occurs from a functional to a parenchymal entity is still lacking.

Bile Acids and Cholemic Nephropathy

Cholemic nephrosis is an old term — now replaced by cholemic nephropathy — that refers to patients who acquire AKI in the context of obstructive jaundice [89]. This condition has been described in patients with cholangiocarcinoma or other causes of mechanical obstruction of the biliary tree and cholestasis [90-93], and can occur concurrently with evidence of acute tubular injury (ATI) and peritubular venular dilatation [91]. Interest in cholemic nephropathy has more recently been renewed following reports of patients with infection or drug-induced cholestasis presenting with AKI and histological evidence of tubular injury with bile cast deposition in the tubular lumen — an entity re-termed bile cast nephropathy [94-99]. Autopsy studies have now also shown histological evidence of tubular injury with intraluminal bile casts in patients with cirrhosis and pronounced elevations of serum bilirubin [100-102], although these should be interpreted with caution, since causality is difficult to ascertain [103]. The question remains as to whether the presence of intratubular bile casts are merely a reflection of decreased GFR and tubular stasis rather than a cause of tubular injury. Notably, bilirubin-stained renal tubular epithelial cell casts are more likely to be found in patients with liver disease and high levels of serum bilirubin than in patients with liver disease without hyperbilirubinemia, supporting an association between severe hyperbilirubinemia and tubular injury [87, 104]. Paradoxically, bilirubin has been shown to possess renoprotective properties [105-108] and the term 'bilirubin cast nephropathy' is therefore discouraged. However, bile acids can elicit tubular damage, tubulointerstitial inflammation, lipid peroxidation, and oxidative stress in the kidney [109-111]. Thus, the more general term 'cholemic nephropathy' has been proposed to describe impaired renal function and histo-morphological changes, such as intratubular cast formation and tubular epithelial cell injury, in patients with hyperbilirrubinemia [99]. The changes in bilirubin excretion that occur in the context of AKI are not negligible; thus, the rise in serum bilirubin that occurs during cholestasis is further exaggerated by AKI itself [112]. This finding further complicates the assessment of AKI in patients with hyperbilirubinemia, as the contributions of functional changes in hepatorenal physiology are difficult to dissect from those resulting from cholemic nephropathy.

Currently, there is no conclusive evidence which demonstrates that cholemic nephropathy can be superimposed onto the deranged renal hemodynamics of HRS-1, and more research is needed to determine the precise contribution of cholemic nephropathy to progressive kidney injury in patients with cirrhosis.

Inflammation

Advanced cirrhosis is associated with increased serum levels of pro-inflammatory cytokines, such as endotoxins, interleukins and TNF [113]. Circulating levels of these cytokines are further increased in patients with SBP or acute-on-chronic liver failure (ACLF) — both of which are common triggers of HRS-1 [114, 115]. The inflammation that occurs in the context of cirrhosis and/or cholestasis might be driven by the translocation of bacteria from the gut into the circulation and release of endotoxins [116]. Of note, a biopsy study showed overexpression of the endotoxin receptor, Toll-like receptor 4 (TLR4), in renal tubules of patients with cirrhosis and AKI [117]. Pro-inflammatory cytokines can cause endothelial dysfunction and tubular injury. Thus, the pathogenesis of AKI in cirrhosis may involve both hemodynamic changes typical of HRS-1 and inflammation-induced ATI (Figure 2).

Diagnosis

No gold standard test exists for the definite diagnosis of HRS-1 and HRS-1 is therefore considered a diagnosis of exclusion. In 1996 the International Club of Ascites (ICA) implemented diagnostic criteria [118]. The original definition of HRS-1 proposed by the ICA comprised a list of major and minor criteria. In 2007, those criteria were revised and among other changes, the minor criteria were eliminated [119]. In 2015, the criteria were again revised to eliminate absolute serum creatinine cut-off values and adopt the standard KDIGO definitions of AKI [120, 121] (Table 1). However, classic phenotypic aspects of HRS-1 such as systemic blood pressure at the low end of the normal range, hyponatremia and oliguria are not included in the current ICA criteria [120]. Thus, although the ICA criteria have proved valuable for clinical and investigational purposes, they do not fully reflect the complexity of actual clinical scenarios resulting from the presence of confounding pathogenic factors. Consequently, sole application of ICA criteria for the diagnosis of HRS-1 is not recommended.

Table 1. Evolution of ICA diagnostic criteria for HRS-1

Category	1996 [118]	2007 [119]	2015 [120]
Major criteria	ESLD or ALD with portal hypertension	ESLD with ascites	ESLD with ascites
	Serum creatinine > 1.5 mg/dL or creatinine clearance < 40 ml/min	Serum creatinine >1.5 mg/dL	Stage ≥2 AKI (>2.0x ↑ in serum creatinine)
	Doubling of serum creatinine to >2.5 mg/dl in <2 weeks	Doubling of serum creatinine to >2.5 mg/dl in <2 weeks	NA
	No sustained improvement in kidney function after 1.5 L of iv volume expansion with normal saline and diuretic withdrawal	No sustained improvement in kidney function after 2 days of iv volume expansion with albumin (1 g/kg/day) and diuretic withdrawal	No sustained improvement in kidney function after 2 days of iv volume expansion with albumin (1 g/kg/day) and diuretic withdrawal
	Absence of shock or ongoing bacterial infection	Absence of shock	Absence of shock
	Absence of nephrotoxin exposure	Absence of nephrotoxin exposure	Absence of nephrotoxin exposure
	NA	Absence of overt hematuria (<50 rbc/hpf)	Absence of overt hematuria (<50 rbc/hpf)
	Absence of overt proteinuria (< 500 mg/day)	Absence of overt proteinuria (< 500 mg/day)	Absence of overt proteinuria (< 500 mg/day)
	Normal kidney ultrasound	Normal kidney ultrasound	Normal kidney ultrasound
Minor criteria	Urine sodium <10 mEq/l; urine volume <500 ml/day; urine osmolality greater than plasma osmolality; absence of overt hematuria (<50 rbc/hpf); serum sodium <130 mEq/L	NA	NA
Other	NA	NA	Introduction of HRS-AKI (or AKI-HRS) and non-HRS-AKI terminology; omission of the term 'HRS type 1'

[a] Multiply by 88.4 to obtain serum creatinine values in µmol/l. AKI, acute kidney injury; ALD, acute liver disease; ESLD, end-stage liver disease; HRS, hepatorenal syndrome; hpf, high powered field; iv, intravenous; NA, not applicable, rbc, red blood cells.

Precipitating Events

Early case reports of HRS-1 described patients with a preceding history of progressive jaundice, gastrointestinal bleeding or LVP, suggesting these conditions could be triggering events [6]. Subsequent studies that have explored risk factors for the development of HRS-1 have consistently shown that SBP is the most common precipitating event [115, 122, 123]. In fact, SBP prophylaxis is associated with a reduction in the subsequent development of HRS-1 among patients with cirrhosis [124]. The recognition that SBP is a triggering factor for HRS-1 was a major stimulant for the eradication of bacterial infection as an exclusion criterion for the diagnosis of HRS-1 [118, 119]. Interestingly, studies that have documented LVP as a precipitating event are sparse [123]. ACLF — a condition that is characterized by acute hepatic or extrahepatic organ failure — is a major driver of hospitalizations among patients with cirrhosis and is often accompanied by AKI [125]. Although the identification of a precipitating event should not be strictly required to diagnose HRS-1, a preceding episode of SBP or ACLF should prompt clinicians to increase their clinical suspicion for HRS-1 if the other elements of the diagnosis are also present.

Change in Kidney Function

Until the latest revision of the definition of HRS-1, the HRS-1 literature was dictated by prior definitions that utilized defined cutoffs in absolute value of serum creatinine level. The most recent version eliminated absolute serum creatinine cut-off values, but its dependence on serum creatinine persists because the KDIGO (Kidney Disease: Improving Global Outcomes) criteria for AKI are based on relative changes in serum creatinine level [120]. However, relative changes in serum creatinine are affected by its absolute values, and those values in turn have important limitations in the context of cirrhosis [126]. First, sarcopenia is a well-described phenomenon in cirrhosis [127], and commonly leads to underestimation of kidney function decline. Furthermore, increased tubular secretion of creatinine has been reported in cirrhosis, and can also contribute to underestimation of loss in GFR [128]. In addition, hyperbilirubinemia is known to interfere with the colorimetric assay for creatinine [129]. Thus, one must remain cognizant of the limitations of serum creatinine measurements when assessing absolute and relative changes in its value. Serum cystatin C correlates with inulin clearance better than serum creatinine and has been proposed to be a more accurate marker of kidney function in cirrhosis [130-134]. However, cystatin C assays are not uniformly available in clinical laboratories and the practicality of implementing its use is questionable. Oliguria is another indicator of kidney dysfunction that might be more sensitive than serum creatinine in the early detection of hepatorenal AKI [135]. However, despite the above-mentioned limitations, measurement of serum creatinine remains the primary method for the assessment of kidney function in patients with cirrhosis. Of note, change in serum creatinine level over time is a clinically useful tool since limitations of absolute creatinine values are mostly overcome when day-to-day changes in serum creatinine level are assessed.

Obligatory Elimination of Volume Depletion

A critical component of the ICA definition of HRS-1 is the exclusion of prerenal azotemia. The current criteria require that patients fail to improve kidney function despite administration of 1 g/kg of intravenous albumin for 24 - 48 hours and withdrawal of diuretics [120]. Although this approach is in general reasonable and practical, the magnitude of volume expansion prescribed is not tailored to the volume status of each patient, and no hemodynamic parameter is used to determine whether the patient has reached optimal intravenous volume expansion. In a single center study of IVC diameter and collapsibility in patients presumed to have presumed HRS-1, we found that up to 44% of patients were either volume-depleted or volume-overloaded [136]. Although this observation requires further validation, it suggests that use of blinded volume expansion is likely to either prevent some patients from achieving optimal volume expansion or worsen hypervolemia, while possibly delaying initiation of vasoconstrictor therapy in others.

Shock

A general notion exists that MAP is generally lower in individuals with cirrhosis than the general population. However, the level at which blood pressure should be considered to be hypotension in patients with cirrhosis is not clearly defined. As a result, variability exists in the threshold at which vasopressors are used to treat shock in these patients. In other words, the definition of shock is in many instances dictated by the medical decision to initiate vasopressor therapy rather than a pre-specified value of blood pressure. This ambiguity could result in an incorrect diagnosis of shock in a patient with low blood pressure and HRS-1, which could affect treatment, since the MAP goal of vasopressor therapy in shock differs from that of HRS-1 (discussed below).

Absence of Nephrotoxins

An ICA criterion for HRS-1 diagnosis requires the absence of recent exposure to potentially nephrotoxic drugs. Infections are not uncommon in patients with decompensated cirrhosis, and consequently these patients often receive antibiotic therapy, particularly for SBP. Infections can precipitate HRS-1 and must be treated. However, some antibiotics, such as fluoroquinolones and cephalosporins are potentially nephrotoxic and can lead to the development of toxic ATN or acute allergic interstitial nephritis (AIN). Although classic cases of AIN are usually accompanied by leukocyturia and/or hematuria, urinary abnormalities can be absent, and some cases can be missed. Furthermore, some antibiotics, such as fluoroquinolones and vancomycin, can cause direct tubular toxicity (that is, toxicity-induced ATN). Therefore, it is often difficult to discern when an antibiotic is the culprit for AKI in cirrhosis, unless an invasive kidney biopsy is performed. Although the ICA criterion correctly points to the need of consideration of a drug-induced form of AKI, the existing diagnostic tools are not sufficiently robust to discard that possibility with certainty.

Absence of Abnormal Renal Imaging

Renal ultrasonography is the modality of choice to rule out anatomical abnormalities, such as hydronephrosis, that would negate a diagnosis of HRS-1 as the primary cause of AKI. In addition, changes in parenchymal echogenicity are indicative of an intrinsic kidney disease, either glomerular, tubular or tubulointerstitial. However, the presence of massive ascites precludes optimal assessment of renal parenchymal echogenicity or corticomedullary differentiation due to the acoustic enhancement produced by the fluid layer (Figure 3). Thus, although renal ultrasonography is the recommended approach for the assessment of AKI in patients with cirrhosis, caution must be taken when interpreting the findings.

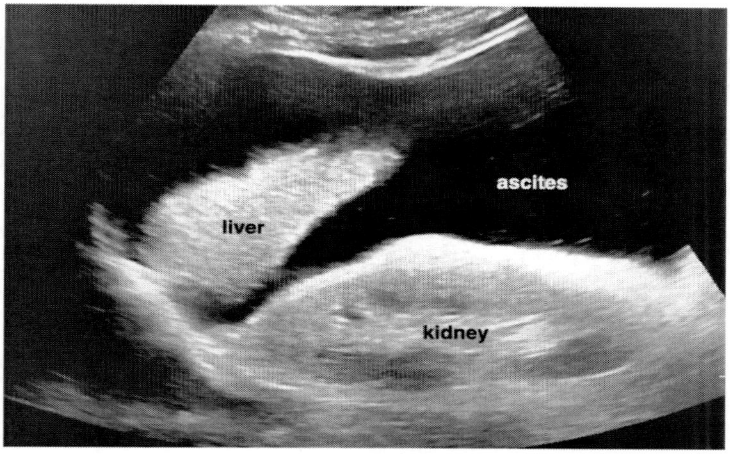

Figure 3. Massive ascites precludes optimal assessment of renal parenchymal echogenicity in patients with cirrhosis. Sagittal view of a right kidney by renal ultrasonography in a patient with cirrhosis, ascites and acute kidney injury. Acoustic enhancement is generated by the anechoic fluid layer (ascites) above the kidney. This artifact limits the possibility of assessing renal parenchymal echogenicity.

Urinary Sodium

Urinary sodium concentration was a minor criterion in the original 1996 ICA definition of HRS-1 [118]. Despite the fact that this criterion was removed in the 2007 version [119] (Table 1), anecdotal evidence suggests it has remained popular in the diagnostic evaluation of AKI in patients with cirrhosis. The most likely reason for its continued popularity is that a low fractional excretion of urinary sodium (FENa; that is, < 1%), and low urinary sodium (that is < 20 mEq/L), are almost universally present in HRS-1, whereas a FENa > 2% or a urinary sodium > 40 mEq/L are suggestive of intrinsic tubular injury, and highly inconsistent with HRS-1 [137] . However, a FENa of < 1% did not accurately establish the diagnosis of HRS-1 in a study of 88 patients who underwent kidney biopsy as part of their pre-transplantation evaluation (11% of whom were considered to have 'biopsy-proven' HRS-1 [137]). However, the FENa does seem to offer diagnostic utility when the cutoff is lowered to < 0.1% [1, 137]. In a similar vein, the fractional excretion of urea (FEUrea) has also been proposed to be valuable for distinguishing HRS-1 from ATN, particularly in the presence of diuretics. A small, single center study from 2018 claimed that a FEUrea > 28.1% offers a positive predictive value of 89% for exclusion of HRS-1 [138]. However, overlap with ATN still exists, since some patients with ATN may present with FEUrea ≤ 28.1%. In summary, while urinary indexes in general should not be ignored in the evaluation of AKI in cirrhosis, as currently outlined in the ICA criteria, they should not be used alone to identify a specific diagnosis.

Urinalysis and Urine Microscopy

The current ICA criteria call for exclusion of HRS-1 when urine microscopy reveals > 50 rbcs per high power field (hpf) or proteinuria (that is, urinary protein excretion >500 mg per day), because those findings might suggest AKI of glomerular etiology. Notably, patients with cirrhosis are at risk of developing secondary IgA nephropathy, hepatitis C-associated membranoproliferative glomerulonephritis and other glomerular pathologies [137, 139, 140], and patients with these glomerular pathologies can present with chronic hematuria and proteinuria (albuminuria), thereby exacerbating the AKI. The absence of 'baseline' urinalysis before development of AKI makes it difficult to determine whether a patient with hematuria and/or proteinuria has HRS-1 in addition to glomerular pathology. Moreover, hospitalized patients with cirrhosis and AKI might have a Foley catheter inserted, which can induce traumatic hematuria and thereby potentially mask true HRS-1. Conversely, the threshold of > 50 rbc/hpf introduces the possibility that a diagnosis of HRS-1 might be falsely assigned to a patient with a hematuric form of AKI, such as acute AIN or acute glomerulonephritis if the urinalysis reveals 10–50 rbc/hpf. In addition, the morphology of urinary rbcs needs to be taken in consideration when performing urine microscopy because the presence of dysmorphic rbcs, in particular acanthocytes, is indicative of glomerular disease, even when found at low abundance (1-5/hpf) [141]. In terms of proteinuria, the ICA criteria require excluding HRS-1 if value is > 500 mg per day. However, quantification of proteinuria in an oliguric patient with AKI using 24-hour urine collection or a random urine protein-to-creatinine ratio lacks accuracy [142]. Practitioners may therefore rely on dipstick proteinuria in this setting — a test that also lacks accuracy for proteinuria quantification. The ICA criteria do not include absence of leukocyturia as an exclusion criterion for HRS-1. Since a urinary tract infection can represent a triggering event for HRS-1, it is appropriate not to rule out HRS-1 in patients who present with leukocyturia. However, if culturing the urine does not yield growth of any bacteria and/or wbc casts are also present, AIN should be considered as a potential cause of AKI. Urinary sediment microscopy is valuable tool to aid the diagnosis [143] and prognosis of AKI [144, 145]. The presence of sheets of "muddy brown" granular casts are highly suggestive of toxic or ischemic ATI, and a scoring system based on the abundance of granular casts and renal tubular epithelial cells has been proposed as a tool to confirm the diagnosis of ATI [143]. Although such urinary cast scores have not been validated in hepatorenal AKI, urine sediment microscopy has proven utility in this setting [34]. The urinary sediment of patients with cirrhosis and AKI contains abundant elements regardless of the etiology of AKI [146] (Figure 4). The coexistence of cholemic nephropathy might also be suggested by the presence of bilirubin-stained tubular epithelial cell casts [97, 147], whereas the presence of white blood cell (wbc) casts and red blood cell (rbc) casts are suggestive of interstitial or glomerular disease, respectively. However, microscopic examination of the urinary sediment to look for casts is not a salient aspect of the current ICA criteria. Therefore, careful inspection of the urinary sediment by an experienced physician can aid interpretation of the etiology of kidney disease in cirrhosis.

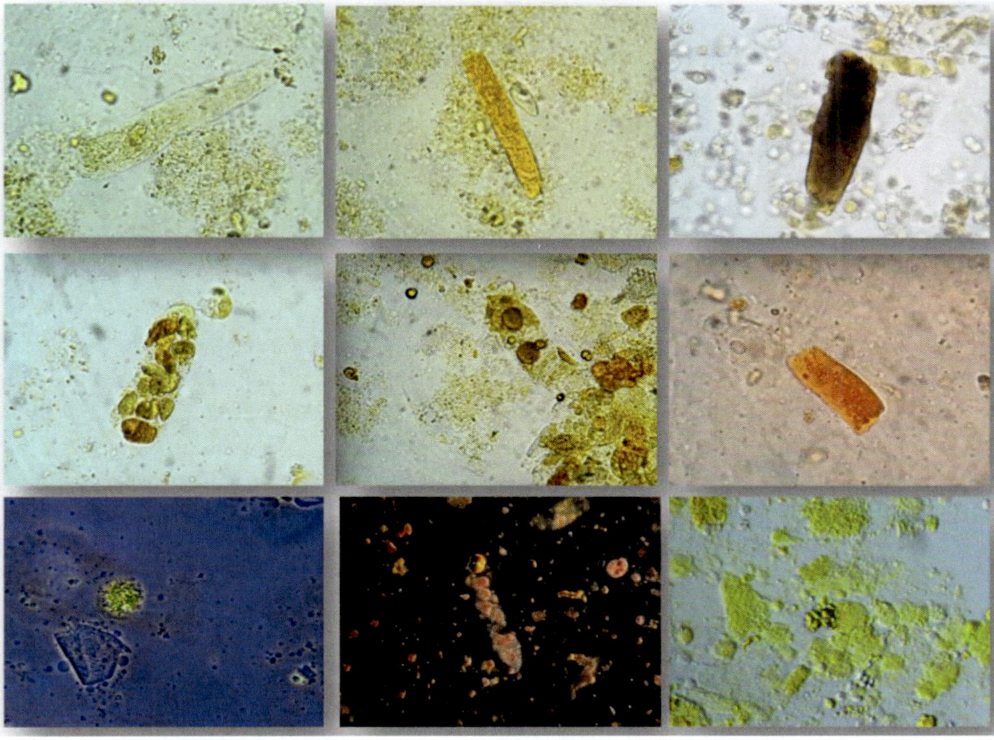

Figure 4. Findings on microscopic examination of the urinary sediment in patients with cirrhosis with acute kidney injury (AKI). Top left: bilirubin-stained hyaline cast. Top center: bilirubin-stained finely granular cast. Top right: "muddy brown" granular cast. Middle left: bilirubin-stained renal tubular epithelial cell (RTEC) cast. Middle center: bilirubin-stained hyaline casts containing leucine crystals. Middle right: Sternheimer-Malbin stained and bilirubin-stained waxy cast. Top and middle row images under bright field illumination, 400X magnification. Bottom left: bilirubin crystal (phase contrast, 400X). Bottom center: Sternheimer-Malbin stained and bilirubin-stained RTEC cast containing a leucine crystal (dark field, 400X). Bottom right: bilirubin-stained amorphous phosphates, debris and leucine crystals (oblique illumination, 400X). Only "muddy brown" granular casts are deemed conclusively indicative of acute tubular injury (ATI) and inconsistent with HRS-1. Waxy casts also denote tubular injury, but they could be of acute (ATI) or chronic (CKD) origin. RTEC casts also suggest ongoing ATI. The remainder of the findings can be present in a urine specimen of a patient with HRS-1 despite the primary functional nature of HRS-1.

Other Biomarkers

The pitfalls of the ICA diagnostic criteria underscore the need to improve our ability to diagnose HRS-1. The limitations of current criteria are highlighted by two retrospective studies which reported that 40 - 60% of cases of AKI in cirrhosis were misdiagnosed as HRS-1 [123, 148]. The field of urinary biomarkers shows promise for the more accurate diagnosis of this entity, and neutrophil gelatinase-associated lipocalin (NGAL) has been investigated as a marker to distinguish HRS-1 from ATI [1, 17, 149-152]. To strengthen the diagnostic accuracy of this approach, a panel of biomarkers that includes NGAL, IL-18, L-fatty acid binding protein and albumin has been proposed [1]. Circulating microRNAs such as miR-21 have also been proposed as biomarkers to distinguish HRS-1 from ATN [153]. Overall, these studies are hampered by the fact that the performance of the biomarkers is adjudicated against diagnosis based on clinical data, the methodology which is inherently vulnerable to misclassification as outlined above. Nonetheless, the ability to incorporate information obtained from urine biomarkers with standard clinical data might improve diagnostic accuracy and help guide therapy.

TREATMENT

Early attempts to treat HRS-1 involved drastic maneuvers intended to restore the deranged hemodynamics of cirrhosis, such as head-out water immersion, portocaval or peritoneovenous shunting, and ascites filtration and reinfusion, with mixed results [154-158]. Subsequently, drugs intended to oppose renal vasoconstriction were tested, also without demonstration of consistent benefit [159-161]. Later, the arrival of vasoconstrictor therapy constituted the first pharmacological intervention with consistent efficacy.

Albumin

Almost all clinical trials that have assessed the efficacy of a vasoconstrictor in patients with HRS-1 have used treatment protocols that include the concomitant use of intravenous albumin to optimize the effective circulatory volume (Table 2). Notably, a study that investigated terlipressin, showed that this vasoconstrictor was more effective when given in combination with albumin than when it was given alone [162].

Table 2. Prospective clinical trials of vasoconstrictors for the treatment of HRS-1

Agent	n	HRS-1 reversal rates[a]	Mean baseline sCr (mg/dL)[b]	Mean baseline total bilirubin (mg/dL)[c]	Ref
Uncontrolled studies					
Ornipressin[d]	8	75%	2.9	6	Guevara et al. (Spain 1998) [188]
Ornipressin with dopamine	9	57%	3.5	NA	Gulberg et al. (Germany 1999) [190]
Midodrine with octreotide	14	71%	3	5	Wong et al. (Canada 2004) [157]
Terlipressin	9	78%	3.9	14	Uriz et al. (Spain 2000) [161]
	12	50%	3.4	6	Mulkay et al. (Belgium 2001) [163]
	7	57%	3.9	15	Saner et al. (Germany 2004) [165]
	13	61%	3.3	NA	Munoz et al. (Mexico 2009) [166]
	8	75%	2.8	8.1	Narahara et al. (Japan 2012) [167]

Agent	n	HRS-1 reversal rates[a]	Mean baseline sCr (mg/dL)[b]	Mean baseline total bilirubin (mg/dL)[c]	Ref
Norepinephrine	12	83%	2.7	17	Duvoux et al. (France 2002) [175]
	30	73%	3.5	3	Gupta et al. (India 2018) [215]
Controlled studies					
Midodrine with octreotide versus dopamine	13	60% versus 0%	5.0 and 3.6	5.4	Angeli et al. (Italy 1999) [155]
Midodrine with octreotide versus noradrenaline	23	73% versus 75%	2.6 and 2.6	8 and 12	Tavakkoli et al. (Iran 2012) [185]
Octreotide versus placebo	14	19% versus 19%	2.2 and 2.4	N/A	Pomier-Layrargues et al. (France 2003) [186]
Terlipressin with albumin versus terlipressin without albumin	21	77% versus 25%	3.6 and 3.4	N/A	Ortega et al. (Spain 2002) [153]
Terlipressin versus albumin alone	14	44% versus 9%	3.6 and 4.1	18 and 11	Martin-Llahi et al. (Spain 2008) [169]
	28	80% versus 19%	2.9 and 2.8	N/A	Neri et al. (Italy 2008) [170]
Terlipressin (bolus) versus terlipressin (infusion)	78	46% versus 56%	3.3 and 3.1	9 and 9	Cavallin et al. (Italy 2016) [216]
Terlipressin versus placebo	112	34% versus 13%	3.9 and 3.8	15 and 16	Sanyal et al. (USA 2008) [172]
	196	24% versus 15%	3.6 and 3.7	11 and 12	Boyer et al. (USA & Canada 2016) [173]
	24	42% versus 0%	2.9 and 2.2	7 and 7	Solanki et al. (India 2003) [162]
	300	29% versus 16%	3.5 and 3.5	14 and 15	Wong et al. (USA & Canada 2020)
Terlipressin versus midodrine with octreotide	49	70% versus 29%	3.7 and 3.8	12 and 11	Cavallin et al. (Italy 2015) [171]
Terlipressin versus norepinephrine	22	83% versus 70%	2.3 and 2.5	4 and 5	Alessandria et al. (Italy 2007) [178]
	40	50% versus 50%	3.3 and 3.0	5 and 8	Sharma et al. (India 2008) [176]
	46	39% versus 43%	3.2 and 3.1	4 and 5	Singh et al. (India 2012) [177]
	51	46% versus 40%	4.5 and 4.7	14 and 15	Badawy et al. (Egypt 2013) [181]
	41	45% versus 48%	3.3 and 3.1	1.9 and 1.7	Goyal et al. (India 2016) [182]
	60	57% versus 53%	3.3 and 3.2	14 and 7	Saif et al. (India 2018) [179]
Terlipressin (infusion) versus norepinephrine	120	40% versus 17%	1.8 and 2.0	22 and 23	Arora et al. (India 2018) [184]

All study protocols included albumin unless otherwise specified. [a]HRS-1 reversal defined as improvement in serum creatinine to a final value ≤ 1.5 mg/dL. [b]Multiply by 88.4 to obtain serum creatinine values in μmol/l.[c]Multiply by 17.104 to obtain total bilirubin levels in μmol/l. [d] only 15-day arm included. NA, not available.

The recommended dose of albumin varies across the literature, but a common approach is to give 25 g of 12.5% albumin intravenously every 6 hours for the first 24 hours followed by 20–25 g daily thereafter, with adjustments made based on the clinical course.

A dose–response relationship between infused albumin and clinical outcome in patients with HRS-1 was suggested by a meta-analysis of 19 clinical studies [163]. Furthermore, the therapeutic efficacy of intravenous albumin in preventing HRS-1 might be partially due to its ability to reduce nitric oxide levels as well as those of other cytokines such as tumor necrosis factor (TNF) [164].

Vasoconstrictor Therapy

Building on the foundation of the arterial underfilling hypothesis, various therapies have been developed to counteract the maladaptive splanchnic vasodilatation that contributes to the development of HRS-1 (Table 2). Studies involving the infusion of vasopressin analogs demonstrated an increase in peripheral vascular resistance [165, 166] and an augmentation in renal blood flow [166] with this approach. As outlined below, other agents have since been tested but because of changes in the definition of HRS-1 over time, participant enrollment in clinical trials in HRS-1 has not been uniform across studies. Thus, the heterogeneity of patient populations between studies must be considered when clinical trial data are reviewed.

Combination Midodrine and Octreotide

A combination of the vasopressor midodrine given orally and the somatostatin analog octreotide given subcutaneously is the most commonly used treatment for HRS-1 in the USA. Its introduction to practice followed a small but seminal non-parallel controlled study, in which three of five (60%) patients treated with midodrine and octreotide demonstrated reversal of HRS-1 compared to none of the eight patients treated with a nonpressor dose of dopamine [167]. An uncontrolled study and 2 retrospective cohort studies subsequently suggested beneficial effect of this therapy [168-170]; however, no large-scale prospective controlled trial supports its current vast use.

Terlipressin

Terlipressin is a vasopressin analog that is less potent than vasopressin but with 2 - 6 times greater affinity for the vascular V1a receptor than for the renal V2 receptor [171, 172]; it has therefore been examined as a treatment for HRS-1 in multiple studies [173-179]. In most countries in Europe and Asia, terlipressin is the standard treatment for HRS-1. In studies outside the USA, treatment of HRS-1 with terlipressin is associated with overall reversal rates of ~ 40 -70% [162, 180-182].

Reversal rates were also higher in a study of patients from Italy treated with terlipressin (70%) than in those treated with midodrine–octreotide combination therapy (28%) [183]. In contrast to European, Latin American and Asian countries, terlipressin is not approved by the FDA for use in the USA. The first clinical trial of terlipressin in the USA was published in 1998 and involved 112 patients [184].

Although HRS-1 reversal was observed more often in the terlipressin arm, the study was deemed non-significant [184]. The subsequent Placebo-Controlled, Double Blind Study to Confirm the Reversal of Hepatorenal Syndrome Type 1 with Terlipressin (REVERSE) trial, which enrolled 196 patients in the USA, again reported a trend for benefit of terlipressin but failed to reach the primary endpoint [185]. A third trial, CONFIRM, which enrolled 300 individuals with HRS-1, was completed in 2019. The primary endpoint of verified HRS-1 reversal was reached by 29% of patients randomized to placebo compared to only 16% of those randomized to placebo [186]. Although the study demonstrated efficacy of terlipressin, it was not powered to assess an effect on survival. Despite its efficacy, terlipressin-treated patients exhibited greater rate of respiratory failure. To some extent, the respiratory failure events were associated with greater exposure to intravenous albumin prior to trial enrollment compared to that observed in previous trials, likely reflecting practice pattern changes. Caution is advised when therapies increasing cardiac preload (albumin) and cardiac afterload (vasoconstrictor) are combined in individuals with HRS-1 at risk for respiratory failure.

Norepinephrine

Norepinephrine is a potent renal vasoconstrictor, and thus its use in HRS-1 might seem counterintuitive. As mentioned earlier, plasma levels of norepinephrine are markedly elevated in patients with HRS-1. However, a supraphysiological dose of norepinephrine increases systemic blood pressure and, by doing so, resets the inciting stimulus of decreased effective circulatory volume and overrides the local vasoconstricting effect of norepinephrine in renal vessels. Interestingly, seminal studies from the 1950s reported transiently improved kidney function and urine volume in patients following administration of norepinephrine [5, 6]. The first prospective report showed that treatment with norepinephrine improved kidney function in 10 of 12 patients [187]. Since then, seven small, randomized head-to-head trials comparing terlipressin, given in divided doses, to continuous infusion of norepinephrine, have uniformly shown comparable efficacy of the 2 agents with no superiority [188-194]. A meta-analysis of four of those trials confirmed the similarity in efficacy rates [195]. In 2018, a study reported superiority of continuous infusion of terlipressin over norepinephrine in a cohort of patients with ACLF [196]. However, the reported rates of HRS-1 reversal and death seem difficult to reconcile with the existing literature. Thus, we suggest that clinicians wait for additional adequately powered multicenter trial data before drawing conclusions about the superiority of terlipressin over norepinephrine.

Another study reported comparable rates of HRS-1 reversal among patients treated with midodrine–octreotide combination therapy and those receiving norepinephrine [197]. However, norepinephrine was effective in improving HRS-1 in patients who did not respond to midodrine–octreotide combination therapy in other studies [148, 193]. Currently, norepinephrine is available in the USA and should be favored over midodrine–octreotide combination therapy on the basis of collective evidence demonstrating its superior efficacy. Logistics related to the need for intensive care represent a barrier to the broad use of norepinephrine, although treatment protocols in step-down units can be implemented. Importantly, adverse effects associated with vasoconstrictor use, such as tachyarrhythmia with noradrenaline or intestinal ischemia with terlipressin, need to be considered carefully when deciding which agent to use.

Targeting a Rise in MAP

Beyond the dispute with regard to the absolute and relative therapeutic efficacies of terlipressin, norepinephrine and midodrine–octreotide combination therapy, an observation across nearly all clinical studies is that an improvement in kidney function in patients with HRS-1 is almost universally accompanied by a concomitant increase in MAP. Of interest, the seminal study of midodrine–octreotide combination therapy was designed to achieve a target increase in MAP of 15 mmHg in the treatment arm only [167]. This is an important aspect of the study design that is often overlooked, because it suggests that the beneficial effect in the treatment arm might be due to the increased MAP rather than a specific effect of the therapy. A placebo-controlled study that tested the efficacy of terlipressin in patients with HRS-1 reported that every 5 mmHg of rise in MAP was associated with an odds ratio for HRS reversal of 9.4 [86]. A pooled analysis of data from 501 patients across 21 studies showed a strong inverse correlation between the magnitude of rise in MAP and the absolute decrease in serum creatinine concentration during vasoconstrictor therapy, irrespective of the vasoconstrictor used [198] (Figure 5). Of note, baseline MAP in patients with HRS-1 might not be particularly low, averaging around 75 mmHg in published studies, and the MAP target in these patients might therefore range from 85 mmHg to 90 mmHg (Figures 5). This target is supported by several independent retrospective studies [148, 199, 200], although the ideal magnitude of rise in MAP to optimize efficacy and safety remains undefined. The signal seems to be close to a 15 mmHg rise in MAP from the baseline value, but prospective data are needed before this target can be strongly advocated. The duration of vasoconstrictor therapy in clinical studies has also varied from ~ 5–14 days. However, most patients that exhibit a favorable response do so within the first 3 days of therapy. Thus, we recommend that patients are treated for a minimum of 3 days and that therapy is extended to 7 days for those who show a favorable response. Variable rates of recurrence of HRS-1 (5 - 60%) have been reported [189, 192, 201, 202], and we recommend that patients who experience recurrence are re-treated.

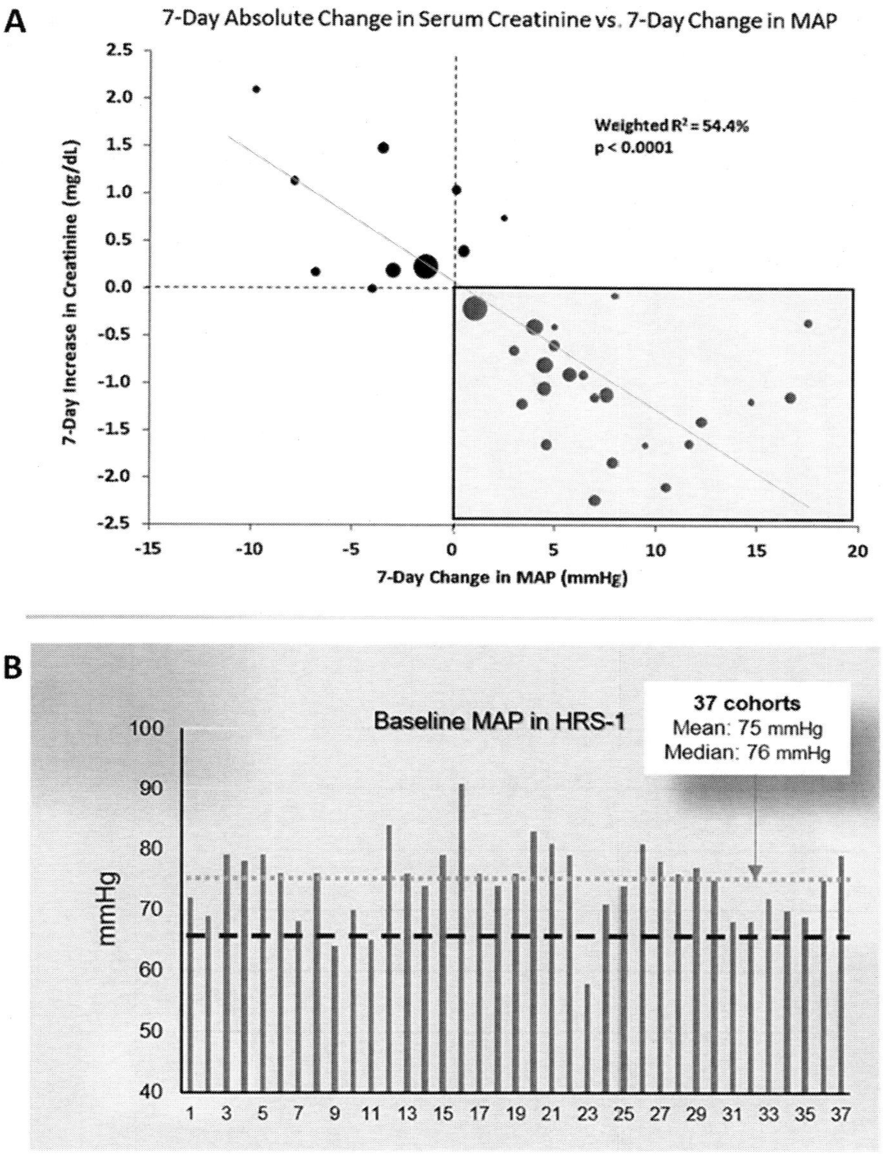

Figure 5. The relationship between mean arterial pressure and kidney function among patients with HRS-1 A) Assessment of the relationship between MAP and improvement in kidney function in the same meta-analysis shows an inverse correlation between the change in MAP and change in serum creatinine level. Multiply by 88.4 to obtain serum creatinine values in μmol/l. The size of data points is proportional to the sample size. B) An assessment of baseline mean arterial pressure (MAP) values reported in a meta-analysis of 37 cohorts across 21 clinical studies of patients with HRS-1 shows that a MAP below 65 mmHg (dashed line) at diagnosis (that is, before initiation of vasoconstrictor therapy) is not the norm (mean MAP 74.6 mmHg). Graph created from previously published data [193]. *Adapted with permission from Velez, JC & Nietert, PJ, Am J Kidney Dis 58, 928-938.*

Targeting Perturbed Renal Autoregulation

The clinical response to a rise in MAP among patients with HRS-1 seems to involve interplay between the SNS and autoregulatory mechanisms of renal blood flow. Alterations in renal autoregulation have long been recognized in rodent models of AKI [203]. However, these alterations seem to be particularly important in the context of HRS-1 in which SNS overactivation co-exists. The interaction between renal autoregulation and SNS activity was demonstrated in a canine model, in which overactivation of the SNS induced a shift-to-the-right in the renal autoregulatory curve [204]. Under normal physiological circumstances, renal blood flow reaches a plateau phase near a renal perfusion pressure of 65 mmHg.

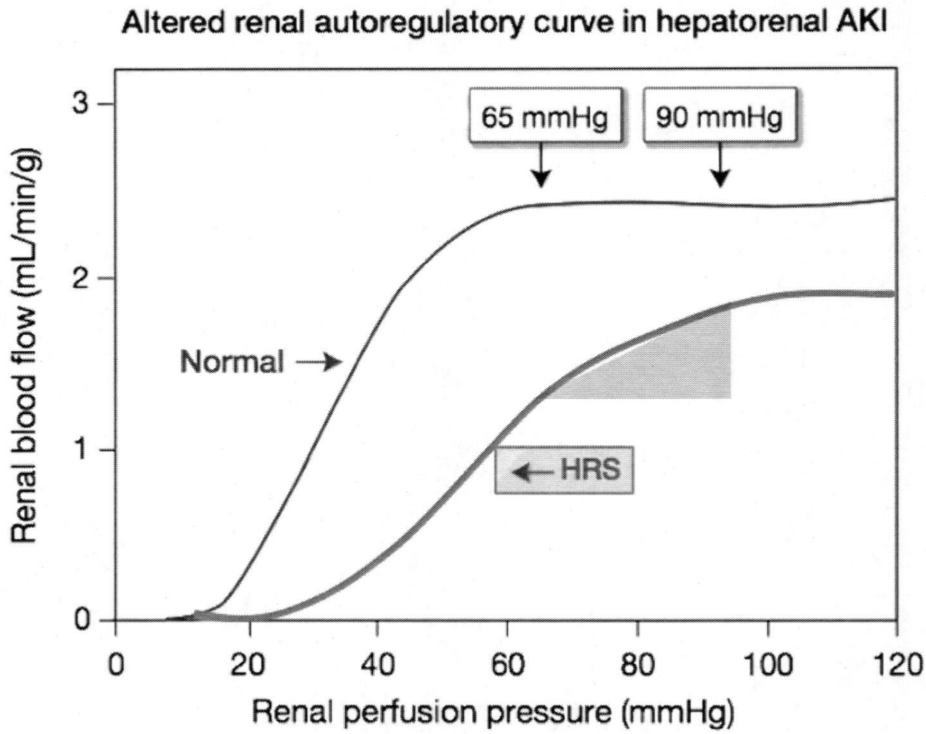

Figure 6. Derangement in renal autoregulation in patients with HRS-1. Under normal physiological circumstances, renal blood flow reaches a plateau near a renal perfusion pressure of 65 mmHg. Overactivation of sympathetic nervous system activity in patients with hepatorenal syndrome type 1 (HRS-1) leads to a continued rise in renal blood flow as renal perfusion pressure increases up to a level around 90 mmHg. The shaded area depicts the '**therapeutic zone**', which represents the levels at which vasoconstrictor therapy might induce arise in mean arterial pressure. Note that the maximum renal blood flow is reduced during acute kidney injury from HRS-1. *Adapted with permission from Velez, JC et al, Nat Rev Nephrol 16:137-155, 2020.*

This threshold is altered in a state of SNS overactivation when renal blood flow continues to rise as renal perfusion pressure (RPP) increases up to ~ 90 mmHg (Figure 6).

This phenomenon was subsequently demonstrated in a cohort of patients with cirrhosis with various degrees of portal hypertension and renal dysfunction [205]. Since MAP augmentation ultimately enhances RPP, it is possible that a simultaneous reduction of IAP via LVP could result in a more effective, yet transient, increase in in RPP as per the following equation:

$$RPP = MAP - IAP \quad (1)$$

Transjugular Intrahepatic Portosystemic Shunt

The contribution of portal hypertension to the development of HRS-1 has prompted the assessment of TIPS as therapy for HRS-1 in small scale studies. One such study reported an improvement in kidney function 30 days after TIPS in 6 of 7 patients [206]. In a cohort of 41 patients with cirrhosis (21 with HRS-1, and 20 with a more chronic form of HRS, HRS type 2), TIPS led to improvement in kidney function, weaning from dialysis and extended survival in 4 of 7 patients [207]. Moreover, improvement in kidney function was observed among 20 patients who underwent TIPS with a baseline serum creatinine > 2.0 mg/dL (176.8 μmol/l) [208]. Periprocedural mortality and worsening of hepatic encephalopathy are potential complications of TIPS. A systematic review of 9 studies showed a pooled rate of 93% of improvement in kidney function and a 46% rate of hepatic encephalopathy [209]. Altogether, a lack of controlled studies limits our ability to draw definite conclusions about the potential role of TIPS as rescue therapy for HRS-1 but it may be worth revisiting this modality for selected patients with HRS-1 who are awaiting liver transplantation.

Liver Transplantation

Liver transplantation is considered the ultimate treatment of choice for HRS-1. An estimated 65-75% of patients experience resolution of HRS-1 after liver transplantation, with lower recovery for patients on dialysis at the time of transplantation [210]. However, the current imbalance between the incidence of HRS-1, the suitability of patients for transplantation and the availability of organs, limit its widespread implementation. For patients who are eligible for liver transplantation, vasoconstrictor therapy is viewed as a 'bridge' therapy until a suitable donor is found. Among patients who are ineligible for liver transplantation, short-term survival is increased in those who respond to vasoconstrictor therapy [211, 212]. In a randomized controlled trial that tested the efficacy of terlipressin, the 3-month survival rate of patients who achieved resolution of HRS-1 was 40% compared to 4% for those who did not respond to treatment [211].

If liver transplantation does not occur within 6 weeks of dialysis-dependence, the likelihood of achieving resolution of AKI post-transplantation is reduced and combined liver-kidney transplantation is recommended [84].

Renal Replacement Therapy

Hemodialysis in a patient with HRS-1 not responsive to vasoconstrictors and deemed ineligible for liver transplantation has in the past been considered futile, with expected mortality exceeding 90% [213, 214]. However, it is not a trivial task for a clinician to deny dialysis to a patient. At best, hemodialysis might extend mean survival from 1 week to 6 months, with a considerable portion of that time spent in a hospital [213]. This prolongation of life might be perceived as futile in a patient who is obtunded, bedbound and severely debilitated. On the other hand, a relevant goal of care for a more functional patient might be to survive a few additional months. Limited data are available to determine whether a specific subset of patients with HRS-1 might benefit from hemodialysis. One study reported that 30-day mortality among patients who received hemodialysis and were on concomitant mechanical ventilation was 100% [215]. Another study found that thrombocytopenia but not HRS-1 was a predictor of mortality in patients with cirrhosis undergoing acute hemodialysis [216]. A study from 2018 reported that among patients with cirrhosis and AKI requiring hemodialysis, the risk of death in those with HRS-1 was comparable to that of patients with ATI [217]. Ultimately, decisions around hemodialysis need to be individualized and should be guided by a multiorgan and functional assessment of the patient rather than solely based on HRS-1 diagnosis.

Clinical Pearls

- Although various non-hemodynamic mechanisms of injury, such as endotoxin-mediated inflammation, bile acid-induced tubular toxicity and true tubular ischemia are implicated in the pathogenesis of hepatorenal syndrome type 1 (HRS-1), renal vasoconstriction and reduced renal blood flow is regarded as the quintessential mechanism of renal dysfunction in HRS-1.
- The differential diagnosis of acute kidney injury (AKI) in patients with cirrhosis is broad and 'pure' HRS-1 likely constitutes a minor subset of these cases; however, different pathogenic mechanisms can coexist and overlap of AKI etiologies is conceivable.
- The current diagnostic ICA criteria for HRS-1 provide a useful foundation to frame the diagnostic approach of AKI in patients with cirrhosis; however, one must remain cognizant of the limitations of those criteria and recognize that key aspects of the HRS-1 'phenotype' are not routinely included and should be carefully considered during clinical evaluation.
- The cornerstone of pharmacological therapy for HRS-1 is the use of vasoconstrictors with a goal-directed approach to target a substantial rise in mean arterial pressure by ~15 mmHg. Liver transplantation is the most effective treatment for HRS-1.
- As kidney function declines and the serum bilirubin increases during the course of HRS-1-associated AKI the likelihood of successful reversal of HRS-1 with a vasoconstrictor decreases; early recognition of HRS-1 is therefore critical to initiate therapy at an early stage of AKI.

Conclusion

HRS-1 is challenging condition that affects patients with cirrhosis and is associated with ominous clinical outcomes.

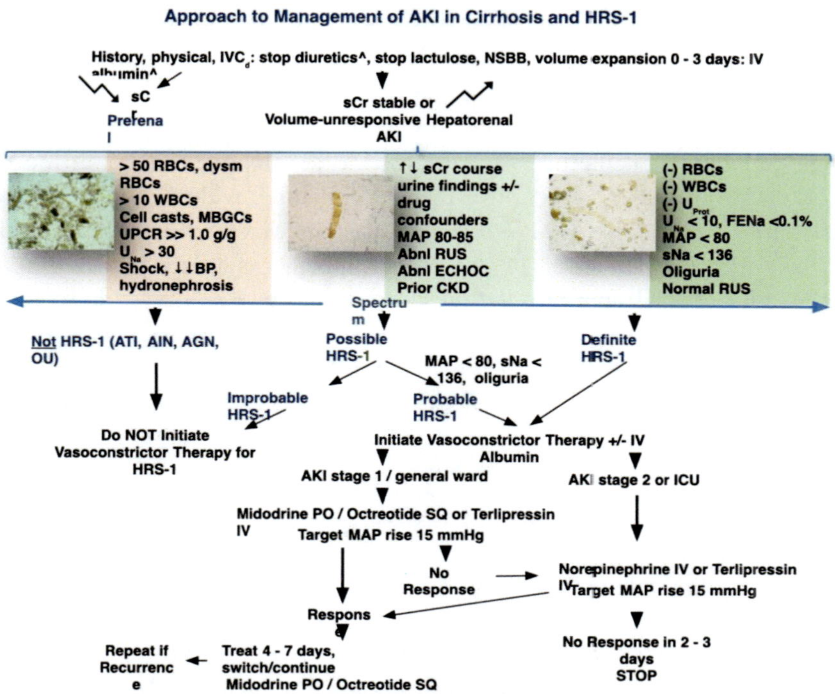

Figure 7. Proposed diagnostic and therapeutic approach to AKI in patients with cirrhosis. This algorithm represents a guide for the methodical collection and integration of data to facilitate clinical reasoning and decision making for patients with cirrhosis and acute kidney injury (AKI); it is not intended to be used as a strict protocol. The guide includes elements of the ICA criteria but also suggests other aspects of clinical evaluation. Initial steps entail careful assessment of volume status, removal of potential offenders and volume expansion through administration of intravenous albumin, as appropriate. For those patients who do not achieve a favorable response to this maneuver, in-depth examination of clinical presentation is required to identify cases of parenchymal or obstructive causes of AKI [that is, not due to hepatorenal syndrome type 1 (HRS-1)]. When all ICA HRS-1 criteria are met, as well as other non-ICA HRS-1 criteria (that is, low urine Na, hyaline casts or bland urinary sediment, hyponatremia, baseline mean arterial pressure (MAP) < 80 mmHg, oliguria), a definite diagnosis of HRS-1 can be made. Acute tubular injury (ATI), rather than HRS-1 is likely when blood pressure (BP) is very low (that is, hypotension is present); if BP is at the upper limit of normal or high (hypertension), other causes of AKI, such as acute glomerulonephritis (AGN) or ATI should be considered. Notably, it is our view that scenarios of uncertainty can be encountered, and this algorithm proposes that the abovementioned non-ICA phenotypic criteria can help determine if a case can be categorized as probable or improbable HRS-1. We recommend treating definite and probable cases of HRS-1 as outlined. Vasoconstrictor therapy (norepinephrine or terlipressin) should be implemented to achieve a prespecified rise in MAP. This step (albumin administration) can be skipped if the patient shows evidence of hypervolemia on initial assessment. IVC_d: inferior vena cava diameter, NSBB: nonselective beta blockers, IV: intravenous, sCr: serum creatinine, RBCs: red blood cells, dysm RBCs: dysmorphic RBCs, WBCs: white blood cells, U_{Na}: urine sodium, S_{Na}: serum sodium, BP: blood pressure, Abnl: abnormal, RUS: renal ultrasound, ECHOC: echocardiogram, U_{Prot}: protein, MAP: mean arterial pressure, sNa: serum sodium, HRS-1: hepatorenal syndrome type 1, AIN: acute interstitial nephritis, OU: obstructive uropathy, PO: per os, SQ: subcutaneous, UPCR: urine protein-to-creatinine ratio, MBGCs: muddy brown granular casts, CKD: chronic kidney disease, FENa: fractional excretion of sodium, ICU: intensive care unit.

The classic view of its pathogenesis focuses on the existence of profound renal vasoconstriction, but likely underestimates the contribution of other non-hemodynamic mechanisms. HRS-1 is difficult to diagnose and treat. The existing diagnostic criteria provide a foundation for the identification of patients with HRS-1, but have several limitations. In addition, the complexity of the disease calls for the development of better tools to aid the diagnosis of HRS-1 and to guide treatment. Available evidence suggests that use of vasoconstrictor therapy to raise MAP is essential to achieve restoration of renal blood flow and improve kidney function. However, the efficacy of this therapeutic approach diminishes with increasing severity of AKI and with the presence of cholestasis. Liver transplantation is the preferred therapy but is not universally available or suitable for all patients. Therefore, newer therapies are urgently needed to improve the care of this vulnerable patient population. Until better diagnostic tools and new therapies are available, critical thinking and careful integration of clinical and laboratorial data is required to optimize the selection of patients who are likely to benefit from vasoconstrictor therapy (Figure 7).

Conflict of Interest

J.C.V. has participated in Speaker Bureau and Advisory Board meetings for Mallinckrodt Pharmaceuticals, the manufacturer of terlipressin, and is a member of the Speaker Bureau of Otsuka Pharmaceuticals (in reference to products not discussed in this article). The other authors declare no competing interests.

References

[1] Belcher JM, Sanyal AJ, Peixoto AJ, Perazella MA, Lim J, Thiessen-Philbrook H, et al. Kidney biomarkers and differential diagnosis of patients with cirrhosis and acute kidney injury. *Hepatology.* 2014;60(2):622-32.

[2] A F. Clinical report on hydro-peritoneum, based on analysis of forty-six cases. *Am J Med Sci.* 1863;45:306-39.

[3] Schmidt CR, Chesky VE. Clinical studies of liver function; the hepatorenal syndrome. *Am J Surg.* 1948;75(6):772-95.

[4] Shear L, Kleinerman J, Gabuzda GJ. Renal Failure in Patients with Cirrhosis of the Liver. I. Clinical and Pathologic Characteristics. *Am J Med.* 1965;39:184-98.

[5] Hecker R, Sherlock S. Electrolyte and circulatory changes in terminal liver failure. *Lancet.* 1956;271(6953):1121-5.

[6] Papper S, Belsky JL, Bleifer KH. Renal failure in Laennec's cirrhosis of the liver. I. Description of clinical and laboratory features. *Ann Intern Med.* 1959;51:759-73.

[7] Epstein M, Berk DP, Hollenberg NK, Adams DF, Chalmers TC, Abrams HL, et al. Renal failure in the patient with cirrhosis. The role of active vasoconstriction. *Am J Med.* 1970;49(2):175-85.

[8] Ring-Larsen H. Renal blood flow in cirrhosis: relation to systemic and portal haemodynamics and liver function. *Scandinavian journal of clinical and laboratory investigation.* 1977;37(7):635-42.

[9] Koppel MH, Coburn JW, Mims MM, Goldstein H, Boyle JD, Rubini ME. Transplantation of cadaveric kidneys from patients with hepatorenal syndrome. Evidence for the functionalnature of renal failure in advanced liver disease. *N Engl J Med.* 1969;280(25):1367-71.

[10] Iwatsuki S, Popovtzer MM, Corman JL, Ishikawa M, Putnam CW, Katz FH, et al. Recovery from "hepatorenal syndrome" after orthotopic liver transplantation. *N Engl J Med.* 1973;289(22):1155-9.

[11] Gines A, Escorsell A, Gines P, Salo J, Jimenez W, Inglada L, et al. Incidence, predictive factors, and prognosis of the hepatorenal syndrome in cirrhosis with ascites. *Gastroenterology.* 1993;105(1):229-36.

[12] Salerno F, Cazzaniga M, Merli M, Spinzi G, Saibeni S, Salmi A, et al. Diagnosis, treatment and survival of patients with hepatorenal syndrome: a survey on daily medical practice. *J Hepatol.* 2011;55(6):1241-8.

[13] Weil D, Levesque E, McPhail M, Cavallazzi R, Theocharidou E, Cholongitas E, et al. Prognosis of cirrhotic patients admitted to intensive care unit: a meta-analysis. *Ann Intensive Care.* 2017;7(1):33.

[14] Butt AK, Khan AA, Alam A, Shah SW, Shafqat F, Naqvi AB. Predicting hospital mortality in cirrhotic patients: comparison of Child-Pugh and Acute Physiology, Age and Chronic Health Evaluation (APACHE III) scoring systems. *Am J Gastroenterol.* 1998;93(12):2469-75.

[15] Shetty S, Nagaraju SP, Shenoy S, Attur RP, Rangaswamy D, Rao IR, et al. Acute kidney injury in patients with cirrhosis of liver: Clinical profile and predictors of outcome. *Indian J Gastroenterol.* 2018;37(3):248-54.

[16] Xiong J, Pu L, Xiong H, Xiang P, Zhang M, Liu J, et al. Evaluation of the criteria of hepatorenal syndrome type of acute kidney injury in patients with cirrhosis admitted to ICU. *Scand J Gastroenterol.* 2018;53(12):1590-6.

[17] Hamdy HS, El-Ray A, Salaheldin M, Lasheen M, Aboul-Ezz M, Abdel-Moaty AS, et al. Urinary Neutrophil Gelatinase-Associated Lipocalin in Cirrhotic Patients with Acute Kidney Injury. *Annals of hepatology.* 2018;17(4):624-30.

[18] Prakash J, Mahapatra AK, Ghosh B, Arora P, Jain AK. Clinical spectrum of renal disorders in patients with cirrhosis of liver. *Ren Fail.* 2011;33(1):40-6.

[19] Velez JCQ, Therapondos G, Juncos LA. Reappraising the spectrum of AKI and hepatorenal syndrome in patients with cirrhosis. *Nat Rev Nephrol.* 2020;16(3):137-55.

[20] Martin PY, Gines P, Schrier RW. Nitric oxide as a mediator of hemodynamic abnormalities and sodium and water retention in cirrhosis. *N Engl J Med.* 1998;339(8):533-41.

[21] Niederberger M, Martin PY, Gines P, Morris K, Tsai P, Xu DL, et al. Normalization of nitric oxide production corrects arterial vasodilation and hyperdynamic circulation in cirrhotic rats. *Gastroenterology.* 1995;109(5):1624-30.

[22] Schrier RW, Arroyo V, Bernardi M, Epstein M, Henriksen JH, Rodes J. Peripheral arterial vasodilation hypothesis: a proposal for the initiation of renal sodium and water retention in cirrhosis. *Hepatology.* 1988;8(5):1151-7.

[23] Wilkinson SP, Williams R. Renin-angiotensin-aldosterone system in cirrhosis. *Gut.* 1980;21(6):545-54.

[24] Bichet DG, Van Putten VJ, Schrier RW. Potential role of increased sympathetic activity in impaired sodium and water excretion in cirrhosis. *N Engl J Med.* 1982;307(25):1552-7.

[25] Ring-Larsen H, Hesse B, Henriksen JH, Christensen NJ. Sympathetic nervous activity and renal and systemic hemodynamics in cirrhosis: plasma norepinephrine concentration, hepatic extraction, and renal release. *Hepatology.* 1982;2(3):304-10.

[26] Salo J, Gines A, Quer JC, Fernandez-Esparrach G, Guevara M, Gines P, et al. Renal and neurohormonal changes following simultaneous administration of systemic vasoconstrictors and dopamine or prostacyclin in cirrhotic patients with hepatorenal syndrome. *J Hepatol.* 1996;25(6):916-23.

[27] Arroyo V, Bernardi M, Epstein M, Henriksen JH, Schrier RW, Rodes J. Pathophysiology of ascites and functional renal failure in cirrhosis. *J Hepatol.* 1988;6(2):239-57.

[28] Fernandez-Seara J, Prieto J, Quiroga J, Zozaya JM, Cobos MA, Rodriguez-Eire JL, et al. Systemic and regional hemodynamics in patients with liver cirrhosis and ascites with and without functional renal failure. *Gastroenterology.* 1989;97(5):1304-12.

[29] Ortiz MC, Garcia-Sanz A, Bentley MD, Fortepiani LA, Garcia-Estan J, Ritman EL, et al. Microcomputed tomography of kidneys following chronic bile duct ligation. *Kidney Int.* 2000;58(4):1632-40.

[30] Kew MC, Brunt PW, Varma RR, Hourigan KJ, Williams HS, Sherlock S. Renal and intrarenal blood-flow in cirrhosis of the liver. *Lancet.* 1971;2(7723):504-10.

[31] Baldus WP, Feichter RN, Summerskill WH, Hunt JC, Wakim KG. The Kidney in Cirrhosis. Ii. Disorders of Renal Function. *Ann Intern Med.* 1964;60:366-77.

[32] Jonassen TE, Marcussen N, Haugan K, Skyum H, Christensen S, Andreasen F, et al. Functional and structural changes in the thick ascending limb of Henle's loop in rats with liver cirrhosis. *Am J Physiol.* 1997;273(2 Pt 2):R568-77.

[33] Horbelt M, Lee SY, Mang HE, Knipe NL, Sado Y, Kribben A, et al. Acute and chronic microvascular alterations in a mouse model of ischemic acute kidney injury. *Am J Physiol Renal Physiol.* 2007;293(3):F688-95.

[34] Allegretti AS, Ortiz G, Wenger J, Deferio JJ, Wibecan J, Kalim S, et al. Prognosis of Acute Kidney Injury and Hepatorenal Syndrome in Patients with Cirrhosis: A Prospective Cohort Study. *Int J Nephrol.* 2015;2015:108139.

[35] Chade AR, Hall JE. Role of the Renal Microcirculation in Progression of Chronic Kidney Injury in Obesity. *Am J Nephrol.* 2016;44(5):354-67.

[36] Levy M, Finestone H, Fechner C. Action of renal vasodilators in dogs following acute biliary obstruction. *J Surg Res.* 1984;36(2):163-71.

[37] Kahng KU, Monaco DO, Schnabel FR, Wait RB. Renal vascular reactivity in the bile duct-ligated rat. *Surgery.* 1988;104(2):250-6.

[38] Chuang CL, Chang CC, Hsu SJ, Huang HC, Lee FY, Huang LJ, et al. Endotoxemia-enhanced renal vascular reactivity to endothelin-1 in cirrhotic rats. *Am J Physiol Gastrointest Liver Physiol.* 2018;315(5):G752-G61.

[39] Chuang CL, Huang HC, Chang CC, Lee FY, Wu JC, Lee JY, et al. Lipopolysaccharide enhanced renal vascular response to endothelin-1 through ETA overexpression in portal hypertensive rats. *Journal of gastroenterology and hepatology.* 2015;30(1):199-207.

[40] Ortiz MC, Manriquez MC, Nath KA, Lager DJ, Romero JC, Juncos LA. Vitamin E prevents renal dysfunction induced by experimental chronic bile duct ligation. *Kidney Int.* 2003;64(3):950-61.

[41] Inan M, Sayek I, Tel BC, Sahin-Erdemli I. Role of endotoxin and nitric oxide in the pathogenesis of renal failure in obstructive jaundice. *Br J Surg.* 1997;84(7):943-7.

[42] Kostreva DR, Castaner A, Kampine JP. Reflex effects of hepatic baroreceptors on renal and cardiac sympathetic nerve activity. *Am J Physiol.* 1980;238(5):R390-4.

[43] Lang F, Tschernko E, Schulze E, Ottl I, Ritter M, Volkl H, et al. Hepatorenal reflex regulating kidney function. *Hepatology.* 1991;14(4 Pt 1):590-4.

[44] Ming Z, Fan YJ, Yang X, Lautt WW. Contribution of hepatic adenosine A1 receptors to renal dysfunction associated with acute liver injury in rats. *Hepatology.* 2006;44(4):813-22.

[45] Ming Z, Lautt WW. Intrahepatic adenosine-mediated activation of hepatorenal reflex is via A1 receptors in rats. *Can J Physiol Pharmacol.* 2006;84(11):1177-84.

[46] Ming Z, Smyth DD, Lautt WW. Decreases in portal flow trigger a hepatorenal reflex to inhibit renal sodium and water excretion in rats: role of adenosine. *Hepatology.* 2002;35(1):167-75.

[47] Lang F, Ottl I, Freudenschuss K, Honeder M, Tschernko E, Haussinger D. Serotoninergic hepatorenal reflex regulating renal glomerular filtration rate. *Pflugers Arch.* 1991;419(1):111-3.

[48] Jalan R, Forrest EH, Redhead DN, Dillon JF, Hayes PC. Reduction in renal blood flow following acute increase in the portal pressure: evidence for the existence of a hepatorenal reflex in man? *Gut.* 1997;40(5):664-70.

[49] DiBona GF, Sawin LL. Hepatorenal baroreflex in cirrhotic rats. *Am J Physiol.* 1995;269(1 Pt 1):G29-33.

[50] Solis-Herruzo JA, Duran A, Favela V, Castellano G, Madrid JL, Munoz-Yague MT, et al. Effects of lumbar sympathetic block on kidney function in cirrhotic patients with hepatorenal syndrome. *J Hepatol.* 1987;5(2):167-73.

[51] Krag A, Gluud LL. Cross-talk between the liver, heart and kidney - another piece in the puzzle. *J Gastrointestin Liver Dis.* 2014;23(2):119-21.

[52] Krag A, Bendtsen F, Henriksen JH, Moller S. Low cardiac output predicts development of hepatorenal syndrome and survival in patients with cirrhosis and ascites. *Gut.* 2010;59(1):105-10.

[53] Moller S, Henriksen JH. Review article: pathogenesis and pathophysiology of hepatorenal syndrome--is there scope for prevention? *Aliment Pharmacol Ther.* 2004;20 Suppl 3:31-41; discussion 2-3.

[54] Ruiz-del-Arbol L, Monescillo A, Arocena C, Valer P, Gines P, Moreira V, et al. Circulatory function and hepatorenal syndrome in cirrhosis. *Hepatology.* 2005;42(2):439-47.

[55] Mandorfer M, Bota S, Schwabl P, Bucsics T, Pfisterer N, Kruzik M, et al. Nonselective beta blockers increase risk for hepatorenal syndrome and death in patients with cirrhosis and spontaneous bacterial peritonitis. *Gastroenterology.* 2014;146(7):1680-90 e1.

[56] Moller S, Iversen JS, Henriksen JH, Bendtsen F. Reduced baroreflex sensitivity in alcoholic cirrhosis: relations to hemodynamics and humoral systems. *Am J Physiol Heart Circ Physiol.* 2007;292(6):H2966-72.

[57] Newton JL, Allen J, Kerr S, Jones DE. Reduced heart rate variability and baroreflex sensitivity in primary biliary cirrhosis. *Liver international: official journal of the International Association for the Study of the Liver.* 2006;26(2):197-202.

[58] Mani AR, Montagnese S, Jackson CD, Jenkins CW, Head IM, Stephens RC, et al. Decreased heart rate variability in patients with cirrhosis relates to the presence and degree of hepatic encephalopathy. *Am J Physiol Gastrointest Liver Physiol.* 2009;296(2):G330-8.

[59] Busk TM, Bendtsen F, Poulsen JH, Clemmesen JO, Larsen FS, Goetze JP, et al. Transjugular intrahepatic portosystemic shunt: impact on systemic hemodynamics and renal and cardiac function in patients with cirrhosis. *Am J Physiol Gastrointest Liver Physiol.* 2018;314(2):G275-G86.

[60] Kazory A, Ronco C. Hepatorenal Syndrome or Hepatocardiorenal Syndrome: Revisiting Basic Concepts in View of Emerging Data. *Cardiorenal Med.* 2019;9(1):1-7.

[61] Zardi EM, Zardi DM, Giorgi C, Chin D, Dobrina A. Portopulmonary hypertension and hepatorenal syndrome. Two faces of the same coin. *Eur J Intern Med.* 2017;43:22-7.

[62] Liberal R, Grant CR, Baptista R, Macedo G. "Porto-pulmonary hypertension: a comprehensive review." *Clin Res Hepatol Gastroenterol.* 2015;39(2):157-67.

[63] Colle IO, Moreau R, Godinho E, Belghiti J, Ettori F, Cohen-Solal A, et al. Diagnosis of portopulmonary hypertension in candidates for liver transplantation: a prospective study. *Hepatology.* 2003;37(2):401-9.

[64] Lebrec D, Capron JP, Dhumeaux D, Benhamou JP. Pulmonary hypertension complicating portal hypertension. *Am Rev Respir Dis.* 1979;120(4):849-56.

[65] Talwalkar JA, Swanson KL, Krowka MJ, Andrews JC, Kamath PS. Prevalence of spontaneous portosystemic shunts in patients with portopulmonary hypertension and effect on treatment. *Gastroenterology.* 2011;141(5):1673-9.

[66] Krowka MJ, Swanson KL, Frantz RP, McGoon MD, Wiesner RH. Portopulmonary hypertension: Results from a 10-year screening algorithm. *Hepatology.* 2006;44(6):1502-10.

[67] Savale L, Weatherald J, Jais X, Vuillard C, Boucly A, Jevnikar M, et al. Acute decompensated pulmonary hypertension. *Eur Respir Rev.* 2017;26(146).

[68] Ruiz-del-Arbol L, Monescillo A, Jimenez W, Garcia-Plaza A, Arroyo V, Rodes J. Paracentesis-induced circulatory dysfunction: mechanism and effect on hepatic hemodynamics in cirrhosis. *Gastroenterology.* 1997;113(2):579-86.

[69] Moreau R, Asselah T, Condat B, de Kerguenec C, Pessione F, Bernard B, et al. Comparison of the effect of terlipressin and albumin on arterial blood volume in patients with cirrhosis and tense ascites treated by paracentesis: a randomised pilot study. *Gut.* 2002;50(1):90-4.

[70] Appenrodt B, Wolf A, Grunhage F, Trebicka J, Schepke M, Rabe C, et al. Prevention of paracentesis-induced circulatory dysfunction: midodrine vs albumin. A randomized pilot study. *Liver Int.* 2008;28(7):1019-25.

[71] Gines P, Arroyo V, Quintero E, Planas R, Bory F, Cabrera J, et al. Comparison of paracentesis and diuretics in the treatment of cirrhotics with tense ascites. Results of a randomized study. *Gastroenterology.* 1987;93(2):234-41.

[72] Gines A, Fernandez-Esparrach G, Monescillo A, Vila C, Domenech E, Abecasis R, et al. Randomized trial comparing albumin, dextran 70, and polygeline in cirrhotic patients with ascites treated by paracentesis. *Gastroenterology.* 1996;111(4):1002-10.

[73] Patel DM, Connor MJ, Jr. Intra-Abdominal Hypertension and Abdominal Compartment Syndrome: An Underappreciated Cause of Acute Kidney Injury. *Adv Chronic Kidney Dis.* 2016;23(3):160-6.

[74] Doty JM, Saggi BH, Blocher CR, Fakhry I, Gehr T, Sica D, et al. Effects of increased renal parenchymal pressure on renal function. *J Trauma.* 2000;48(5):874-7.

[75] Chang Y, Qi X, Li Z, Wang F, Wang S, Zhang Z, et al. Hepatorenal syndrome: insights into the mechanisms of intra-abdominal hypertension. *Int J Clin Exp Pathol.* 2013;6(11):2523-8.

[76] Cade R, Wagemaker H, Vogel S, Mars D, Hood-Lewis D, Privette M, et al. Hepatorenal syndrome. Studies of the effect of vascular volume and intraperitoneal pressure on renal and hepatic function. *Am J Med.* 1987;82(3):427-38.

[77] Savino JA, Cerabona T, Agarwal N, Byrne D. Manipulation of ascitic fluid pressure in cirrhotics to optimize hemodynamic and renal function. *Ann Surg.* 1988;208(4):504-11.

[78] Umgelter A, Reindl W, Franzen M, Lenhardt C, Huber W, Schmid RM. Renal resistive index and renal function before and after paracentesis in patients with hepatorenal syndrome and tense ascites. *Intensive Care Med.* 2009;35(1):152-6.

[79] Seethapathy H, Sharma S, Zhao S, Chung RT, Connor MJ, Jr., Leaf DE, et al. Acute Kidney Injury Following Paracentesis Among Inpatients With Cirrhosis. *Kidney Int Rep.* 2020;5(8):1305-8.

[80] de Cleva R, Silva FP, Zilberstein B, Machado DJ. Acute renal failure due to abdominal compartment syndrome: report on four cases and literature review. *Rev Hosp Clin Fac Med Sao Paulo.* 2001;56(4):123-30.

[81] Huggins JT, Doelken P, Walters C, Rockey DC. Point-of-Care Echocardiography Improves Assessment of Volume Status in Cirrhosis and Hepatorenal Syndrome. *Am J Med Sci.* 2016;351(5):550-3.

[82] Mandal AK, Lansing M, Fahmy A. Acute tubular necrosis in hepatorenal syndrome: an electron microscopy study. *Am J Kidney Dis.* 1982;2(3):363-74.

[83] Kanel GC, Peters RL. Glomerular tubular reflux--a morphologic renal lesion associated with the hepatorenal syndrome. *Hepatology.* 1984;4(2):242-6.

[84] Hussain SM, Sureshkumar KK. Refining the Role of Simultaneous Liver Kidney Transplantation. *J Clin Transl Hepatol.* 2018;6(3):289-95.

[85] Sharma P, Goodrich NP, Zhang M, Guidinger MK, Schaubel DE, Merion RM. Short-term pretransplant renal replacement therapy and renal nonrecovery after liver transplantation alone. *Clin J Am Soc Nephrol.* 2013;8(7):1135-42.

[86] Nazar A, Pereira GH, Guevara M, Martin-Llahi M, Pepin MN, Marinelli M, et al. Predictors of response to therapy with terlipressin and albumin in patients with cirrhosis and type 1 hepatorenal syndrome. *Hepatology.* 2010;51(1):219-26.

[87] Poloni JAT, Perazella MA, Keitel E, Marroni CA, Leite SB, Rotta LN. Utility of a urine sediment score in hyperbilirubinemia/hyperbilirubinuria. *Clin Nephrol.* 2019.

[88] Varga ZV, Erdelyi K, Paloczi J, Cinar R, Zsengeller ZK, Jourdan T, et al. Disruption of Renal Arginine Metabolism Promotes Kidney Injury in Hepatorenal Syndrome in Mice. *Hepatology.* 2018;68(4):1519-33.

[89] Holmes TW, Jr. The histologic lesion of cholemic nephrosis. *J Urol.* 1953;70(5):677-85.

[90] Betjes MG, Bajema I. The pathology of jaundice-related renal insufficiency: cholemic nephrosis revisited. *J Nephrol.* 2006;19(2):229-33.

[91] Uslu A, Tasli FA, Nart A, Postaci H, Aykas A, Bati H, et al. Human kidney histopathology in acute obstructive jaundice: a prospective study. *European journal of gastroenterology & hepatology.* 2010;22(12):1458-65.

[92] Mairiang P, Bhudhisawasdi V, Borirakchanyavat V, Sitprija V. Acute renal failure in obstructive jaundice in cholangiocarcinoma. *Arch Intern Med.* 1990;150(11):2357-60.

[93] Uslu A, Cayci M, Nart A, Karaca C, Zalluhoglu N, Gurkan A, et al. Renal failure in obstructive jaundice. *Hepatogastroenterology.* 2005;52(61):52-4.

[94] Tabatabaee SM, Elahi R, Savaj S. Bile cast nephropathy due to cholestatic jaundice after using stanozolol in 2 amateur bodybuilders. *Iran J Kidney Dis.* 2015;9(4):331-4.

[95] Aniort J, Poyet A, Kemeny JL, Philipponnet C, Heng AE. Bile Cast Nephropathy Caused by Obstructive Cholestasis. *Am J Kidney Dis.* 2017;69(1):143-6.

[96] Sequeira A, Gu X. Bile cast nephropathy: an often forgotten diagnosis. *Hemodial Int.* 2015;19(1):132-5.

[97] Luciano RL, Castano E, Moeckel G, Perazella MA. Bile acid nephropathy in a bodybuilder abusing an anabolic androgenic steroid. *Am J Kidney Dis.* 2014;64(3):473-6.

[98] Kritmetapak K, Sathidatekoonchorn T, Papanrueng W. Bile cast nephropathy in a patient with cholangiocarcinoma - a case report. *Clin Case Rep.* 2018;6(5):779-83.

[99] Krones E, Pollheimer MJ, Rosenkranz AR, Fickert P. Cholemic nephropathy - Historical notes and novel perspectives. *Biochim Biophys Acta.* 2018;1864(4 Pt B):1356-66.

[100] Nayak SL, Kumar M, Bihari C, Rastogi A. Bile Cast Nephropathy in Patients with Acute Kidney Injury Due to Hepatorenal Syndrome: A Postmortem Kidney Biopsy Study. *J Clin Transl Hepatol.* 2017;5(2):92-100.

[101] van Slambrouck CM, Salem F, Meehan SM, Chang A. Bile cast nephropathy is a common pathologic finding for kidney injury associated with severe liver dysfunction. *Kidney Int.* 2013;84(1):192-7.

[102] Foshat M, Ruff HM, Fischer WG, Beach RE, Fowler MR, Ju H, et al. Bile Cast Nephropathy in Cirrhotic Patients: Effects of Chronic Hyperbilirubinemia. *Am J Clin Pathol.* 2017;147(5):525-35.

[103] Heyman SN, Darmon D, Ackerman Z, Rosenberger C, Rosen S. Bile cast nephropathy. *Kidney Int.* 2014;85(2):479.

[104] Rivera M, Alghamdi A, Velez JC. Assessment of utility of urine sediment microscopy in hepatorenal acute kidney injury. *J Am Soc Nephrol.* 2018;29(A):F0004.

[105] Kirkby K, Baylis C, Agarwal A, Croker B, Archer L, Adin C. Intravenous bilirubin provides incomplete protection against renal ischemia-reperfusion injury in vivo. *Am J Physiol Renal Physiol.* 2007;292(2):F888-94.

[106] Adin CA, Croker BP, Agarwal A. Protective effects of exogenous bilirubin on ischemia-reperfusion injury in the isolated, perfused rat kidney. *Am J Physiol Renal Physiol.* 2005;288(4):F778-84.

[107] Barabas K, Milner R, Farese J, Baylis C, Croker B, Archer L, et al. Hyperbilirubinemia's protective effect against cisplatin nephrotoxicity in the Gunn rat. *Anticancer Drugs.* 2008;19(5):495-502.

[108] Oh SW, Lee ES, Kim S, Na KY, Chae DW, Kim S, et al. Bilirubin attenuates the renal tubular injury by inhibition of oxidative stress and apoptosis. *BMC Nephrol.* 2013;14:105.

[109] Fickert P, Krones E, Pollheimer MJ, Thueringer A, Moustafa T, Silbert D, et al. Bile acids trigger cholemic nephropathy in common bile-duct-ligated mice. *Hepatology.* 2013;58(6):2056-69.

[110] Kaler B, Karram T, Morgan WA, Bach PH, Yousef IM, Bomzon A. Are bile acids involved in the renal dysfunction of obstructive jaundice? An experimental study in bile duct ligated rats. *Ren Fail.* 2004;26(5):507-16.

[111] Ljubuncic P, Tanne Z, Bomzon A. Evidence of a systemic phenomenon for oxidative stress in cholestatic liver disease. *Gut.* 2000;47(5):710-6.

[112] Fulop M, Brazeau P. Impaired renal function exaggerates hyperbilirubinemia in bile duct-ligated dogs. *Am J Dig Dis.* 1970;15(12):1067-72.

[113] Adebayo D, Morabito V, Davenport A, Jalan R. Renal dysfunction in cirrhosis is not just a vasomotor nephropathy. *Kidney Int.* 2015;87(3):509-15.

[114] Garg H, Kumar A, Garg V, Sharma P, Sharma BC, Sarin SK. Clinical profile and predictors of mortality in patients of acute-on-chronic liver failure. *Digestive and liver disease: official journal of the Italian Society of Gastroenterology and the Italian Association for the Study of the Liver.* 2012;44(2):166-71.

[115] Hampel H, Bynum GD, Zamora E, El-Serag HB. Risk factors for the development of renal dysfunction in hospitalized patients with cirrhosis. *Am J Gastroenterol.* 2001;96(7):2206-10.

[116] Wilkinson SP, Moodie H, Stamatakis JD, Kakkar VV, Williams R. Endotoxaemia and renal failure in cirrhosis and obstructive jaundice. *Br Med J.* 1976;2(6049):1415-8.

[117] Shah N, Mohamed FE, Jover-Cobos M, Macnaughtan J, Davies N, Moreau R, et al. Increased renal expression and urinary excretion of TLR4 in acute kidney injury associated with cirrhosis. *Liver international: official journal of the International Association for the Study of the Liver.* 2013;33(3):398-409.

[118] Arroyo V, Gines P, Gerbes AL, Dudley FJ, Gentilini P, Laffi G, et al. Definition and diagnostic criteria of refractory ascites and hepatorenal syndrome in cirrhosis. International Ascites Club. *Hepatology.* 1996;23(1):164-76.

[119] Salerno F, Gerbes A, Gines P, Wong F, Arroyo V. Diagnosis, prevention and treatment of hepatorenal syndrome in cirrhosis. *Gut.* 2007;56(9):1310-8.

[120] Angeli P, Gines P, Wong F, Bernardi M, Boyer TD, Gerbes A, et al. Diagnosis and management of acute kidney injury in patients with cirrhosis: revised consensus recommendations of the International Club of Ascites. *J Hepatol.* 2015;62(4):968-74.

[121] Wong F, Angeli P. New diagnostic criteria and management of acute kidney injury. *J Hepatol.* 2017;66(4):860-1.

[122] Follo A, Llovet JM, Navasa M, Planas R, Forns X, Francitorra A, et al. Renal impairment after spontaneous bacterial peritonitis in cirrhosis: incidence, clinical course, predictive factors and prognosis. *Hepatology.* 1994;20(6):1495-501.

[123] Watt K, Uhanova J, Minuk GY. Hepatorenal syndrome: diagnostic accuracy, clinical features, and outcome in a tertiary care center. *Am J Gastroenterol.* 2002;97(8):2046-50.

[124] Fernandez J, Navasa M, Planas R, Montoliu S, Monfort D, Soriano G, et al. Primary prophylaxis of spontaneous bacterial peritonitis delays hepatorenal syndrome and improves survival in cirrhosis. *Gastroenterology.* 2007;133(3):818-24.

[125] Davenport A, Sheikh MF, Lamb E, Agarwal B, Jalan R. Acute kidney injury in acute-on-chronic liver failure: where does hepatorenal syndrome fit? *Kidney Int.* 2017;92(5):1058-70.

[126] Regner KR, Singbartl K. Kidney Injury in Liver Disease. *Crit Care Clin.* 2016;32(3):343-55.

[127] Montano-Loza AJ, Duarte-Rojo A, Meza-Junco J, Baracos VE, Sawyer MB, Pang JX, et al. Inclusion of Sarcopenia Within MELD (MELD-Sarcopenia) and the Prediction of Mortality in Patients With Cirrhosis. *Clin Transl Gastroenterol.* 2015;6:e102.
[128] Sansoe G, Ferrari A, Castellana CN, Bonardi L, Villa E, Manenti F. Cimetidine administration and tubular creatinine secretion in patients with compensated cirrhosis. *Clin Sci* (Lond). 2002;102(1):91-8.
[129] Daugherty NA, Hammond KB, Osberg IM. Bilirubin interference with the kinetic Jaffe method for serum creatinine. *Clin Chem.* 1978;24(2):392-3.
[130] Gomaa SH, Shamseya MM, Madkour MA. Clinical utility of urinary neutrophil gelatinase-associated lipocalin and serum cystatin C in a cohort of liver cirrhosis patients with renal dysfunction: a challenge in the diagnosis of hepatorenal syndrome. *European journal of gastroenterology & hepatology*. 2019.
[131] Woitas RP, Stoffel-Wagner B, Flommersfeld S, Poege U, Schiedermaier P, Klehr HU, et al. Correlation of serum concentrations of cystatin C and creatinine to inulin clearance in liver cirrhosis. *Clin Chem.* 2000;46(5):712-5.
[132] Gerbes AL, Gulberg V, Bilzer M, Vogeser M. Evaluation of serum cystatin C concentration as a marker of renal function in patients with cirrhosis of the liver. *Gut.* 2002;50(1):106-10.
[133] Demirtas S, Bozbas A, Akbay A, Yavuz Y, Karaca L. Diagnostic value of serum cystatin C for evaluation of hepatorenal syndrome. *Clin Chim Acta.* 2001;311(2):81-9.
[134] Ahn HS, Kim YS, Kim SG, Kim HK, Min SK, Jeong SW, et al. Cystatin C is a good predictor of hepatorenal syndrome and survival in patients with cirrhosis who have normal serum creatinine levels. *Hepatogastroenterology.* 2012;59(116):1168-73.
[135] Amathieu R, Al-Khafaji A, Sileanu FE, Foldes E, DeSensi R, Hilmi I, et al. Significance of oliguria in critically ill patients with chronic liver disease. *Hepatology.* 2017;66(5):1592-600.
[136] Velez JCQ, Petkovich B, Karakala N, Huggins JT. Point-of-Care Echocardiography Unveils Misclassification of Acute Kidney Injury as Hepatorenal Syndrome. *Am J Nephrol.* 2019:1-8.
[137] Alsaad AA, Wadei HM. Fractional excretion of sodium in hepatorenal syndrome: Clinical and pathological correlation. *World J Hepatol.* 2016;8(34):1497-501.
[138] Patidar KR, Kang L, Bajaj JS, Carl D, Sanyal AJ. Fractional excretion of urea: A simple tool for the differential diagnosis of acute kidney injury in cirrhosis. *Hepatology.* 2018;68(1):224-33.
[139] Newell GC. Cirrhotic glomerulonephritis: incidence, morphology, clinical features, and pathogenesis. *Am J Kidney Dis.* 1987;9(3):183-90.
[140] Wadei HM, Geiger XJ, Cortese C, Mai ML, Kramer DJ, Rosser BG, et al. Kidney allocation to liver transplant candidates with renal failure of undetermined etiology: role of percutaneous renal biopsy. *Am J Transplant.* 2008;8(12):2618-26.
[141] Kohler H, Wandel E, Brunck B. Acanthocyturia--a characteristic marker for glomerular bleeding. *Kidney Int.* 1991;40(1):115-20.
[142] Nguyen MT, Maynard SE, Kimmel PL. Misapplications of commonly used kidney equations: renal physiology in practice. *Clin J Am Soc Nephrol.* 2009;4(3):528-34.
[143] Perazella MA, Coca SG, Kanbay M, Brewster UC, Parikh CR. Diagnostic value of urine microscopy for differential diagnosis of acute kidney injury in hospitalized patients. *Clin J Am Soc Nephrol.* 2008;3(6):1615-9.

[144] Perazella MA, Coca SG, Hall IE, Iyanam U, Koraishy M, Parikh CR. Urine microscopy is associated with severity and worsening of acute kidney injury in hospitalized patients. *Clin J Am Soc Nephrol.* 2010;5(3):402-8.

[145] Chawla LS, Dommu A, Berger A, Shih S, Patel SS. Urinary sediment cast scoring index for acute kidney injury: a pilot study. *Nephron Clin Pract.* 2008;110(3):c145-50.

[146] Eknoyan G. Letter: Renal disorders in hepatic failure. *Br Med J.* 1974;2(5920):670.

[147] Elsom K. Renal function in obstructive jaundice. *Arch Intern Med.* 1937;60(6):1028-33.

[148] Velez JC, Kadian M, Taburyanskaya M, Bohm NM, Delay TA, Karakala N, et al. Hepatorenal Acute Kidney Injury and the Importance of Raising Mean Arterial Pressure. *Nephron.* 2015;131(3):191-201.

[149] Puthumana J, Ariza X, Belcher JM, Graupera I, Gines P, Parikh CR. Urine Interleukin 18 and Lipocalin 2 Are Biomarkers of Acute Tubular Necrosis in Patients With Cirrhosis: A Systematic Review and Meta-analysis. *Clin Gastroenterol Hepatol.* 2017;15(7):1003-13 e3.

[150] Fagundes C, Pepin MN, Guevara M, Barreto R, Casals G, Sola E, et al. Urinary neutrophil gelatinase-associated lipocalin as biomarker in the differential diagnosis of impairment of kidney function in cirrhosis. *J Hepatol.* 2012;57(2):267-73.

[151] Verna EC, Brown RS, Farrand E, Pichardo EM, Forster CS, Sola-Del Valle DA, et al. Urinary neutrophil gelatinase-associated lipocalin predicts mortality and identifies acute kidney injury in cirrhosis. *Digestive diseases and sciences.* 2012;57(9):2362-70.

[152] Huelin P, Sola E, Elia C, Sole C, Risso A, Moreira R, et al. Neutrophil Gelatinase-Associated Lipocalin for Assessment of Acute Kidney Injury in Cirrhosis: A Prospective Study. *Hepatology.* 2019.

[153] Watany MM, Hagag RY, Okda HI. Circulating miR-21, miR-210 and miR-146a as potential biomarkers to differentiate acute tubular necrosis from hepatorenal syndrome in patients with liver cirrhosis: a pilot study. *Clin Chem Lab Med.* 2018;56(5):739-47.

[154] Bichet DG, Groves BG, Schrier RW. Effect of head-out water immersion on hepatorenal syndrome. *Am J Kidney Dis.* 1984;3(4):258-63.

[155] Yersin B, Burnier M, Magnenat P. Improvement of renal failure with repeated head-out water immersions in patients with hepatorenal syndrome associated with alcoholic hepatitis. *Am J Nephrol.* 1995;15(3):260-5.

[156] Ariyan S, Sweeney T, Kerstein MD. The hepatorenal syndrome: recovery after portacaval shunt. *Ann Surg.* 1975;181(6):847-9.

[157] Pladson TR, Parrish RM. Hepatorenal syndrome. Recovery after peritoneovenous shunt. *Arch Intern Med.* 1977;137(9):1248-9.

[158] Landini S, Coli U, Fracasso A, Morachiello P, Righetto F, Scanferla F, et al. Spontaneous ascites filtration and reinfusion (SAFR) as ambulatory chronic treatment for hepatorenal syndrome. *Trans Am Soc Artif Intern Organs.* 1985;31:439-43.

[159] Cobden I, Shore A, Wilkinson R, Record CO. Captopril in the hepatorenal syndrome. *Journal of clinical gastroenterology.* 1985;7(4):354-60.

[160] Zipser RD, Kronborg I, Rector W, Reynolds T, Daskalopoulos G. Therapeutic trial of thromboxane synthesis inhibition in the hepatorenal syndrome. *Gastroenterology.* 1984;87(6):1228-32.

[161] Fevery J, Van Cutsem E, Nevens F, Van Steenbergen W, Verberckmoes R, De Groote J. Reversal of hepatorenal syndrome in four patients by peroral misoprostol (prostaglandin E1 analogue) and albumin administration. *J Hepatol.* 1990;11(2):153-8.

[162] Ortega R, Gines P, Uriz J, Cardenas A, Calahorra B, De Las Heras D, et al. Terlipressin therapy with and without albumin for patients with hepatorenal syndrome: results of a prospective, nonrandomized study. *Hepatology.* 2002;36(4 Pt 1):941-8.

[163] Salerno F, Navickis RJ, Wilkes MM. Albumin treatment regimen for type 1 hepatorenal syndrome: a dose-response meta-analysis. *BMC Gastroenterol.* 2015;15:167.

[164] Chen TA, Tsao YC, Chen A, Lo GH, Lin CK, Yu HC, et al. Effect of intravenous albumin on endotoxin removal, cytokines, and nitric oxide production in patients with cirrhosis and spontaneous bacterial peritonitis. *Scand J Gastroenterol.* 2009;44(5):619-25.

[165] Therapondos G, Stanley AJ, Hayes PC. Systemic, portal and renal effects of terlipressin in patients with cirrhotic ascites: pilot study. *Journal of gastroenterology and hepatology.* 2004;19(1):73-7.

[166] Lenz K, Hortnagl H, Druml W, Reither H, Schmid R, Schneeweiss B, et al. Ornipressin in the treatment of functional renal failure in decompensated liver cirrhosis. Effects on renal hemodynamics and atrial natriuretic factor. *Gastroenterology.* 1991;101(4):1060-7.

[167] Angeli P, Volpin R, Gerunda G, Craighero R, Roner P, Merenda R, et al. Reversal of type 1 hepatorenal syndrome with the administration of midodrine and octreotide. *Hepatology.* 1999;29(6):1690-7.

[168] Skagen C, Einstein M, Lucey MR, Said A. Combination treatment with octreotide, midodrine, and albumin improves survival in patients with type 1 and type 2 hepatorenal syndrome. *Journal of clinical gastroenterology.* 2009;43(7):680-5.

[169] Wong F, Pantea L, Sniderman K. Midodrine, octreotide, albumin, and TIPS in selected patients with cirrhosis and type 1 hepatorenal syndrome. *Hepatology.* 2004;40(1):55-64.

[170] Esrailian E, Pantangco ER, Kyulo NL, Hu KQ, Runyon BA. Octreotide/Midodrine therapy significantly improves renal function and 30-day survival in patients with type 1 hepatorenal syndrome. *Digestive diseases and sciences.* 2007;52(3):742-8.

[171] Jamil K, Pappas SC, Devarakonda KR. In vitro binding and receptor-mediated activity of terlipressin at vasopressin receptors V1 and V2. *J Exp Pharmacol.* 2018;10:1-7.

[172] Bernadich C, Bandi JC, Melin P, Bosch J. Effects of F-180, a new selective vasoconstrictor peptide, compared with terlipressin and vasopressin on systemic and splanchnic hemodynamics in a rat model of portal hypertension. *Hepatology.* 1998;27(2):351-6.

[173] Uriz J, Gines P, Cardenas A, Sort P, Jimenez W, Salmeron JM, et al. Terlipressin plus albumin infusion: an effective and safe therapy of hepatorenal syndrome. *J Hepatol.* 2000;33(1):43-8.

[174] Solanki P, Chawla A, Garg R, Gupta R, Jain M, Sarin SK. Beneficial effects of terlipressin in hepatorenal syndrome: a prospective, randomized placebo-controlled clinical trial. *Journal of gastroenterology and hepatology.* 2003;18(2):152-6.

[175] Mulkay JP, Louis H, Donckier V, Bourgeois N, Adler M, Deviere J, et al. Long-term terlipressin administration improves renal function in cirrhotic patients with type 1 hepatorenal syndrome: a pilot study. *Acta Gastroenterol Belg*. 2001;64(1):15-9.

[176] Moreau R, Durand F, Poynard T, Duhamel C, Cervoni JP, Ichai P, et al. Terlipressin in patients with cirrhosis and type 1 hepatorenal syndrome: a retrospective multicenter study. *Gastroenterology*. 2002;122(4):923-30.

[177] Saner F, Kavuk I, Lang H, Biglarnia R, Fruhauf NR, Schafers RF, et al. Terlipressin and gelafundin: safe therapy of hepatorenal syndrome. *Eur J Med Res.* 2004;9(2):78-82.

[178] Munoz LE, Alcala EG, Cordero P, Martinez MA, Vazquez NY, Galindo S, et al. Reversal of hepatorenal syndrome in cirrhotic patients with terlipressin plus albumin. First experience in Mexico. *Annals of hepatology.* 2009;8(3):207-11.

[179] Narahara Y, Kanazawa H, Sakamoto C, Maruyama H, Yokosuka O, Mochida S, et al. The efficacy and safety of terlipressin and albumin in patients with type 1 hepatorenal syndrome: a multicenter, open-label, explorative study. *J Gastroenterol.* 2012;47(3):313-20.

[180] Gluud LL, Christensen K, Christensen E, Krag A. Terlipressin for hepatorenal syndrome. *Cochrane Database Syst Rev.* 2012(9):CD005162.

[181] Martin-Llahi M, Pepin MN, Guevara M, Diaz F, Torre A, Monescillo A, et al. Terlipressin and albumin vs albumin in patients with cirrhosis and hepatorenal syndrome: a randomized study. *Gastroenterology.* 2008;134(5):1352-9.

[182] Neri S, Pulvirenti D, Malaguarnera M, Cosimo BM, Bertino G, Ignaccolo L, et al. Terlipressin and albumin in patients with cirrhosis and type I hepatorenal syndrome. *Digestive diseases and sciences.* 2008;53(3):830-5.

[183] Cavallin M, Kamath PS, Merli M, Fasolato S, Toniutto P, Salerno F, et al. Terlipressin plus albumin versus midodrine and octreotide plus albumin in the treatment of hepatorenal syndrome: A randomized trial. *Hepatology.* 2015.

[184] Sanyal AJ, Boyer T, Garcia-Tsao G, Regenstein F, Rossaro L, Appenrodt B, et al. A randomized, prospective, double-blind, placebo-controlled trial of terlipressin for type 1 hepatorenal syndrome. *Gastroenterology.* 2008;134(5):1360-8.

[185] Boyer TD, Sanyal AJ, Wong F, Frederick RT, Lake JR, O'Leary JG, et al. Terlipressin Plus Albumin Is More Effective Than Albumin Alone in Improving Renal Function in Patients With Cirrhosis and Hepatorenal Syndrome Type 1. *Gastroenterology.* 2016;150(7):1579-89 e2.

[186] Wong F, Pappas SC, Curry MP, Reddy KR, Rubin RA, Porayko MK, et al. Terlipressin plus Albumin for the Treatment of Type 1 Hepatorenal Syndrome. *N Engl J Med.* 2021;384(9):818-28.

[187] Duvoux C, Zanditenas D, Hezode C, Chauvat A, Monin JL, Roudot-Thoraval F, et al. Effects of noradrenalin and albumin in patients with type I hepatorenal syndrome: a pilot study. *Hepatology.* 2002;36(2):374-80.

[188] Sharma P, Kumar A, Shrama BC, Sarin SK. An open label, pilot, randomized controlled trial of noradrenaline versus terlipressin in the treatment of type 1 hepatorenal syndrome and predictors of response. *Am J Gastroenterol.* 2008;103(7):1689-97.

[189] Singh V, Ghosh S, Singh B, Kumar P, Sharma N, Bhalla A, et al. Noradrenaline vs. terlipressin in the treatment of hepatorenal syndrome: a randomized study. *J Hepatol.* 2012;56(6):1293-8.

[190] Alessandria C, Ottobrelli A, Debernardi-Venon W, Todros L, Cerenzia MT, Martini S, et al. Noradrenalin vs terlipressin in patients with hepatorenal syndrome: a prospective, randomized, unblinded, pilot study. *J Hepatol.* 2007;47(4):499-505.

[191] Saif RU, Dar HA, Sofi SM, Andrabi MS, Javid G, Zargar SA. Noradrenaline versus terlipressin in the management of type 1 hepatorenal syndrome: A randomized controlled study. *Indian J Gastroenterol.* 2018;37(5):424-9.

[192] Ghosh S, Choudhary NS, Sharma AK, Singh B, Kumar P, Agarwal R, et al. Noradrenaline vs terlipressin in the treatment of type 2 hepatorenal syndrome: a randomized pilot study. *Liver international: official journal of the International Association for the Study of the Liver.* 2013;33(8):1187-93.

[193] Badawy SS MN, Ahmed A. Norepinephrine versus terlipressin in patients with type 1 hepatorenal syndrome refractory to treatment with octreotide, midodrine, and albumin: a prospective randomized comparative study. *Egypt J Cardiothorac Anesth.* 2013;7:13-8.

[194] Goyal O, Sidhu SS, Sehgal N, Puri S. Noradrenaline is as Effective as Terlipressin in Hepatorenal Syndrome Type 1: A Prospective, Randomized Trial. *J Assoc Physicians India.* 2016;64(9):30-5.

[195] Nassar Junior AP, Farias AQ, LA DA, Carrilho FJ, Malbouisson LM. Terlipressin versus norepinephrine in the treatment of hepatorenal syndrome: a systematic review and meta-analysis. *PLoS One.* 2014;9(9):e107466.

[196] Arora V, Maiwall R, Vijayaraghavan R, Jindal A, Saggere Muralikrishna S, Kumar G, et al. Terlipressin is superior to noradrenaline in the management of acute kidney injury in acute on chronic liver failure. *Hepatology.* 2018.

[197] Tavakkoli H, Yazdanpanah K, Mansourian M. Noradrenalin versus the combination of midodrine and octreotide in patients with hepatorenal syndrome: randomized clinical trial. *International journal of preventive medicine.* 2012;3(11):764-9.

[198] Velez JC, Nietert PJ. Therapeutic response to vasoconstrictors in hepatorenal syndrome parallels increase in mean arterial pressure: a pooled analysis of clinical trials. *Am J Kidney Dis.* 2011;58(6):928-38.

[199] Maddukuri G, Cai CX, Munigala S, Mohammadi F, Zhang Z. Targeting an early and substantial increase in mean arterial pressure is critical in the management of type 1 hepatorenal syndrome: a combined retrospective and pilot study. *Digestive diseases and sciences.* 2014;59(2):471-81.

[200] Cai CX, Maddukuri G, Jaipaul N, Zhang Z. A Treat-to-Target Concept to Guide the Medical Management of Hepatorenal Syndrome. *Digestive diseases and sciences.* 2015;60(5):1474-81.

[201] Alessandria C, Ottobrelli A, Debernardi-Venon W, Todros L, Cerenzia MT, Martini S, et al. Noradrenalin vs terlipressin in patients with hepatorenal syndrome: a prospective, randomized, unblinded, pilot study. *J Hepatol.* 2007;47(4):499-505.

[202] Sanyal AJ, Boyer TD, Frederick RT, Wong F, Rossaro L, Araya V, et al. Reversal of hepatorenal syndrome type 1 with terlipressin plus albumin vs. placebo plus albumin in a pooled analysis of the OT-0401 and REVERSE randomised clinical studies. *Aliment Pharmacol Ther.* 2017;45(11):1390-402.

[203] Kelleher SP, Robinette JB, Conger JD. Sympathetic nervous system in the loss of autoregulation in acute renal failure. *Am J Physiol.* 1984;246(4 Pt 2):F379-86.

[204] Persson PB, Ehmke H, Nafz B, Kirchheim HR. Sympathetic modulation of renal autoregulation by carotid occlusion in conscious dogs. *Am J Physiol.* 1990;258(2 Pt 2):F364-70.

[205] Stadlbauer V, Wright GA, Banaji M, Mukhopadhya A, Mookerjee RP, Moore K, et al. Relationship between activation of the sympathetic nervous system and renal blood flow autoregulation in cirrhosis. *Gastroenterology.* 2008;134(1):111-9.

[206] Guevara M, Gines P, Bandi JC, Gilabert R, Sort P, Jimenez W, et al. Transjugular intrahepatic portosystemic shunt in hepatorenal syndrome: effects on renal function and vasoactive systems. *Hepatology.* 1998;28(2):416-22.

[207] Brensing KA, Textor J, Perz J, Schiedermaier P, Raab P, Strunk H, et al. Long term outcome after transjugular intrahepatic portosystemic stent-shunt in non-transplant cirrhotics with hepatorenal syndrome: a phase II study. *Gut.* 2000;47(2):288-95.

[208] Anderson CL, Saad WE, Kalagher SD, Caldwell S, Sabri S, Turba UC, et al. Effect of transjugular intrahepatic portosystemic shunt placement on renal function: a 7-year, single-center experience. *J Vasc Interv Radiol.* 2010;21(9):1370-6.

[209] Song T, Rossle M, He F, Liu F, Guo X, Qi X. Transjugular intrahepatic portosystemic shunt for hepatorenal syndrome: A systematic review and meta-analysis. *Digestive and liver disease: official journal of the Italian Society of Gastroenterology and the Italian Association for the Study of the Liver.* 2018;50(4):323-30.

[210] Wong F, Leung W, Al Beshir M, Marquez M, Renner EL. Outcomes of patients with cirrhosis and hepatorenal syndrome type 1 treated with liver transplantation. *Liver transplantation: official publication of the American Association for the Study of Liver Diseases and the International Liver Transplantation Society.* 2015;21(3):300-7.

[211] Boyer TD, Sanyal AJ, Garcia-Tsao G, Regenstein F, Rossaro L, Appenrodt B, et al. Impact of liver transplantation on the survival of patients treated for hepatorenal syndrome type 1. *Liver transplantation: official publication of the American Association for the Study of Liver Diseases and the International Liver Transplantation Society.* 2011;17(11):1328-32.

[212] Heidemann J, Bartels C, Berssenbrugge C, Schmidt H, Meister T. Hepatorenal syndrome: outcome of response to therapy and predictors of survival. *Gastroenterol Res Pract.* 2015;2015:457613.

[213] Capling RK, Bastani B. The clinical course of patients with type 1 hepatorenal syndrome maintained on hemodialysis. *Ren Fail.* 2004;26(5):563-8.

[214] Wong LP, Blackley MP, Andreoni KA, Chin H, Falk RJ, Klemmer PJ. Survival of liver transplant candidates with acute renal failure receiving renal replacement therapy. *Kidney Int.* 2005;68(1):362-70.

[215] Witzke O, Baumann M, Patschan D, Patschan S, Mitchell A, Treichel U, et al. Which patients benefit from hemodialysis therapy in hepatorenal syndrome? *Journal of gastroenterology and hepatology.* 2004;19(12):1369-73.

[216] Keller F, Heinze H, Jochimsen F, Passfall J, Schuppan D, Buttner P. Risk factors and outcome of 107 patients with decompensated liver disease and acute renal failure (including 26 patients with hepatorenal syndrome): the role of hemodialysis. *Ren Fail.* 1995;17(2):135-46.

[217] Allegretti AS, Parada XV, Eneanya ND, Gilligan H, Xu D, Zhao S, et al. Prognosis of Patients with Cirrhosis and AKI Who Initiate RRT. *Clin J Am Soc Nephrol.* 2018;13(1):16-25.

In: Issues in Kidney Disease – Acute Kidney Injury
Editors: S. Z. Fadem and A. Arslan Yousuf Awan ISBN: 978-1-68507-002-1

Chapter 16

ACUTE KIDNEY INJURY IN MALIGNANCY

Omar Mamlouk, MD, Harini Bejjanki, MD and Biruh Workeneh*, MD

The University of Texas MD Anderson Cancer Center, Houston, TX, USA

ABSTRACT

Acute kidney injury (AKI) is a common complication in patients with malignancy. The incidence and severity depend on the cancer type, treatment regimen, and the patient's comorbidities. The presence of CKD is also a determinant of AKI. The development of AKI can impact survival because of direct complications and because it influences decisions about continuing cancer treatment. The diagnosis, including novel biomarkers, are discussed. Renal toxicity associated with chemotherapy and novel therapies are also discussed. Finally, the treatment and prognosis of the unique syndromes associated with AKI in patients with malignancy are reviewed in this chapter.

Keywords: acute kidney injury, tumor lysis syndrome, thrombotic microangiopathy, renal toxicity, cisplatin, immunotherapy, surgical complication

INTRODUCTION

Cancer is a significant public health burden and the 2nd leading cause of death in the United States, with estimated new cancer cases of 1.76 million and cancer-related death of 0.6 million in 2019 [1]. Acute kidney injury (AKI) is a common complication in patients with malignancy. The incidence and severity depend on the cancer type, treatment regimen, and the patient's comorbidities [2, 3]. The presence of CKD is also a determinant of AKI. The development of AKI can impact survival because of direct complications and because it influences decisions about continuing cancer treatment. Therefore, this topic is essential and timely for clinical

* Corresponding Author's E-mail: btworkeneh@mdanderson.org.

trainees and practicing oncologists and nephrologists. Furthermore, the rapid pace of drug discovery results in emerging information about novel agents' effects on renal function. We will review the diagnosis, treatment, and prognosis of the unique syndromes associated with AKI in patients with malignancy [1, 4].

DEFINITION

AKI is a syndrome manifested by a decrease in the glomerular filtration rate (GFR) and subsequent dysregulation of the body electrolytes and volume, and abnormal retention of nitrogenous waste products when a sudden change in kidney function occurs. The Kidney Disease Improving Global Outcome (KDIGO) definition has unified the definition of AKI and includes patients with cancer. The definition is based on the change of serum creatinine and urine output:

- Rise in serum creatinine ≥0.3 mg/dL within 48 hours
- Rise in serum creatinine ≥1.5 times baseline, which is known or presumed to have occurred within the prior seven days
- Urine output < 0.5 ml/kg/hour for six hours [5]

The pursuit of other, more reliable markers of AKI has been elusive. Markers that have been explored in cancer patients include the functional marker, cystatin-c. In cancer patients, the cystatin-c level can be influenced by tumor burden, the presence of inflammation, or cancer therapy. To date, the current data is not supportive of using the change in cystatin levels to define AKI. However, it can be useful as an early marker to predict AKI, especially in critical care patients [6-8].

Novel tubular injury markers, such as neutrophil gelatinase-associated lipocalin (NGAL) and kidney molecule-1 (KIM-1), are still under investigation to validate their use in various AKI settings. Moreover, these markers might be influenced by malignancies, such as NGAL in ovarian and chronic myeloid leukemia [9, 10]. Their use in cancer patients so far has been limited to being a potential early prediction marker of kidney injury associated with nephrotoxic chemotherapy agents, such as cisplatin [11, 12]. More details about novel tubular injury biomarkers are discussed in Chapter 4.

EPIDEMIOLOGY

Incidence

AKI is more common in cancer patients than in the general population for multiple factors, including old age, cancer itself, and the nephrotoxicity and complications associated with its treatment (chemotherapy, immunotherapy, stem cell transplant, tumor lysis, and sepsis) [2]. The incidence of AKI in cancer patients varies based on the criteria used to define AKI (Risk, Injury, Failure, Loss, End-stage renal disease; RIFLE, Acute Kidney Injury Network; AKIN, or KDIGO) and patient risk factors. The reported overall risk of developing AKI during a hospitalization ranged from 12 to 21% [2, 13, 14]. Moreover, the cumulative incidence over a more extended period has been reported to range 9.3- 25.7% over 1.85-5 years of follow-up [14, 15]. Furthermore, when analyzed by cancer type, hematological, gastrointestinal, liver, and kidney cancers tend to have the highest rate of AKI [13, 14]. Of the majority of the reported AKI, 50-75% are mild, RIFLE risk category or KDIGO grade 1, and only 4-5% of the patients with AKI have required renal replacement therapy [2, 13, 14]. The rate increases to 8-52% as the severity and incidence of AKI increases up to 68% in critical care patients, particularly in hematologic cancers [16-19].

Risk Factors

Multiple risk factors are associated with this increased risk of AKI across different care levels. Table 1 summarizes these factors that include sepsis, diabetes, chronic kidney disease, chemotherapy, antibiotics, angiotensin receptor blockers (ARB), angiotensin-converting enzyme inhibitors (ACEI), diuretics, hyponatremia, tumor lysis syndrome, hypo-albuminemia, history of stem cell transplant, older age (> 65-year-old), certain geographical areas, and a higher per capita gross domestic product [2, 13, 15, 18].

Table 1. Risk factors associated with acute kidney injury in cancer patient

Risk factors		
Age > 65-year-old	Neutropenia and sepsis	Hypovolemia
Congestive heart failure	Liver cirrhosis	Chronic kidney disease
Diabetes Mellitus	Nephrectomy for renal cell cancer	Liver cancer
Hematological Malignancies	Metastatic disease	Hematological stem cell transplant
Chemotherapy	Antibiotics and nephrotoxins	Tumor lysis syndrome
Certain geographical area and higher income	Hyponatremia	Hypercalcemia

Prognosis

Compared to cancer patients with no AKI, AKI is associated with an increased length of stay, treatment cost, lower hematological malignancy remission, and higher mortality rates (1.7-6.5-fold increase); and in some studies, this was correlated with the degree of kidney injury [2, 16, 18-20]. Regarding kidney outcome post-AKI, it is overall positive with close to 60% recovery upon hospital discharge [13]. Significantly, 13-23% of those who survive critical illness with severe AKI require long-term renal replacement therapy [14, 19, 21]. We will discuss in more detail disease-specific kidney recovery and the risk of CKD post-AKI [22-25].

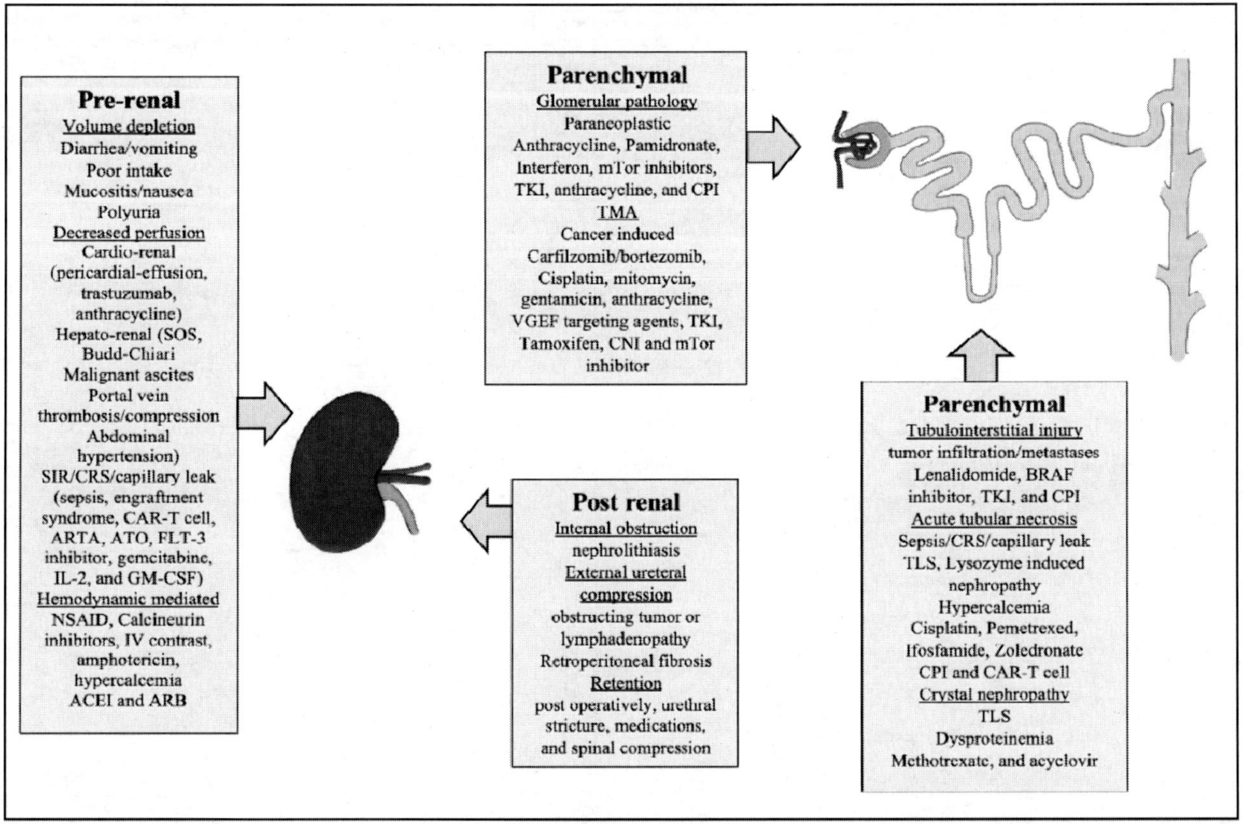

SOS, sinusoidal obstruction syndrome; SIR, systemic inflammation reaction; CRS, cytokine release syndrome; CAR-T, chimeric antigen receptor- T lymphocyte; ATRA, All-Trans Retinoic Acid; ATO, Arsenic trioxide; FLT-3, fms like tyrosine kinase-3; IL-2, interlukin-2; GM-CSF, granulocyte-macrophage colony stimulating factor; NSAID, non-steroidal anti-inflammatory drug; IV, intravenous; ACEI, angiotensin converting enzyme inhibitor; ARB angiotensin II receptor blocker; mTor, mammalian target of rapamycin; TKI, tyrosine kinase inhibitor; CPI, checkpoint inhibitors; TMA, thrombotic microangiopathy; VGEF, vascular endothelial growth factor; CNI, calcineurin inhibitor; TLS, tumor lysis syndrome.

Figure 1. AKI etiologies in cancer patients.

ETIOLOGY

Evaluating a cancer patient with acute kidney injury starts with a detailed history, followed by physical examination and necessary laboratory/imaging investigations. The traditional approach of classifying AKI into pre-renal, intrinsic, and post-renal etiologies applies to patients with malignancy and is the one we will use in this chapter. However, it is useful to frame AKI further as follows: directly related to malignancy; direct effects of chemotherapy; complications of treatment and other factors. Extra attention needs to be paid to the cancer status and stage, as well as cancer treatment history, dose, and duration. Like the non-cancer population, hypovolemia and acute tubular necrosis (ATN) remain the most common etiologies, with sepsis and nephrotoxin being leading causes of ATN [16, 26]. Cancer-specific etiologies are summarized in Figure 1.

PRE-RENAL ETIOLOGY

Pre-renal etiology is common, accounting for 40-50% of total AKI cases, and can be classified based on the pathophysiology into three major categories: hypovolemia, decreased kidney perfusion, and altered glomerular hemodynamics [16, 27]. Cancer patients are susceptible to hypovolemia as a consequence of cancer/chemotherapy-related nausea, vomiting, poor appetite, mucositis (5-fluorouracil, methotrexate, cytarabine, and head and neck radiation therapy), diarrhea, severe anemia/hemorrhage, and diuresis (osmotic diuresis, diabetes insipidus, and diuretics use).

Decreased kidney perfusion can be observed in multiple syndromes and can be further divided into cardio-renal, systemic inflammatory response, hepato-renal, and abdominal compartment syndromes. The cardio-renal syndrome includes malignant and medication-related pericardial tamponade, and chemotherapy-associated cardiotoxicity (anthracycline, trastuzumab, and checkpoint inhibitor). The systemic inflammatory response syndrome (SIRS) is associated with diffuse endothelial injury in patients with sepsis, capillary leak syndrome, differentiation syndrome (all-Trans Retinoic Acid and arsenic trioxide in acute myeloid leukemia and acute promyeloid leukemia), cytokine release syndrome (immunotherapy, chimeric antigen receptor T lymphocyte, CAR-T cell, and interleukin-2), engraftment syndrome (post stem cell transplant), and granulocyte-macrophage colony-stimulating factor [28]. The third subtype is hepato-renal like syndrome and includes hepatic sinusoidal obstruction after stem-cell transplant, massive malignant ascites, Budd-Chiari syndrome, liver cirrhosis, and intrahepatic inferior vena cava compression/thrombosis. Lastly, abdominal compartment syndrome is defined as intra-abdominal hypertension, with pressure >12 mmHg and new organ impairment. It can be associated with pre-renal like syndrome in the setting of renal artery vasoconstriction with activated renin-angiotensin system and renal venous congestion in the setting of impaired venous drainage from vein compression that leads subsequently to decrease in the glomerular filtration. Patients with compartment syndrome are usually critically ill with oliguric AKI, tense abdomen, on ventilation support, and a provoking factor related to massive malignant ascites, large intra-abdominal tumor, post tumor resection, ileus, pancreatitis, or massive volume fluid resuscitation in septic patients [29].

Alteration of glomerular hemodynamics can be observed with certain drugs that interfere with afferent and efferent arteriole dilation through different mechanisms. Non-steroidal anti-inflammatory drugs for pain control, calcineurin inhibitor for graft versus host disease (GVHD) in post allogeneic stem cell transplant, and intravenous contrast activate renin-angiotensin-aldosterone system (RAAS) and inhibit endothelial cell mediators (like nitric oxide and prostaglandin E2). Intravenous (IV) vasopressor can also decrease glomerular filtration by activating vascular smooth muscle alpha 1 adrenoreceptor and subsequently increasing the vascular tone. Moreover, arteriolar vascular tone is increased with the use of amphotericin and in hypercalcemia as they can cause depolarization dependent calcium influx through calcium channels in the vascular smooth muscles surrounding the afferent arterioles. Regarding efferent arterioles, medication like ARB and ACEI inhibit their vasodilation by blocking angiotensin II.

The diagnosis of pre-renal AKI can be made based on a patient's clinical presentation (history and examination). Urinalysis, microscopy, and urine electrolytes can differentiate pre-renal from ATN in conditions that can overlap with ATN. Bland urinalysis with no tubular cells, no granular casts, and no significant proteinuria (< 0.5 g/24hours) support pre-renal etiology. Also, in severe AKI and particularly with oliguria, a fraction excretion sodium < 1% supports a pre-renal diagnosis [30, 31]. Other diagnostic tools are disease-specific and include complete blood count (CBC), cytokines level, liver enzymes, coagulation profile, serum albumin, abdominal ultrasound, liver Doppler sonogram, cardiac echogram, and abdominal pressure measurement (with urinary bladder catheter).

The treatment for pre-renal AKI is correcting the underlying condition. For example, in volume depletion, crystalloid with saline or balanced solutions is indicated, while in SIRS we provide supportive care with as-needed volume expansion/diuresis, IV pressors, antibiotics, and corticosteroids. Other anti-inflammatory medications, like tocilizumab, may have a role, in addition to corticosteroids, in treatment of cytokine release syndrome (CRS) related to CAR-T cell infusion. Patients with cardio-renal syndrome may require more aggressive diuretic therapy to improve cardiac output or inotropic support. For patients with hepato-renal syndrome, holding diuretics, IV pressors/midodrine with octreotide, paracentesis, anticoagulation, tumor resection/chemotherapy/radiation therapy, and defibrotide (SOS) are all therapeutic options. Abdominal compartment syndrome can be relieved by abdominal decompression with large-volume paracentesis, nasogastric tube or laparotomy, and tumor resection. In altered glomerular hemodynamic related AKI, discounting the offending medication and treatment of hypercalcemia as needed.

The prognosis is dependent on the ability to treat the associated comorbid condition, ranging from full recovery in patients with hypovolemia to poor prognosis in patients with advanced liver disease or septic shock with multi-organ failure.

Parenchymal AKI

Monoclonal gammopathy, including multiple myeloma-related kidney disease, sepsis-associated ATN, nephrotoxins associated acute kidney injury, glomerulonephritis, and renal vascular diseases are associated with acute kidney injury in cancer and are discussed elsewhere (please refer to chapter 7-13). We will review specific conditions that are associated with cancer/cancer therapy with intra-renal pathology.

TUMOR LYSIS SYNDROME (TLS)

TLS describes the metabolic derangement caused by tumor breakdown following anti-tumor therapy or rarely following corticosteroids treatment or even spontaneously. Because of the rapid destruction of a massive amount of tumor cells, there is an abrupt release of intracellular ions (including phosphorus and potassium). The nucleic acid that gets catabolized to uric acid overwhelms the body's homeostatic mechanisms. This metabolic derangement can be classified as a laboratory TLS and as a clinical TLS when associated with life-threatening complications. AKI associated with clinical TLS is attributed to urate precipitation in kidney interstitium leading to vasoconstriction, inflammation, and calcium-phosphate tubular deposition. TLS most frequently occurs in patients with hematologic malignancy following chemotherapy, notably with non-Hodgkin lymphoma (Burkitt lymphoma subtype) and acute lymphoblastic leukemia (ALL), with an incidence ranging 16-42% while on prophylactic allopurinol (6% of which had clinical TLS) [32, 33]. TLS is less frequently associated with anaplastic large cell lymphoma, acute myeloid leukemia (AML), chronic lymphocytic leukemia (CLL), and multiple myeloma (MM) and rarely associated with solid tumors [34, 35].

The diagnosis of TLS is based on high pre-test probability, taking into account the cancer type, patient risk factors, presence of metabolic disturbances (laboratory TLS), and clinical manifestations (clinical TLS). The Cairo-Bishop laboratory criteria require two or more of the following laboratory changes within 3 days before or 7 days after cytotoxic therapy (on adequate IV hydration and hypouricemic agent):

- Serum uric acid $\geq$ 8 mg/dL (or 25% increase from baseline)
- Serum potassium $\geq$ 6 mEq/L (or 25% increase from baseline)
- Serum phosphorus $\geq$ 4.5 mg/dL (or 25% increase from baseline)
- Serum calcium $\leq$ 7 mg/dL (or 25% decrease from baseline)

Clinical TLS diagnosis requires meeting the laboratory criteria above plus at least one of the following that is not attributed to the therapeutic agent: increase in AKI (creatinine > 1.5 times the baseline criteria), cardiac arrhythmia, and seizure. Each element has grade 0-5 based on the severity [36].

Stratifying risk, based on the following multiple factors, can assist in prophylaxis treatment choice. Tumor-related factors include high proliferative rate, chemo-sensitivity, and large tumor burden (tumor > 10 cm in diameter, WBC > 50,000 per microL, LDH > 2x baseline pre-treatment, organ/bone marrow infiltration). Patient characteristics that raise risk for TLS include hypovolemia, underlying CKD, concomitant nephrotoxins, volume depletion, lymphatic/leukemic infiltration of the kidney and hyperuricemia at baseline. Treatment-related factors include rituximab, fludarabine, lenalidomide, docetaxel (in solid tumors), and targeted therapy with Venetoclax (B-Cell Lymphoma 2 inhibitor), Obinutuzumab (anti-CD20 monoclonal antibody), CAR-T cell, and Dinaciclib (Cyclin-dependent kinase inhibitor).

A consensus expert opinion proposed a guideline for prophylaxis therapy to decrease the risk of TLS based on the above risk stratification [37]. In high-risk patients (TLS risk > 5%), rasburicase is administered (0.2 mg/kg daily with uric acid level monitoring or a single dose of 3 mg) in addition to aggressive IV hydration (2-3 L/m^2 daily) to achieve a urine output of at least 80 ml/m^2 per hour). In intermediate-risk patients (1-5% risk) with low pre-treatment uric acid (< 8 mg/dL), allopurinol (or febuxostat if cannot tolerate allopurinol) is administered with aggressive IV hydration, as opposed to low-risk category patients (<1% risk) where only IV hydration and monitoring. Despite prophylactic therapy, around 3-5% of high-risk patients still develop TLS. There is no benefit of urine alkalization, rather there is a potential for harm with calcium phosphate deposition in kidney tubules.

Allopurinol inhibits xanthine oxidase blocking the conversion of xanthine to uric acid, for which it helps to decrease the new formation of uric acid. It does not reduce the level of already formed uric acid in contrast with rasburicase, a recombinant version of urate oxidase that metabolizes the insoluble uric acid to allantoin, which is excreted in the urine. The recommended allopurinol dose is 100 mg every 8 hours, with the need for reduction to ≤ 100 mg/day in patients with severe kidney impairment. Reviewing patients' medications before starting the cancer therapy is vital due to the risk of interaction with purine analog drugs and other medications, including diuretics, and measuring G6PD is recommended before the administration of rasburicase due to the associated hemolysis risk in patients with G6PD deficiency.

Interventions for active TLS need to be implemented urgently. Transfer patients who develop tumor lysis to an intensive care unit for continuous cardiac monitoring and frequent laboratory check (serum electrolytes, uric acid, and creatinine every 4-6 hours) [38]. Start aggressive IV hydration with as-needed diuretics to avoid hypervolemia. Administer rasburicase (0.2 mg/kg) with repeated doses as needed. Administer oral potassium and phosphate binders, limiting dietary potassium and phosphate in patients with hyperkalemia and hyperphosphatemia, and administering IV dextrose with insulin, nebulized albuterol, and IV calcium gluconate to decrease the risk of hyperkalemia associated dysrhythmia. Avoid calcium supplement to decrease the risk of calcium phosphate precipitation in the tissues, unless the patient has symptomatic hypocalcemia. Renal replacement therapy (RRT) is required in around 5% of patients despite rasburicase use and for indications similar to non-TLS related AKI, including severe oliguria with hypervolemia, persistent hyperkalemia, symptomatic hypocalcemia secondary to hyperphosphatemia, or calcium phosphate product 70 mg^2/dl^2. Continuous renal replacement therapy may be preferred over conventional hemodialysis due to higher phosphate clearance, and since the rapid lowering of phosphate and uric acid with early initiation is associated with an excellent kidney prognosis.

Hypercalcemia of Malignancy

A total serum calcium level > 10.5 mg/dl is reported in 20-30% of cancer patients and is the most common etiology of hypercalcemia in all hospitalized patients. It is commonly associated with multiple myeloma, breast, kidney, and lung (especially squamous cell) cancers [39]. Its clinical presentation is influenced by the severity and the rate of onset of hypercalcemia. Generally, patients have nonspecific symptoms, including nausea, poor appetite, constipation, abdominal pain, polyuria, and generalized weakness. However, in severe hypercalcemia (level > 14 mg/dL), patients can present with neurological manifestations, like altered mental status and confusion [40]. Additionally, hypercalcemia can present with kidney manifestations, including pre-renal acute kidney injury secondary to direct renal vasoconstriction and hypovolemia in the setting of inadequate fluid intake, polyuria from downregulation of aquaporin 2 water channels, and activation of the calcium-sensing receptor of Henle's thick ascending loop, leading to inhibition of sodium-potassium-chloride transporter. The other kidney manifestation is intra-renal kidney injury that is mediated by calcium deposition in the tubules and interstitium (nephrocalcinosis).

Hypercalcemia of malignancy can be attributed to a few causes. Humoral hypercalcemia of malignancy, which is the most common etiology of hypercalcemia and accounts for approximately 80% of the cases [41]. It is associated mainly with non-metastatic solid cancer. However, it occurs less frequently with hematological cancers (NHL, non-Hodgkin lymphoma, CML, chronic myeloid leukemia, and CLL, chronic lymphoid leukemia). It is related to the secretion of parathyroid hormone-related peptide (PTHrP) directly by the tumor. PTHrP has some homology to parathyroid hormone (PTH) and can act like PTH by binding to PTH1 receptors leading to bone resorption and calcium reabsorption in distal tubules. However, it does not stimulate the production of 1,25 vitamin D, and accordingly, these patients are expected to have high PTHrP, very low PTH, and low to normal 1,25 hydroxyvitamin D. This is in contrast to hypercalcemia associated with 1,25 dihydroxyvitamin D that is produced by the tumor and mainly observed in Hodgkin lymphoma patients, and to a lesser degree with non-Hodgkin lymphoma, and rarely with solid tumors. The activated vitamin D (calcitriol) is produced from 25 hydroxyvitamin D, independently of PTH, in extrarenal cells (lymphoma cells and macrophages). Therefore, PTHrP is expected to be low; PTH is very low, and 1,25 hydroxyvitamin D is high.

Local cytokine release from osteolytic metastases is the second most common etiology in cancer patients, accounting for approximately 20% of the cases [41]. It is observed in MM and breast cancer patients with metastatic bone disease, as the tumor cell produces local cytokines that activate osteoclasts and leads to bone resorption and hypercalcemia. These cytokines include receptor activator of nuclear factor kappa-beta ligand (RANKL), interleukin-3 and -6 in MM and PTHrP in breast cancer, with PTHrP being secreted locally and not expected to be elevated in the serum. Hence, PTHrP is expected to be low; PTH is very low; and 1,25 hydroxyvitamin D low to normal. Ectopic PTH secretion is a rare etiology in cancer patients and is described in solid organ cancer patients (ovarian, lung, pancreatic, and gastric carcinoma) after ruling out parathyroid adenoma. Cancer patients are also at increased risk of developing primary hyperparathyroidism. Therefore, it should always be ruled in hypercalcemic patients by measuring PTH level. For example, having high PTH and PTHrP inpatient levels with humoral hypercalcemia of malignancy would suggest coexisting primary hyperparathyroidism.

Cancer diagnosis is usually, but not always, established before developing hypercalcemia and therefore, the diagnosis is made based on the type of cancer, the presence/absence of bone metastasis, PTH, PTHrP, and 1,25 dihydroxyvitamin D levels. Generally, the kidney function recovers as serum calcium level decreases. However, hypercalcemia is associated with poor prognosis. In a patient with humoral hypercalcemia of malignancy, the PTHrP level can be a tumor response marker and may predict the response and the risk recurrence of hypercalcemia after therapy.

The clinical manifestations of hypercalcemia can be severe. Typically, when total albumin corrected calcium level is > 14 mg/dl, or there is an acute rise in serum calcium, there can be marked change in sensorium, requiring hospitalization and aggressive therapy. The workup and treatment can be initiated as an outpatient in asymptomatic mild and chronic moderate hypercalcemia (12-14 mg/dl). Initial therapy should start with aggressive IV hydration for volume expansion and natriuresis using normal saline at a rate of 200-300 ml/hr to achieve a goal of > 100 ml/hr of urine output. Loop diuretics should not be administered routinely but restricted to patients with hypervolemia. Nonetheless, IV hydration rarely normalizes moderate to severe hypercalcemia and should be administered concurrently with calcitonin (for rapid calcium reduction) and bisphosphonate (for sustained reduction). Calcitonin helps to decrease serum calcium by reducing bone resorption and calcium excretion. However, tachyphylaxis can develop for which its administration is limited to 48 hours and with a recommended dose of 4-8 international unit/kg every 6-12 hours, intramuscularly or subcutaneously. Bisphosphonates are analogs of inorganic pyrophosphate; they lower calcium level by binding to the surface of bone hydroxyapatite and suppress osteoclast-mediated bone resorption. The three potent intravenous bisphosphonate drugs that show efficacy in hypercalcemia treatment are zoledronic acid, pamidronate, and ibandronate. The choice of drug is made based on its potency and risk of toxicity. When compared to pamidronate (90 mg), zoledronic acid (4 mg) is more efficacious in normalizing calcium level (87% vs. 70%), is sustained for a longer duration (32 vs. 18 days), and has a similar incidence of severe nephrotoxicity (grade 3 and 4) [42]. Furthermore, Ibandronate has comparable efficacy to pamidronate (76 vs. 77%); however, it is sustained for a longer duration (14 vs. 4 days) [43].

A practical approach for bisphosphonate dosing is to use 4 mg of zoledronic acid, 60-90 mg of pamidronate, or 2-6 mg of ibandronate and not to repeat the doses sooner than 7 days. The higher doses are recommended in patients with severe hypercalcemia and the lower doses, along with longer infusion duration, for patients with decreased kidney function to minimize the risk of side effects. It is generally recommended to avoid IV bisphosphonate administration in patients with eGFR < 30 ml/min. Nonetheless, few studies reported successful use with advanced kidney impairment for patients on hemodialysis [42]. Flu-like symptoms are the most common side effect, and less common but serious side effects include osteonecrosis of the jaw, atypical fractures, and nephrotoxicity. Acute kidney injury and proteinuria are reported with zoledronic acid (mainly ATN) and pamidronate (FSGS and minimal change disease). In a cohort of patients treated with repeated doses of zoledronic acid, AKI developed around 2 months after therapy initiation with a mean of 2.4 doses, and approximately one-third of the patients required hemodialysis. Most of the patients did not have full kidney recovery [44].

Denosumab can be used in treatment of hypercalcemia when it is refractory to bisphosphonate or as an alternative to bisphosphonate in patients with a significant reduction in kidney function. As discussed earlier, RANKL plays an essential role in patients with bone metastases associated hypercalcemia. By binding to RANKL, denosumab prevents the activation of RANK receptors on the osteoclast surface. The recommended dose is 120 mg subcutaneously every 4 week and lower starting dose of 0.3 mg/kg is suggested in patients with reduced kidney function as prolonged hypocalcemia requiring IV calcium replacement was reported in patients with decreased kidney function or vitamin D deficiency. Therefore, it is crucial to measure and replete vitamin 25 D before administration of denosumab [45].

Glucocorticoids are primarily used in the patient with high 1,25 dihydroxyvitamin D secreted by the tumor as it suppresses the conversion of 25 hydroxyvitamin D to 1,25 dihydroxyvitamin D in macrophages over 2-5 days of therapy. There is no consensus about the optimal dose and duration of corticosteroids, and a suggested regimen is 200-300 mg of IV hydrocortisone for 3-5 days followed by oral prednisone at a dose of 10-30 mg/day [46]. In severe hypercalcemia, hemodialysis with low calcium bath (≤1 mmol/) can be used to lower calcium rapidly, especially in patients with significant oliguric acute kidney injury and when IV hydration and zoledronic acid use is not feasible.

Acute Kidney Injury in Hematopoietic Cell Transplant Recipients

AKI is a common complication following hematopoietic cell transplant (HCT), affecting 76% of the patients following myeloablative allogeneic transplant. The AKI incidence varies based on the source of the cells (autologous vs. allogeneic), with the lowest incidence being associated with autologous HCT (23%), followed by non-myeloablative allogeneic HCT (43%), and myeloablative allogeneic HCT (76%), and with an overall risk of needing hemodialysis ranging from 2-5% [47, 48]. This is partially related to allogeneic HCT recipients receiving calcineurin inhibitors post HCT to decrease the risk of graft-versus-host disease (GVHD), and patients with myeloablative HCT receiving a high dose of conditioning chemotherapy, while the non-myeloablative HCT recipients, that generally are older and with a comorbid condition, receiving reduced intensity of the conditioning regimen.

The etiology for AKI post SCT is multifactorial and can be divided into pre-renal factor (hypovolemia), overlapping pre- and intra-renal factors (sepsis, engraftment syndrome, sinusoidal obstruction syndrome, and calcineurin inhibitor), intra-renal factors (chemotherapy, anti-microbial, acute GVHD, thrombotic microangiopathy, BK and CMV related nephropathy, and ABO incompatibility/TLS pigment related nephropathy), and post renal factors (BK virus associated hydronephrosis, hemorrhagic cystitis, and urine retention.)

Acute tubular injury is the most common intrarenal etiology that usually occurs within the first few weeks of transplant and is associated with sepsis, pancytopenia, and antimicrobial therapy (including acyclovir, amphotericin, and aminoglycoside). Hepatic sinusoidal obstruction syndrome (SOS) is another common AKI etiology that develops early, within the first 4 weeks, post HCT. It is attributed to pretransplant conditioning therapy causing hepatic vein endothelial injury; hence, it is mainly observed in myeloablative HCT. Risk factors include allogeneic myeloablative HCT (higher risk compared to autologous HCT), pre-existing liver disease, low functional status, high dose of pre-transplant radiation, cyclophosphamide, and inotuzumab ozogamicin therapy [49]. Ursodeoxycholic acid and heparin are used as a prophylaxis to decrease the risk of SOS. Patients usually develop sudden weight gain (> 2-5% of pre-transplant weight), hepatomegaly, ascites, and elevated serum total bilirubin (> 2 mg/dL); having 2 or more of these clinical findings support the SOS diagnosis. Liver Doppler is not diagnostic; however, it might show a reversal of flow in the portal vein waveform. AKI is a common complication in SOS; approximately half of the patients will develop acute kidney injury (hepato-renal like syndrome), and one fourth might require hemodialysis. SOS is treated based on its severity and is classified based on 5 factors: total bilirubin, serum aspartate aminotransferase, weight gain, kidney function, and disease progression. In mild-to-moderate SOS, supportive care is provided by controlling the abdominal discomfort with paracentesis and analgesics, as well as achieving euvolemia with fluid restriction and diuretics as needed. In severe SOS, the same steps as above are followed, and defibrotide is added as it demonstrates good outcomes with more than 30% expected survival by day 100 post-HCT [50].

Other less common etiology of kidney impairment post SCT and associated with subacute to chronic kidney disease is thrombotic microangiopathy (TMA). It is typically diagnosed between day 20 to100 after transplant and most commonly involves the kidneys, and occasionally involves the lung and the gastrointestinal tract. The kidney involvement manifests as hypertension, acute kidney injury, proteinuria, and with variable incidence (< 10% and up to 64%) in allogeneic HCT due to the lack of standard HCT-TMA diagnostic criteria [51].

The etiology for TMA associated HCT is likely multifactorial as multiple factors contributing to endothelial injury and thrombi formation, including radiation therapy, HLA mismatch, a calcineurin inhibitor, GVHD, viral infection (CMV and HHV6), and complement dysregulation.

The diagnosis is based on either microangiopathy diagnosed on tissue biopsy or meeting a laboratory criterion. One of the widely used criteria by Jodele et al. [52] is based on these laboratory findings: the presence of schistocytes, elevated LDH, proteinuria ≥ 30 mg/dl or hypertension, de novo thrombocytopenia, decreased hemoglobin, and elevated serum c5b-9. Elevated creatinine, elevated c5b-9, proteinuria, and high TMA index (LDH/platelet counts) ≥ 20 are among the risk factors that are associated with poor overall prognosis.

Generally, treatment of TMA associated with HCT includes providing supportive care and treating the underlying associated risk factors; for example, switching calcineurin inhibitor to different, non-CNI, immunosuppressant for GVHD prevention, as decreasing CNI dose or switching from one CNI class to another may not be effective, and by treating the systemic viral infection and GVHD. Other therapeutic options to date did not show significant success in the management of HCT-associated TMA, and this includes the lack of supportive evidence for using plasma exchange, and the limited evidence of success that was based on small studies with the use of anti CD20 antibody (rituximab) and anti-complement c5 therapy (eculizumab) [53, 54].

Based on research in children, the proposed eculizumab regimen starts with an induction phase when eculizumab is given weekly, and with a dose adjustment based on TMA clinical response and CH50 level to achieve a level of less than 10% of a lower limit of normal. Once this response is sustained for 4-6 weeks, transition to the maintenance phase occurs and subsequently to medication discontinuation if there is no relapse [54]. At present, there are ongoing trials about using new promising anti-complement therapy in TMA treatment, including OMS721 (IV) and ACH-4471 (oral).

Another rare kidney complication (< 5%) that is predominantly present in allogeneic HCT is glomerular disease associated with HCT. It manifests as nephrotic syndrome after tapering or discontinuation of immunosuppressive therapy and within 8 weeks of GVHD. It is attributed to likely an immune dysregulation with donor lymphocytes reacting toward specific antigens of kidney recipients and its most common kidney pathology are membranous nephropathy and minimal change disease [55]. The kidney outcome in these patients is variable, with most cases achieving remission upon restarting immunosuppression (glucocorticoids ± CNI) or rituximab [56]. An additional rare kidney complication to keep in mind in HCT recipients is Polyomavirus BK related. It predominantly manifests as hemorrhagic cystitis and rarely as BK related nephropathy (interstitial nephritis and tubular injury) and ureteric stenosis.

The overall kidney prognosis of AKI post HCT is positive as majority of AKIs recover, 20-30% develop CKD, and 0.4-4.4% develop end-stage renal disease [57, 58]. Nonetheless, the overall mortality rate increases two fold following AKI, and 7 folds in severe kidney impairment requiring renal replacement, with around 80% death within 2 months of HCT [59].

MALIGNANCY INDUCED TMA

TMA is a clinical disorder defined by the presence of microangiopathic hemolytic anemia, thrombocytopenia, and microthrombi formation in the microcirculation that can potentially be life-threatening and is associated with organs damage, most notably the central nervous system and the kidney. TMA is divided into primary type (acquired and hereditary) and secondary that is associated with infection, pregnancy, transplant, pregnancy-associated, autoimmune, severe hypertension, drugs, and cancer as discussed in the section on TMA associated with cancer and cancer therapy.

It can be challenging to determine whether the observed TMA in cancer patients is secondary to cancer itself or its treatment. However, there are some clinical features that can help to differentiate between the two. Drug-induced TMA is more common, occurs generally in patients with minimal residual tumor or in remission, and has clinical features of renal-limited disease. On the contrary, cancer-induced TMA tends to occur in disseminated tumor cells and resembles thrombotic thrombocytopenic purpura (TTP) and disseminated intravascular coagulation (DIC) [60].

Cancer-induced TMA is common in patients with mucin-producing adenocarcinoma, disseminated malignancy, and malignancy invading the bone marrow. It can affect up to 5.7% of patients with metastatic adenocarcinoma and accounts for more than two-thirds of cases. Gastric adenocarcinoma is the most commonly associated cancer, followed by breast, prostate, and lung adenocarcinomas [61].

It is hypothesized that the bone marrow endothelial cells get injured secondary to mucin, direct tumor invasion, abnormal angiogenesis, or secondary myelofibrosis. This injury can lead to the formation of large von Willebrand factor (VWF) and a possible decrease in a disintegrin and metalloproteinase with a thrombospondin type 1 motif, member 13 (ADAMTS13) activity, however, with no evidence of ADAMTS13 enzyme deficiency contributing to the development of cancer-induced TMA [62]. As there is no evidence of ADAMTS13 deficiency, the response to plasma exchange or immunosuppressive therapy was not significant. There are reports of TMA improvement with cancer remission. Nonetheless, the overall prognosis remains poor [63].

In comparison, drug-induced TMA is divided into two categories: First, immune-mediated TMA occurs after exposure to any drug under than three weeks, is attributed to antibody development causing direct endothelial injury, and includes only few medications (gemcitabine, oxaliplatin, and possibly CPI). The second category comprises non-immune mediated TMA that is generally dose-related, occurs after weeks to months of therapy, and is attributed to the drug's direct endothelial injury. This category includes most of the cancer therapies associated with TMA (bevacizumab, sunitinib, ponatinib, bortezomib, carfilzomib, ixazomib, mitomycin, pentostatin, and vincristine), and immunosuppressive medications (cyclosporine, tacrolimus, sirolimus, and IVIG). In both categories, there is a thrombi formation that can be associated with microangiopathic hemolytic anemia, hypertension, and possible organ ischemia, including kidney injury and proteinuria.

Cancer therapy-induced TMA can be further divided based on manifestation, onset, clinical presentation, and prognosis into two types [60]. Type 1 that usually has delayed onset (6 months to years), most often is cumulative dose-related, its associated acute kidney injury can be permanent and irreversible, usually has hypertension and hematological manifestations, and has poor kidney and overall prognosis despite therapy; hence reintroducing the medication is not recommended. Type 1 includes mitomycin, gemcitabine, cisplatin, and pegylated liposomal doxorubicin.

On the contrary, Type 2 can occur after any dose, is dose independent, the hematological manifestation presents in around half of the patients, and almost all patients have hypertension with variable proteinuria (with or without kidney injury). It has good prognosis and with high chance of recovery upon drug discontinuation and therefore, re-challenge can be considered. It includes VGEF pathway inhibitors, such as tyrosine kinase inhibitor, sunitinib, sorafenib, pazopanib, axitinib, and bevacizumab. The diagnosis of drug-induced TMA is a clinical one and is made based on history of the drug exposure, correlation with the development of clinical syndrome (proteinuria, hypertension, and/or AKI), resolution of the clinical syndrome upon holding or discontinuation of the drug, and laboratory findings of microangiopathic hemolytic anemia (MAHA): thrombocytopenia, anemia, high LDH, and schistocytes.

Other laboratory tests should be considered, including a coagulation profile to rule out DIC, Coombs test to rule out autoimmune hemolysis, and ADAMTS13 to rule out severe deficiency (< 10%) that would rather suggest a diagnosis of TTP. Keeping in mind that TMA can be kidney limited with no laboratory finding of MAHA and only acute or subacute kidney injury, a kidney biopsy is not required for the diagnosis and is considered if the diagnosis is not clear and to exclude other etiologies. Intravascular fibrin thrombi with mucoid changes are suggestive of acute TMA. At the same time, glomerular basement membrane double contours with no immune complex and intimal proliferation of the arterioles suggest chronic TMA [64].

The most crucial step in drug-induced TMA therapy is to discontinue the offending drug and provide supportive care with antihypertensive medications, platelet transfusion, and hemodialysis, if indicated. There is no substantial evidence that supports the use of plasma exchange therapy or other immunosuppression therapy in the treatment of drug-induced TMA; however, limited evidence based on case reports demonstrate good outcome with the use of anti-complement therapy (eculizumab) and immunosuppressive therapy (rituximab) in these patients. It might be reasonable to consider these when there are no signs of kidney recovery despite the discontinuation of the offending drug and possibly if there is evidence of a complement dysregulation (eculizumab).

Malignancy Associated Glomerulopathy

The pathogenesis of malignancy associated glomerulopathy is unclear and postulated to be related to possible immune dysregulation associated with malignancy, overexpression of vascular endothelial grow factor, and to antibody formation against circulating or deposited tumor antigen or a cross-reactive glomerulus antigen [65]. In solid tumor associated glomerular disease, membranous nephropathy is the most common paraneoplastic glomerulopathy and should be suspected in patients with nephrotic syndrome and who are at risk of developing malignancy, as most of the cancer diagnoses are made within 1 year of membranous nephropathy diagnosis. Similar to other etiologies of secondary membranous nephropathy, glomerular staining is classically positive to IgG1, IgG2, and IgG3, and without PLA2R staining, THD7A staining or antibody serology. However, up to 40% and 2% of the patients were found to have positive PLA2R antibody and THSD7A antibody, respectively; this was attributed to a possible coincidental association [66]. Other reported paraneoplastic pathologies in solid tumors include minimal change disease, membranoproliferative glomerulonephritis (MPGN), rapid progressive glomerulonephritis (RPGN), and IgA nephropathy.

Similarly, Paraneoplastic glomerulopathy has a well-known association with hematological malignancies. It is more common with chronic lymphoid neoplasms as opposed to acute lymphocytic and acute myeloid leukemias, where it is rarely reported [65].

Minimal change disease is the most common pathology (reported in 1%) in patients with Hodgkin lymphoma and usually present around the time of lymphoma diagnosis. Focal segmental glomerulosclerosis (FSGS) is reported as well in patients with Hodgkin lymphoma but less commonly.

By comparison, MPGN is the most commonly reported pathology in patients with chronic lymphocytic leukemia that is often associated with monoclonal, and in some cases, mixed cryoglobulinemia. Other less common pathology in CLL is membranous nephropathy. In regard to myeloid malignancies, paraneoplastic glomerulopathy is not uncommon in myeloproliferative disorders, with exception of chronic myeloid leukemia, as it is being reported in around 4% of patients with FSGS and mesangial proliferative glomerulopathy being the predominant pathologies. The glomerulopathy presents at a later stage of disease and is associated with poor kidney prognosis [67].

Furthermore, myelodysplastic syndrome (MDS) has reported to be commonly associated with glomerulopathy, as well, with an incidence as high as 27%. The glomerulopathy in MDS patients are variable and includes membranous nephropathy, mesangial proliferative GN, IgA nephropathy, and MPGN. Paraneoplastic glomerular pathologies associated with solid and hematological malignancies are summarized in Table 2 [61, 68].

Table 2. Glomerular pathology associated with malignancy (paraneoplastic)

Kidney pathology	Malignancy
Membranous nephropathy	Lung, colon, stomach, pancreas, prostate, breast, head/neck, teratoma, ovarian, cervical, endometrial, melanoma, basal cell and SCC, thymoma, Hodgkin and non-Hodgkin lymphoma, CLL, AML, and CML
Minimal change disease	Lung, colon, bladder, pancreas, renal cell, ovarian, mesothelioma, thymoma, Hodgkin and non-Hodgkin lymphoma, CLL, and CML
Focal segmental glomerulosclerosis	Lung, renal cell, breast, esophageal, thymoma, Hodgkin and non-Hodgkin lymphoma, CLL, and T cell leukemia
IgA nephropathy	Lung, pancreatic, renal cell, head/neck, Hodgkin and non-Hodgkin lymphoma, and cutaneous T cell lymphoma
Crescentic glomerulonephritis	Lung, colon, prostate, gastric, thymoma, Hodgkin lymphoma, and CLL
Membranoproliferative glomerulonephritis	Lung, renal cell, breast, esophageal, gastric, melanoma, thymoma, Hodgkin and non-Hodgkin lymphoma, CLL, CML, and MGUS
Thrombotic microangiopathy	Lung, colon, gastric, prostate, ovarian, renal cell, hepatocellular, pancreatic, neuroendocrine tumor, non-Hodgkin lymphoma, ALL, and MDS

SCC, squamous cell carcinoma; CLL, chronic lymphocytic leukemia; AML; acute myelogenous leukemia; CML; chronic myelogenous leukemia; MGUS, monoclonal gammopathy of unclear significance; MDS; myelodysplastic syndrome.

The diagnosis should be suspected in patients with biopsy proven glomerulonephritis, having an active malignancy, and having kidney manifestations that usually remit when cancer is in remission and relapse with cancer recurrence. Malignancy associated glomerulonephritis is primarily treated by focusing on the underlying malignancy, and in some situations (untreatable/unresectable tumor, severe AKI (RPGN), or in certain malignancies, like CML) by adding immunosuppressive medication as it was associated with improved the kidney function; however, this was based on a limited evidence from case reports [65].

Infiltrative Disease Associated AKI

Cancer associated kidney infiltrative disease is a rare etiology for AKI, accounting for ≤1% of AKI despite the fact that evidence of kidney infiltration occurs in up to 90% of patients with hematological malignancies [69]. It is most commonly associated with chronic lymphocytic leukemia (CLL) and acute lymphoblastic leukemia (ALL), and its clinical presentation can vary from no symptoms (most commonly) to severe acute kidney injury (rarely) [70]. Symptomatic patients might present with flank pain, abdominal distention, hypertension, or hematuria. The AKI etiology is possibly related to acute tubular injury secondary to tubular compression and disruption of microcirculation by the infiltrative tumor, and a component of tumor lysis upon initiating therapy. It is usually diagnosed based on the patient clinical history and a kidney imaging finding of symmetrical and enlarged kidneys bilaterally. A kidney biopsy can be useful to evaluate the extent of infiltration and therefore the prognosis, as well as to differentiate the subtype of malignancy that can guide the therapy. The overall kidney prognosis is dependent on treating the underlying leukemia/lymphoma and with expectation that the kidney recovers rapidly, as soon as within few days of starting therapy [69].

AKI Post Nephrectomy

Nephrectomy remains the gold standard therapy for localized renal cancer lesions and has a very good prognosis approaching 95% or 5 years survival for stage 1 cancer (< 7 cm). AKI is a common complication post nephrectomy and its incidence varies widely among the studies. It can be as high as 40%, with majority being a mild injury (stage 1 AKI) [71]. Perioperative AKI is a major concern in cancer patients who frequently undergo cytoreductive or curative surgeries and include major surgeries defined as intra-thoracic or intra-abdominal. In particular, radical nephrectomy is associated with high rates of AKI (OR of 3.5), but the renal prognosis after surgery is in large part related to the health of the remaining kidney. Additional risk factors for AKI include a history of CKD, male gender, obesity, hypertension, hypoalbuminemia, and prolonged surgical/ischemia time [71, 72]. The etiology for AKI is attributed to surgical factors, mainly ischemic kidney injury and reduction in kidney mass, as well as secondary FSGS that contributes to long term reduction in kidney function.

Treatment comprises providing supportive kidney care, shorter ischemia/procedure time if possible, blood pressure control, and pre-operative referral to nephrology. Nonetheless, AKI post nephrectomy increases the risk of CKD by more than 4 folds (20-50% post nephrectomy); it increases the risk of hospitalization, length of stay, and mortality [71].

CONVENTIONAL CHEMOTHERAPY ASSOCIATED NEPHROTOXICITY

Multiple conventional chemotherapy agents are associated with acute kidney injury that is related to tubulointerstitial injury and less often, a glomerulus lesion or TMA. Risk factors include high or cumulative drug dose, hypovolemia, old age, kidney impairment, concurrent use of other nephrotoxins, hypoalbuminemia, and genetic factors (in CYP450 enzyme and transport proteins). Three chemotherapy agents with widely studied nephrotoxicity are briefly discussed and nephrotoxicity associated with other chemotherapy agents are summarized in Table 3 [73-75].

Cisplatin is a platinum-based chemotherapy that inhibits DNA replication and is used in treatment of a broad spectrum of malignancies. Its class includes carboplatin and oxaliplatin that are much less nephrotoxic. It is transported into the tubular cells by the basolateral membrane organic cation transporter 2 (OCT2) in segment 3 (S3) of the proximal tubules and cause direct tubular injury. Other associated kidney impairment mechanisms include increasing expression of inflammatory cytokines (high IL6 and TNF alpha), vasoconstriction, and TMA. AKI is a common complication and is reported in up to half of patients treated with cisplatin, and this varies based on the frequency of administration and dosage of cisplatin, with around 30% of patients receiving a single dose of > 50 mg/m^2 who develop AKI. It is typically mild to moderate in severity, non-oliguric, occurs day 5-7 of therapy, and with urinalysis showing no hematuria or significant proteinuria. Aggressive IV hydration and decreasing cisplatin dose or switching to other platinum-based chemotherapy, if feasible, can decrease the risk of its nephrotoxicity. AKI usually recovers within a few weeks; nonetheless, cisplatin has been associated with permanent injury and progression to a higher stage of CKD.

Ifosfamide (IFO) is an alkylating agent that interferes with DNA synthesis and used in treatment of multiple tumors, including testicular cancer and sarcoma. Despite the structural similarity, and unlike cyclophosphamide, IFO is transported into the proximal tubule cells by OCT2 and subsequently metabolized to a nephrotoxic metabolite, chloroacetaldehyde. The onset of nephrotoxicity is variable as it can occur during or many months after completing IFO therapy. Moreover, the incidence of nephrotoxicity varies; this is mainly related to the total cumulative dose and the coadministration with cisplatin. When compared to a high dose, a dose < 84 g/m^2 in general is associated with a transient, mild to moderate, and a relatively low incidence of nephrotoxicity (10 vs. 40%). So far there is no proven intervention to decrease the nephrotoxicity aside from limiting the cumulative dose. Furthermore, a long-term side effect with a gradual decline in kidney function is observed with IFO use.

Methotrexate is a weak organic acid antimetabolite that competitively inhibits dihydrofolate reductase and subsequently DNA synthesis. Around 2% of patients receiving high dose methotrexate (>0.5 gram/m^2) develop nephrotoxicity that is attributed to the direct tubular injury and intratubular crystal formation. The AKI is typically nonoliguric; patients recover within 10- 14 days of injury. The cornerstone for prevention and early treatment of nephrotoxicity is by IV hydration, urine alkalization (goal urine PH > 7), and administration of Leucovorin. Additionally, hemodialysis can remove methotrexate; however, its therapeutic role is limited due to significant post-dialysis rebound. This is in contrast to Glucarpidase, a carboxypeptidase enzyme that is highly effective in rapidly reducing methotrexate level (98% reduction) and is FDA approved for treatment of toxic blood levels in the setting of nephrotoxicity.

Table 3. Conventional chemotherapy associated nephrotoxicity

Chemotherapy class Drug	Kidney manifestation	Reported Kidney pathology
Platinum based		
Cisplatin Carboplatin Oxaliplatin	Non oliguric AKI, proximal tubulopathy, RTA, HTN, and electrolytes disturbances (Low Na, K, and Mg)	ATN and TMA
Alkylating agent		
Ifosfamide	AKI, proximal tubulopathy, RTA, DI	ATN, TMA, glomerular disease, and interstitial nephritis
Melphalan	AKI and nephrotic syndrome	Glomerulosclerosis and
Nitrosoureas	Subacute and chronic kidney disease	chronic interstitial nephritis
Antimetabolites		
Methotrexate	Non oliguric AKI	ATN and crystalline nephropathy
Azacitadine	AKI, tubulopathy and polyuria	ATN
5-FU	AKI and electrolytes disturbances (low Na and K)	
Gemcitabine	KI, HTN and proteinuria	ATN and TMA
Pemetrexed	AKI, RTA, and DI	ATN and interstitial edema
Antitumor antibiotic		
Anthracycline	AKI and nephrotic syndrome	MCD, FSGS, and TMA
Bleomycin and Mitomycin	AKI, HTN and proteinuria	TMA
Other		
Taxanes	AKI and electrolytes disturbances (low Na and K)	ATN and TMA
Tamoxifen	Hypertension and proteinuria	

5-FU, 5-fluorouracil; RTA, renal tubular acidosis; Na, sodium; K, potassium; Mg, magnesium; DI, diabetes insipidus; FSGS, focal segmental glomerulosclerosis; GN, glomerulonephritis; MCD, minimal change disease; ATN, acute tubular necrosis; TMA, thrombotic microangiopathy

Cancer Immunotherapy Associated Nephrotoxicity

Immune checkpoint inhibitors (CPIs) are monoclonal antibodies that harness the immune system against tumor cells by releasing the breaks off their regulators, such as cytotoxic T lymphocyte-associated antigen 4 (CTLA-4), programmed cell death protein-1 (PD-1), and its ligand (PD-L1). Ipilimumab was the first FDA approved CPI in 2011 for treatment of melanoma, and since then, 6 other CPIs were approved for treatment of various malignancies, including non-small lung cancer, advanced renal cell carcinoma, and urothelial cancer as they demonstrated significant improvement in cancer overall and progression free survival. However, they have been associated with off target immune related adverse events (IrAEs) that involve almost every organ, including the kidneys.

There are multiple postulated mechanisms for the observed nephrotoxicity, including the loss of tolerance with reactivation of drug specific T cells, formation of T cells against tumor antigen that cross react with kidney antigen, local increase of pro-inflammatory cytokines, and generation of autoantibodies [76]. AKI is a relatively common nephrotoxic side effect with a variable incidence of 1-29%; however, most studies report around 3% rate with an increase to 5% in patients receiving combination CPI therapies (CTLA-4 with PD-1/PDL-1 inhibitors), and with only 0.6% severe injury (KDIGO stage 3) [77]. In regard to kidney allograft recipients, acute rejection was reported in 44% of the patients; this includes antibody, cell-mediated and mixed rejections [78].

The CPI associated AKI was more reported with the use of combination CPIs, proton pump inhibitors (PPI), and with lower eGFR level prior to starting CPI [79]. It usually presents at a median of 12-14 weeks of drug initiation; however, it is widely variable and ranges from few weeks to more than 1 year. Most of the patients have sub-nephrotic range proteinuria and approximately half of them have pyuria. Other reported kidney related adverse events include acute kidney allograft rejection (with median of 24 days of the 1st dose), electrolytes disturbances, nephrotic syndrome. and tubulopathy. In patients with AKI, acute tubulointerstitial nephritis is the most common reported biopsy proven pathology, and other reported pathologies are less frequent and include acute tubular injury, IgA nephropathy, membranous nephropathy, FSGS, minimal change disease, TMA, and pauci-immune glomerulonephritis (ANCA- and +). Table 4 summarizes the reported kidney pathology associated with CPI [80].

CPI-related nephrotoxicity should be suspected in all patients with sustained AKI or a recent exposure to CPI (up to 6 months of last CPI dose). In general, a kidney biopsy is recommended, when no contraindication exists, in order to identify the associated kidney pathology, especially in patients with microscopic hematuria, nephrotic range proteinuria, severe AKI, or sustained injury, despite holding CPI and 1-2-week trial of corticosteroids.

Table 4. FDA approved Checkpoint inhibitors and other immunotherapies and their associated nephrotoxicity

FDA approved immune checkpoint inhibitors			
PD-1 inhibitors	pembrolizumab	nivolumab	cemiplimab
PD-L1 inhibitors	atezolizumab	avelumab	durvalumab
CTLA-4 inhibitors	Ipilimumab		
Nephrotoxicity associated with checkpoint inhibitors and other immunotherapies			
CPI	Kidney pathology		
Nivolumab	ATIN, FSGS, Membranous nephropathy, IgA/immune complex nephropathy, Pauci-immune GN.		
Pembrolizumab	ATIN, MCD IgA/immune complex nephropathy, Pauci-immune GN, TMA, ATN		
Ipilimumab	ATIN, MCD, IgA nephropathy, pauci-immune GN, TMA, and lupus nephropathy		
Nephrotoxicity associated with other immunotherapies			
Chimeric antigen receptor T cell	Pre-renal, ATN, and tumor lysis syndrome		
Interlukin-2	Pre-renal (Capillary leak syndrome and hypotension) and ATN		
Interferon alpha	TMA and FSGS		

FDA, food and drug administration; PD-1, programmed death-1; PDL-1, programmed death-ligand-1; CTLA-4, cytotoxic T lymphocyte associated protein-4; CPI, checkpoint inhibitor; ATIN; acute interstitial nephritis; FSGS, focal segmental glomerulosclerosis; GN, glomerulonephritis; MCD, minimal change disease; ATN, acute tubular necrosis; TMA, thrombotic microangiopathy.

After ruling out reversible etiology (hypovolemia or obstruction) and holding CPI, it is recommended, based on multiple observational studies, to start patients on corticosteroids as a favorable kidney outcome was observed with 87% chance of kidney recovery (including partial and complete) [79]. Suggested dose is 1 mg/kg of prednisone with a slow taper over 8-12 weeks based on kidney response. Other immunosuppressants, including infliximab and rituximab were used in addition to corticosteroids in patients with refractory AIN and renal vasculitis, respectively, and with reported partial to complete response. Re-challenge with CPI may be considered after kidney recovery as the risk of subsequent kidney injury is relatively low (23%) and with the majority having subsequent kidney recovery (only 3% did not recover). Conversely, kidney transplant patients have poor kidney and overall prognosis, as 83% of patients with acute graft rejection develop allograft failure and 44% die [78].

Chimeric antigen receptor T-cell (CAR-T) is another novel and relatively new immunotherapy that is created by genetically engineering patients' T lymphocytes in vitro to express certain receptors that bind and target a specific protein (tumor antigen). Tisagenlecleucel and Axicabtagene ciloleucel are the two FDA approved CAR-T cell therapies for treatment of relapse/aggressive diffuse large B cell lymphoma. AKI is a common side effect observed with CAR-T cell therapy and reported in up to 30% of patients. Most of these cases have mild injury (grade 1 AKI) and recover completely within 30 days of injury. The risk factors for AKI include grade 3-4 cytokine release syndrome and history of stem cell transplant, and the reported underlying etiology for AKI is hypovolemia and acute tubular injury [81].

In contrast, Interlukin-2 (IL-2) and interferon alpha (IFN-α) are immunotherapeutic drugs that were used since 1980s in the treatment of various cancers, including metastatic melanoma and renal cell carcinoma; however, there have been concern for their systemic toxicity and loss of efficacy [76]. Their anti-tumor effect is related to activation of immune cells (T cells, natural killer cells and macrophages) to attack cancer cells and inhibiting angiogenesis (IFN-α). Nephrotoxicity is reported with both medications and attributed to pre-renal and acute tubular injury with IL-2, and TMA and FSGS with IFN- α. Nonetheless, the overall kidney outcome is favorable with most cases having partial to complete recovery upon discontinuation of the drug and providing support kidney care.

POST-RENAL ETIOLOGY

Post renal etiology is an important cause to consider, especially in patients with regionally advanced cancer in the abdomen and pelvis (bladder, prostate, cervical cancer, and lymphoma), history of metastatic disease with retroperitoneal lymphadenopathy or fibrosis, history of pelvic radiation, and in recipient of HCT with BK infection. Another susceptible population includes those who are at risk for bladder retention from medication, post operatively, infection, urethral stricture, and spinal cord compression/infraction. Kidney ultrasound is the preferred diagnostic imaging to evaluate for hydronephrosis and bladder retention as it has negative predictive value of 98% to detect hydronephrosis [82]; however, the hydronephrosis might be absent on ultrasound early in the course of obstruction or in hypovolemia. Computed tomography (CT) scan is considered in patients with suspected nephrolithiasis or ureteral obstruction to help determining the etiology. Treatment involves addressing the underlying etiology, providing supportive care, and placing Foley catheter if indicated. If the obstruction is present, a stent or percutaneous nephrostomy tube might be required, depending on the location of obstruction. Kidney function in general is expected to recover fully unless there is a delay in therapy as it can lead to irreversible damage.

RENAL REPLACEMENT THERAPY IN MALIGNANCY

The rate of AKI requiring renal replacement therapy in patients with malignancy ranges 9-30%, which reflects the wide spectrum of illness and cancer-specific risk and exposures that occur. The mortality for those needing dialysis is high, and the need for dialysis in critical illness is in excess of 60% [83, 84]. To our knowledge, there are no large trials testing which mode of dialysis therapy (intermittent of continuous) confers greater benefit in cancer patients, but retrospective analysis suggests RRT modality is not associated with outcome in critical illness [19]. It can be reasonably extrapolated from prospective studies in non-cancer populations that there is no difference in renal recovery or mortality between patients initiated on CRRT vs intermittent HD [85]. However, KDIGO recommendations consider using CRRT, rather than standard intermittent RRT, for hemodynamically unstable patients and patients with acute cerebral injury or edema [5].

There are special considerations in patients with myeloma because kidney involvement is part of the natural history of the disease. In patients with AKI related to cast nephropathy, the clinical strategy has been to clear pathogenic light chains from circulation as quickly as possible with the aim of recovering renal function [86]. Since the introduction of bortezomib-based chemotherapy, there have been two notable prospective studies examining high-cutoff dialysis (HCO-HD) in patients with myeloma. The EuLITE study enrolled 90 subjects with newly diagnosed myeloma, light chains >500mg/L and AKI requiring dialysis [87]. There were no statistical differences in dialysis independence at day 30 and long-term renal recovery in the patients treated with HCO-HD. The MYRE study included 98 patients with new or untreated myeloma who were randomized to conventional HD and HCO-HD, which showed no difference in dialysis dependence by day 30 [88]. In this study, however, 35% of the HF-HD were able to discontinue maintenance hemodialysis at 6 months compared to 57% in the HCO-HD ($p = 0.04$). It is important to note that in both studies, patients received Bortezomib based chemotherapy, which by its virtue is highly effective at reducing light chain burden.

Generally, if the current illness is deemed reversible, then RRT should be considered. However, frequently the role of renal replacement therapy in cancer patients, particularly in advanced disease, is fraught with ethical issues and should ultimately be grounded in ethical principles of avoiding harm, patient autonomy, and beneficence [89]. Clinicians should avail themselves of the evidence and recommendations from practice guidelines, such as the Shared Decision-Making in the Appropriate Initiation of and Withdrawal from Dialysis [90]. Good communication is essential to developing shared decision-making, and clinicians should always inquire from patients and family how they want prognosis, goals of care, and end-of-life issues discussed with them [91]. Early involvement of palliative care should be considered because dialysis in advanced disease is an end-of-life complication of end-of-life disease. An ethics consultation may also be wise whenever tension is detected, or a consensus does not seem to be reached among family or among the family and treatment team about the merits of renal replacement therapy.

REFERENCES

[1] Siegel RL, Miller KD, Jemal A. Cancer statistics, 2019. *CA Cancer J Clin.* 2019;69(1):7-34.

[2] Salahudeen AK, Doshi SM, Pawar T, Nowshad G, Lahoti A, Shah P. Incidence rate, clinical correlates, and outcomes of AKI in patients admitted to a comprehensive cancer center. *Clin J Am Soc Nephrol.* 2013;8(3):347-54.

[3] Rosner MH, Perazella MA. Acute Kidney Injury in Patients with Cancer. *N Engl J Med.* 2017;377(5):500-1.

[4] Lam AQ, Humphreys BD. Onco-nephrology: AKI in the cancer patient. *Clin J Am Soc Nephrol.* 2012;7(10):1692-700.

[5] Kellum J, Lameire N, Aspelin P, Barsoum R, Burdmann E, Goldstein S, et al. Kidney disease: Improving global outcomes (KDIGO) acute kidney injury work group. KDIGO clinical practice guideline for acute kidney injury. *Kidney International Supplements;* 2012. p. 1-138.

[6] Bagshaw SM, Bellomo R. Cystatin C in acute kidney injury. *Curr Opin Crit Care.* 2010;16(6):533-9.

[7] Lagos-Arevalo P, Palijan A, Vertullo L, Devarajan P, Bennett MR, Sabbisetti V, et al. Cystatin C in acute kidney injury diagnosis: early biomarker or alternative to serum creatinine? *Pediatr Nephrol.* 2015;30(4):665-76.

[8] Jones M, Denieffe S, Griffin C, Tinago W, Fitzgibbon MC. Evaluation of cystatin C in malignancy and comparability of estimates of GFR in oncology patients. *Pract Lab Med.* 2017;8:95-104.

[9] Lim R, Ahmed N, Borregaard N, Riley C, Wafai R, Thompson EW, et al. Neutrophil gelatinase-associated lipocalin (NGAL) an early-screening biomarker for ovarian cancer: NGAL is associated with epidermal growth factor-induced epithelio-mesenchymal transition. *Int J Cancer.* 2007;120(11):2426-34.

[10] Villalva C, Sorel N, Bonnet ML, Guilhot J, Mayeur-Rousse C, Guilhot F, et al. Neutrophil gelatinase-associated lipocalin expression in chronic myeloid leukemia. *Leuk Lymphoma.* 2008;49(5):984-8.

[11] Tanase DM, Gosav EM, Radu S, Costea CF, Ciocoiu M, Carauleanu A, et al. The Predictive Role of the Biomarker Kidney Molecule-1 (KIM-1) in Acute Kidney Injury (AKI) Cisplatin-Induced Nephrotoxicity. *Int J Mol Sci.* 2019;20(20).

[12] Córdova-Sánchez BM, Ruiz-García EB, López-Yañez A, Barragan-Dessavre M, Bautista-Ocampo AR, Meneses-García A, et al. Plasma neutrophil gelatinase-associated lipocalin and factors related to acute kidney injury and mortality in critically ill cancer patients. *Ecancer medical science.* 2019;13:903.

[13] Jin J, Wang Y, Shen Q, Gong J, Zhao L, He Q. Acute kidney injury in cancer patients: A nationwide survey in China. *Sci Rep.* 2019;9(1):3540.

[14] Christiansen CF, Johansen MB, Langeberg WJ, Fryzek JP, Sørensen HT. Incidence of acute kidney injury in cancer patients: a Danish population-based cohort study. *Eur J Intern Med.* 2011;22(4):399-406.

[15] Kitchlu A, McArthur E, Amir E, Booth CM, Sutradhar R, Majeed H, et al. Acute Kidney Injury in Patients Receiving Systemic Treatment for Cancer: A Population-Based Cohort Study. *J Natl Cancer Inst.* 2019;111(7):727-36.

[16] Canet E, Zafrani L, Lambert J, Thieblemont C, Galicier L, Schnell D, et al. Acute kidney injury in patients with newly diagnosed high-grade hematological malignancies: impact on remission and survival. *PLoS One.* 2013;8(2):e55870.

[17] Bird GT, Farquhar-Smith P, Wigmore T, Potter M, Gruber PC. Outcomes and prognostic factors in patients with haematological malignancy admitted to a specialist cancer intensive care unit: a 5 yr study. *Br J Anaesth.* 2012;108(3):452-9.

[18] Lahoti A, Kantarjian H, Salahudeen AK, Ravandi F, Cortes JE, Faderl S, et al. Predictors and outcome of acute kidney injury in patients with acute myelogenous leukemia or high-risk myelodysplastic syndrome. *Cancer.* 2010;116(17):4063-8.

[19] Darmon M, Vincent F, Canet E, Mokart D, Pène F, Kouatchet A, et al. Acute kidney injury in critically ill patients with haematological malignancies: results of a multicentre cohort study from the Groupe de Recherche en Réanimation Respiratoire en Onco-Hématologie. *Nephrol Dial Transplant.* 2015;30(12):2006-13.

[20] Chertow GM, Burdick E, Honour M, Bonventre JV, Bates DW. Acute kidney injury, mortality, length of stay, and costs in hospitalized patients. *J Am Soc Nephrol.* 2005;16(11):3365-70.

[21] Park MR, Jeon K, Song JU, Lim SY, Park SY, Lee JE, et al. Outcomes in critically ill patients with hematologic malignancies who received renal replacement therapy for acute kidney injury in an intensive care unit. *J Crit Care.* 2011;26(1):107.e1-6.

[22] Shimoi T, Ando M, Munakata W, Kobayashi T, Kakihana K, Ohashi K, et al. The significant impact of acute kidney injury on CKD in patients who survived over 10 years after myeloablative allogeneic SCT. *Bone Marrow Transplant.* 2013;48(1):80-4.

[23] Hingorani S. Renal Complications of Hematopoietic-Cell Transplantation. *N Engl J Med.* 2016;374(23):2256-67.

[24] Perazella MA. Onco-nephrology: renal toxicities of chemotherapeutic agents. *Clin J Am Soc Nephrol.* 2012;7(10):1713-21.

[25] Porta C, Cosmai L, Gallieni M, Pedrazzoli P, Malberti F. Renal effects of targeted anticancer therapies. *Nat Rev Nephrol.* 2015;11(6):354-70.

[26] Harris KP, Hattersley JM, Feehally J, Walls J. Acute renal failure associated with haematological malignancies: a review of 10 years experience. *Eur J Haematol.* 1991;47(2):119-22.

[27] Kemlin D, Biard L, Kerhuel L, Zafrani L, Venot M, Teixeira L, et al. Acute kidney injury in critically ill patients with solid tumours. *Nephrol Dial Transplant.* 2018;33(11):1997-2005.

[28] Lahoti A, Humphreys B. *AKI associated with malignancies: Onconephrology Curriculum* [online curriculum]. American Society of Nephrology; 2016. https://www.asn-online.org/education/distancelearning/curricula/onco/Chapter3.pdf.

[29] Mohmand H, Goldfarb S. Renal dysfunction associated with intra-abdominal hypertension and the abdominal compartment syndrome. *J Am Soc Nephrol.* 2011;22(4):615-21.

[30] Schrier RW. Diagnostic value of urinary sodium, chloride, urea, and flow. *J Am Soc Nephrol.* 2011;22(9):1610-3.

[31] Kanbay M, Kasapoglu B, Perazella MA. Acute tubular necrosis and pre-renal acute kidney injury: utility of urine microscopy in their evaluation- a systematic review. *Int Urol Nephrol.* 2010;42(2):425-33.

[32] Hande KR, Garrow GC. Acute tumor lysis syndrome in patients with high-grade non-Hodgkin's lymphoma. *Am J Med.* 1993;94(2):133-9.

[33] Wössmann W, Schrappe M, Meyer U, Zimmermann M, Reiter A. Incidence of tumor lysis syndrome in children with advanced stage Burkitt's lymphoma/leukemia before and after introduction of prophylactic use of urate oxidase. *Ann Hematol.* 2003;82(3):160-5.

[34] Kalemkerian GP, Darwish B, Varterasian ML. Tumor lysis syndrome in small cell carcinoma and other solid tumors. *Am J Med.* 1997;103(5):363-7.

[35] Baeksgaard L, Sørensen JB. Acute tumor lysis syndrome in solid tumors--a case report and review of the literature. *Cancer Chemother Pharmacol.* 2003;51(3):187-92.

[36] Cairo MS, Bishop M. Tumour lysis syndrome: new therapeutic strategies and classification. *Br J Haematol.* 2004;127(1):3-11.

[37] Cairo MS, Coiffier B, Reiter A, Younes A, Panel TE. Recommendations for the evaluation of risk and prophylaxis of tumour lysis syndrome (TLS) in adults and children with malignant diseases: an expert TLS panel consensus. *Br J Haematol.* 2010;149(4):578-86.

[38] Howard SC, Jones DP, Pui CH. The tumor lysis syndrome. *N Engl J Med.* 2011;364(19):1844-54.

[39] Stewart AF. Clinical practice. Hypercalcemia associated with cancer. *N Engl J Med.* 2005;352(4):373-9.

[40] Rosner MH, Dalkin AC. Onco-nephrology: the pathophysiology and treatment of malignancy-associated hypercalcemia. *Clin J Am Soc Nephrol.* 2012;7(10):1722-9.

[41] Horwitz M. Non-parathyroid hypercalcemia. In: *Primer on the Metabolic Bone Diseases and Disorders of Mineral Metabolism,* 9th ed, Bilezikian JP (Ed), Wiley-Blackwell, Hoboken, NJ 2018. p.639.

[42] Major P, Lortholary A, Hon J, Abdi E, Mills G, Menssen HD, et al. Zoledronic acid is superior to pamidronate in the treatment of hypercalcemia of malignancy: a pooled analysis of two randomized, controlled clinical trials. *J Clin Oncol.* 2001;19(2):558-67.

[43] Pecherstorfer M, Steinhauer EU, Rizzoli R, Wetterwald M, Bergström B. Efficacy and safety of ibandronate in the treatment of hypercalcemia of malignancy: a randomized multicentric comparison to pamidronate. *Support Care Cancer.* 2003;11(8):539-47.

[44] Chang JT, Green L, Beitz J. Renal failure with the use of zoledronic acid. *N Engl J Med.* 2003;349(17):1676-9; discussion -9.

[45] Cicci JD, Buie L, Bates J, van Deventer H. Denosumab for the management of hypercalcemia of malignancy in patients with multiple myeloma and renal dysfunction. *Clin Lymphoma Myeloma Leuk.* 2014;14(6):e207-11.

[46] Santarpia L, Koch CA, Sarlis NJ. Hypercalcemia in cancer patients: pathobiology and management. *Horm Metab Res.* 2010;42(3):153-64.

[47] Parikh CR, Sandmaier BM, Storb RF, Blume KG, Sahebi F, Maloney DG, et al. Acute renal failure after nonmyeloablative hematopoietic cell transplantation. *J Am Soc Nephrol.* 2004;15(7):1868-76.

[48] Parikh CR, Schrier RW, Storer B, Diaconescu R, Sorror ML, Maris MB, et al. Comparison of ARF after myeloablative and nonmyeloablative hematopoietic cell transplantation. *Am J Kidney Dis.* 2005;45(3):502-9.

[49] Corbacioglu S, Jabbour EJ, Mohty M. Risk Factors for Development of and Progression of Hepatic Veno-Occlusive Disease/Sinusoidal Obstruction Syndrome. *Biol Blood Marrow Transplant.* 2019;25(7):1271-80.

[50] Richardson PG, Riches ML, Kernan NA, Brochstein JA, Mineishi S, Termuhlen AM, et al. Phase 3 trial of defibrotide for the treatment of severe veno-occlusive disease and multi-organ failure. *Blood.* 2016;127(13):1656-65.

[51] Khosla J, Yeh AC, Spitzer TR, Dey BR. Hematopoietic stem cell transplant-associated thrombotic microangiopathy: current paradigm and novel therapies. *Bone Marrow Transplant.* 2018;53(2):129-37.

[52] Jodele S, Laskin BL, Dandoy CE, Myers KC, El-Bietar J, Davies SM, et al. A new paradigm: Diagnosis and management of HSCT-associated thrombotic microangiopathy as multi-system endothelial injury. *Blood Rev.* 2015;29(3):191-204.

[53] Au WY, Ma ES, Lee TL, Ha SY, Fung AT, Lie AK, et al. Successful treatment of thrombotic microangiopathy after haematopoietic stem cell transplantation with rituximab. *Br J Haematol.* 2007;137(5):475-8.

[54] Jodele S, Fukuda T, Vinks A, Mizuno K, Laskin BL, Goebel J, et al. Eculizumab therapy in children with severe hematopoietic stem cell transplantation-associated thrombotic microangiopathy. *Biol Blood Marrow Transplant.* 2014;20(4):518-25.

[55] Srinivasan R, Balow JE, Sabnis S, Lundqvist A, Igarashi T, Takahashi Y, et al. Nephrotic syndrome: an under-recognised immune-mediated complication of non-myeloablative allogeneic haematopoietic cell transplantation. *Br J Haematol.* 2005;131(1):74-9.

[56] Reddy P, Johnson K, Uberti JP, Reynolds C, Silver S, Ayash L, et al. Nephrotic syndrome associated with chronic graft-versus-host disease after allogeneic hematopoietic stem cell transplantation. *Bone Marrow Transplant.* 2006;38(5):351-7.

[57] Choi M, Sun CL, Kurian S, Carter A, Francisco L, Forman SJ, et al. Incidence and predictors of delayed chronic kidney disease in long-term survivors of hematopoietic cell transplantation. *Cancer.* 2008;113(7):1580-7.

[58] Touzot M, Elie C, van Massenhove J, Maillard N, Buzyn A, Fakhouri F. Long-term renal function after allogenic haematopoietic stem cell transplantation in adult patients: a single-centre study. *Nephrol Dial Transplant.* 2010;25(2):624-7.

[59] Parikh CR, McSweeney P, Schrier RW. Acute renal failure independently predicts mortality after myeloablative allogeneic hematopoietic cell transplant. *Kidney Int.* 2005;67(5):1999-2005.

[60] Izzedine H, Escudier B, Lhomme C, Pautier P, Rouvier P, Gueutin V, et al. Kidney diseases associated with anti-vascular endothelial growth factor (VEGF): an 8-year observational study at a single center. *Medicine* (Baltimore). 2014;93(24):333-9.

[61] Lechner K, Obermeier HL. Cancer-related microangiopathic hemolytic anemia: clinical and laboratory features in 168 reported cases. *Medicine* (Baltimore). 2012;91(4):195-205.

[62] Brain MC, Azzopardi JG, Baker LR, Pineo GF, Roberts PD, Dacie JV. Microangiopathic haemolytic anaemia and mucin-forming adenocarcinoma. *Br J Haematol.* 1970;18(2):183-93.

[63] von Bubnoff N, Sandherr M, Schneller F, Peschel C. Thrombotic thrombocytopenic purpura in metastatic carcinoma of the breast. *Am J Clin Oncol.* 2000;23(1):74-7.

[64] Lusco MA, Fogo AB, Najafian B, Alpers CE. AJKD Atlas of Renal Pathology: Thrombotic Microangiopathy. *Am J Kidney Dis.* 2016;68(6):e33-e4.

[65] Lien YH, Lai LW. Pathogenesis, diagnosis and management of paraneoplastic glomerulonephritis. *Nat Rev Nephrol.* 2011;7(2):85-95.

[66] Zaghrini C, Seitz-Polski B, Justino J, Dolla G, Payré C, Jourde-Chiche N, et al. Novel ELISA for thrombospondin type 1 domain-containing 7A autoantibodies in membranous nephropathy. *Kidney Int.* 2019;95(3):666-79.

[67] Said SM, Leung N, Sethi S, Cornell LD, Fidler ME, Grande JP, et al. Myeloproliferative neoplasms cause glomerulopathy. *Kidney Int.* 2011;80(7):753-9.

[68] Jhaveri KD, Shah HH, Calderon K, Campenot ES, Radhakrishnan J. Glomerular diseases seen with cancer and chemotherapy: a narrative review. *Kidney Int.* 2013;84(1):34-44.

[69] Obrador GT, Price B, O'Meara Y, Salant DJ. Acute renal failure due to lymphomatous infiltration of the kidneys. *J Am Soc Nephrol.* 1997;8(8):1348-54.

[70] Richmond J, Sherman RS, Diamond HD, Craver LF. Renal lesions associated with malignant lymphomas. *Am J Med.* 1962;32:184-207.

[71] Rajan S, Babazade R, Govindarajan SR, Pal R, You J, Mascha EJ, et al. Perioperative factors associated with acute kidney injury after partial nephrectomy. *Br J Anaesth.* 2016;116(1):70-6.

[72] Xu L, Li C, Zhao L, Zhou B, Luo C, Man X, et al. Acute kidney injury after nephrectomy: a new nomogram to predict postoperative renal function. *BMC Nephrol.* 2020;21(1):181.

[73] Malyszko J, Tesarova P, Capasso G, Capasso A. The link between kidney disease and cancer: complications and treatment. *Lancet.* 2020;396(10246):277-87.

[74] Sprangers B, Cosmai L, Porta C. Chemotherapy and Radiation Related Kidney Diseases-Conventional Chemotherapy. *Onco-Nephrology.* 1 ed2019. p. 128-53.

[75] Olabisi O, Bonventre J. Acute Kidney Injury in Cancer Patients. *Onconephrology* 2015. p. 1-24.

[76] Perazella MA, Shirali AC. Nephrotoxicity of Cancer Immunotherapies: Past, Present and Future. *J Am Soc Nephrol.* 2018;29(8):2039-52.

[77] Cortazar FB, Marrone KA, Troxell ML, Ralto KM, Hoenig MP, Brahmer JR, et al. Clinicopathological features of acute kidney injury associated with immune checkpoint inhibitors. *Kidney Int.* 2016;90(3):638-47.

[78] Manohar S, Thongprayoon C, Cheungpasitporn W, Markovic SN, Herrmann SM. Systematic Review of the Safety of Immune Checkpoint Inhibitors Among Kidney Transplant Patients. *Kidney Int Rep.* 2020;5(2):149-58.

[79] Cortazar FB, Kibbelaar ZA, Glezerman IG, Abudayyeh A, Mamlouk O, Motwani SS, et al. Clinical Features and Outcomes of Immune Checkpoint Inhibitor-Associated AKI: A Multicenter Study. *J Am Soc Nephrol.* 2020;31(2):435-46.

[80] Mamlouk O, Selamet U, Machado S, Abdelrahim M, Glass WF, Tchakarov A, et al. Nephrotoxicity of immune checkpoint inhibitors beyond tubulointerstitial nephritis: single-center experience. *J Immunother Cancer.* 2019;7(1):2.

[81] Gutgarts V, Jain T, Zheng J, Maloy MA, Ruiz JD, Pennisi M, et al. Acute Kidney Injury after CAR-T Cell Therapy: Low Incidence and Rapid Recovery. *Biol Blood Marrow Transplant.* 2020;26(6):1071-6.

[82] Ellenbogen PH, Scheible FW, Talner LB, Leopold GR. Sensitivity of gray scale ultrasound in detecting urinary tract obstruction. *AJR Am J Roentgenol.* 1978;130(4):731-3.

[83] Soares M, Salluh JI, Carvalho MS, Darmon M, Rocco JR, Spector N. Prognosis of critically ill patients with cancer and acute renal dysfunction. *J Clin Oncol.* 2006;24(24):4003-10.

[84] Lameire N, Vanholder R, Van Biesen W, Benoit D. Acute kidney injury in critically ill cancer patients: an update. *Crit Care.* 2016;20(1):209.

[85] Palevsky PM, Zhang JH, O'Connor TZ, Chertow GM, Crowley ST, Choudhury D, et al. Intensity of renal support in critically ill patients with acute kidney injury. *N Engl J Med.* 2008;359(1):7-20.

[86] Hutchison CA, Cockwell P, Stringer S, Bradwell A, Cook M, Gertz MA, et al. Early reduction of serum-free light chains associates with renal recovery in myeloma kidney. *J Am Soc Nephrol.* 2011;22(6):1129-36.

[87] Hutchison CA, Cockwell P, Moroz V, Bradwell AR, Fifer L, Gillmore JD, et al. High cutoff versus high-flux haemodialysis for myeloma cast nephropathy in patients receiving bortezomib-based chemotherapy (EuLITE): a phase 2 randomised controlled trial. *Lancet Haematol.* 2019;6(4):e217-e28.

[88] Bridoux F, Carron PL, Pegourie B, Alamartine E, Augeul-Meunier K, Karras A, et al. Effect of High-Cutoff Hemodialysis vs Conventional Hemodialysis on Hemodialysis Independence Among Patients With Myeloma Cast Nephropathy: A Randomized Clinical Trial. *JAMA.* 2017;318(21):2099-110.

[89] Germain MJ. *Ethics of RRT, Initiation, and Withdrawal in Cancer Patients.* American Society of Nephrology 2016.

[90] Patel SS, Holley JL. Withholding and withdrawing dialysis in the intensive care unit: benefits derived from consulting the renal physicians association/american society of nephrology clinical practice guideline, shared decision-making in the appropriate initiation of and withdrawal from dialysis. *Clin J Am Soc Nephrol.* 2008;3(2):587-93.

[91] Brown EA, Bekker HL, Davison SN, Koffman J, Schell JO. Supportive Care: Communication Strategies to Improve Cultural Competence in Shared Decision Making. *Clin J Am Soc Nephrol.* 2016;11(10):1902-8.

In: Issues in Kidney Disease – Acute Kidney Injury
Editors: S. Z. Fadem and A. Arslan Yousuf Awan
ISBN: 978-1-68507-002-1

Chapter 17

PRINCIPLES OF DRUG THERAPY IN PATIENTS WITH ACUTE KIDNEY INJURY

Chandan Vangala*, MD

Selzman Institute for Kidney Health, Section of Nephrology, Department of Medicine,
Baylor College of Medicine, Houston, TX, USA
Michael E. DeBakey VA Medical Center, Houston, TX, USA

ABSTRACT

The clinical course of acute kidney injury (AKI) often necessitates determining complex dosing strategies for several different treatment responses: supportive care with no kidney replacement therapy, intermittent hemodialysis, urgent peritoneal dialysis, prolonged intermittent renal replacement therapy, and continuous renal replacement therapy. Depending on the method employed, current estimations of kidney function during AKI are broad or possibly even inaccurate. Further complicating matters, limited contemporary data exist regarding medication dosing in patients receiving kidney replacement therapy. Consequently, nephrologists must be keenly aware of theoretical concepts influencing free drug availability and the impact of treatment plans to medication dosing. Strategies for optimizing dosing include multidisciplinary communication and treatment plans, as well as implementation of accessible tools (nomograms, forecasting software programs) for adjusting dosing during AKI. Future study is focused on improving these tools to accommodate a wide array of diverse clinical scenarios and improving estimations of dynamic kidney function.

Keywords: Acute Kidney Injury, AKI, Continuous Renal Replacement Therapy, CRRT, Prolonged Intermittent Renal Replacement Therapy, PIRRT, hemodialysis, HD, dosing, pharmacokinetics

---

* Corresponding Author's E-mail: vangala@bcm.edu.

INTRODUCTION

Generating an intended and effective pharmacodynamic response while minimizing risk of toxicities is increasingly difficult when clinical pathology produces conditions and characteristics in a state of flux. Acute kidney injury (AKI) is a dynamic and common component of critical illness that impacts free drug availability through several mechanisms. Consequently, dosing medications amidst acute changes in kidney function is challenging. No commonly agreed upon method exists for accurately estimating kidney function during an AKI. Since creatinine-based estimates of glomerular filtration rate (eGFR) are determined in steady state, only broad estimates can be determined from creatinine levels. Additional layers of complexity complicate matters when one appreciates varying consequences that can result from the clinical context typically surrounding AKI as a part of critical illness. Easily appreciated is the decreased clearance attributed to reduced glomerular filtration and tubular secretion of drugs. While the majority of drugs have some component of drug elimination affected by kidney function, important oversights include the non-renal elimination as well as fluctuating volume of distribution and protein binding.

FUNCTIONAL ASSESSMENT

Current assessment is rather facile and wrought with opportunity for error, particularly concerning with administration of medications that have narrow therapeutic indices and lack practically available drug monitoring. Simply put, if the creatinine is increasing rapidly, any pharmacotherapy typically should assume an eGFR of 0 milliliters per minute (ml/min). Conversely, when creatinine values are dropping, practitioners should assume that the calculated eGFR underestimates the true filtration rate. Estimating creatinine clearance with short interval (4 hours) urine collection has been described [1], but these assessments are onerous and have substantial opportunity for error. As a result, they are not regularly incorporated into practice.

Studies that examine pharmacodynamic and pharmacokinetic drug properties in the setting of reduced kidney function are limited. Practitioners are even less informed when administering medications while kidney function is dynamically changing. Kinetic GFR is a more recently coined calculation that utilizes age, sex, race, baseline creatinine value, two recorded creatinine values, and time between values to estimate current eGFR during dynamic clinical scenarios. This data is not any more than what is frequently appreciated during most acute care clinical assessments, and the lack of additional data or labs required makes this calculation particularly attractive. In observational studies, kinetic GFR has been associated with AKI, renal recovery, delayed graft function, and need for kidney replacement therapy [2-5]. While these studies validate the predictive nature of kinetic GFR, further studies are needed to understand the accuracy of these estimations.

Novel markers of kidney injury have also been suggested [6]. Most notably, the presence of a combination of cell cycle arrest biomarkers (tissue inhibitor of metalloproteinase-2 and insulin-like growth factor-binding protein 7) in the urine, have been implemented in post-surgical cases [7]. However, these lab values have largely been studied to provide earlier recognition of kidney injury. While a recent study has suggested that sequential values may provide prognostic value with regards to resuscitation efforts in septic patients [8], no work has thoroughly examined dense, longitudinal data that follows any of these markers over the course of acute kidney injury. Thus, their utility in drug dosing is limited other than to alert providers of the potential need to avoid potential nephrotoxic medications as feasible and to be prepared to adjust dosing in the future.

THEORETICAL DETERMINANTS OF DRUG CONCENTRATION

AKI has complex, downstream sequelae that alter the quantities of free drug available to work at intended sites. While understanding of pharmacokinetic concepts is warranted, this chapter will only provide an overview with the understanding that limited quantifiable data exists with regards to the determinants of drug disposition in patients with AKI. For example, the degree to which sepsis-induced AKI alters bioavailability, volume of distribution, and metabolism of certain drugs is unknown, but the reader should have a general understanding of the clinical pathology's impact on these concepts.

Bioavailability

Bioavailability refers to the proportion of the administered drug that reaches the systemic circulation as an active moiety. Simply put, drugs administered via intravenous routes are completely bioavailable. Absorption via alternative means may be impacted by downstream effects of kidney injury. Edema, commonly encountered in patients with AKI, can impact topical, subcutaneous, intramuscular, and enteral routes. Additionally, enterally-administered drugs are subject to first-pass metabolism via gastrointestinal flora and enzymes, as well as hepatic enzymes, all of which may be functionally impacted by uremic toxins, especially if kidney dysfunction persists for an extended period of time. Patients with AKI are often critically ill, and in these clinical scenarios, drug transit via enteral means is highly unpredictable due to delayed gastric emptying, damaged epithelial barrier function, abnormal colonization, and other gut dysfunction.

Volume of Distribution

The volume of distribution (V_d) is a theoretical volume of fluid into which a drug dose would achieve the observed plasma concentration. The V_d is calculated by dividing the total amount of drug in the body by the plasma drug concentration. The desired serum concentration multiplied by the V_d determines the loading dose for medications.

Efforts to expand the effective circulation of a patient with AKI and critical illness are common. Whether the clinical scenario is post-operative care in the surgical intensive care unit or sepsis in the medical intensive care unit, crystalloids and colloids increase the volume of distribution for administered drugs. Thus, drugs such as aminoglycosides, which have small V_d tend to have more dramatic shifts in plasma concentration with volume resuscitation. Combined with the increased V_{d},, the considerable quantities of intravenous fluids frequently have a dilutional impact on assessments of creatinine, resulting in underdosing of medications [9].

By contrast, critical illness frequently results in inflammation-related hypoalbuminemia. Protein-binding limits free drug available to enact intended pharmacodynamic impact on target sites. Theoretically, critical illness-related hypoalbuminemia would then decrease the V_d.

Lastly, patients with critical illness experience significant alterations in pH, which can impact whether drugs exist in ionized or un-ionized forms. Ionization impacts the lipid solubility of the drug, which in turn affects the V_d.

Elimination

Drugs that are primarily cleared via glomerular filtration and tubular secretion are obviously impacted by reductions in kidney function, but frequently overlooked is the impact of AKI on non-renal clearance. The half-lives of non-renally cleared drugs are also extended due to the impact of uremic toxin retention on enzymatic activity. More specifically, uremic toxin accumulation reduces transcriptional activity and resulting expression of cytochrome p450 enzymes [10]. Additionally, uremia inhibits drug transporters at various sites [11]. The inhibition of intestinal drug transport would assume more limited plasma accrual; however, the decrease in hepatic sinusoidal drug transport would also change access to metabolizing enzymes. Somewhat expectedly, kidney replacement therapy would then stand to impact non-renal clearance. CYP3A4, a group of enzymes estimated to be responsible for more than half of all drug metabolism, increases its activity by 27% post dialysis, and its activity is inversely related to blood urea nitrogen values [12].

While the number of mechanisms in which drug availability are affected by AKI is numerous, there are a few mechanisms that bear the brunt of influence: increased V_d via extracellular fluid expansion; increased proportion of freely available drug due to hypoalbuminemia; and reduced drug metabolism and clearance.

Dosing in AKI Independent of Kidney Replacement Therapy

The V_d is commonly believed to be increased in AKI; however, practical considerations related to V_d are uncommonly employed in clinical practice. Per the Kidney Disease Improving Global Outcomes (KDIGO) clinical update in patients with acute and chronic kidney disease, the significantly increased V_d, particularly among hydrophilic drugs, warrants a 25-50% greater increase in loading doses [13]. Commonly used classes of hydrophilic antimicrobials include beta-lactams, cephalosporins, carbapenems, glycopeptides, and aminoglycosides [14].

Dynamic volume status and unpredictable kidney function render estimating maintenance dosing rather imprecise. In general, doses are lowered based on the assessment of the degree of functional decline, a rather difficult valuation as already noted. However, due to non-renal clearance, the dosing of many key drugs should mimic that of patients with normal kidney function. Therapeutic drug monitoring should be enacted when feasible, as the number of shifting factors that can influence plasma concentration are often too difficult to appreciate throughout a clinical course. All too often, such monitoring is not readily available or timely, requiring vigilant monitoring of drug pharmacodynamic effect and potential side effects.

Dosing in AKI Receiving Kidney Replacement Therapy

Based on the theoretical determinants of drug concentration already discussed, the drugs least likely to be affected by kidney replacement therapy are large molecules with increased V_d that are considerably protein-bound or drugs that typically experience non-renal elimination. Theoretical understanding has also shaped simulation studies that can assist when real-world data is unavailable. Many dosing recommendations in AKI requiring kidney replacement therapy are derived from studies in patients with ESKD. Importantly, one should note that these two clinical conditions are not equivalent. Residual or recovering kidney function is more commonly encountered in AKI, and consideration of this additional mechanism of clearance should encourage practitioners to err on the side of higher dosing regimens. Yet, no universally applicable guide regarding residual kidney function exists due to the diversity of pharmacokinetic properties of each drug. Additionally, non-renal elimination in AKI receiving kidney replacement therapy is not perfectly comparable to that of patients with ESKD. For example, while initially quite significant, non-renal elimination of vancomycin only approaches that of patients with ESKD after several days of continuous veno-venous hemofiltration [15]. Lastly, AKI is typically found in critical illness with acute inflammation, stressors, and more frequent kidney replacement therapy, all of which impact free drug availability. Dosing in patients with ESKD is assumed to be at steady state with thrice/weekly dialysis.

When feasible, drug dosing for patients experiencing acute kidney injury should ideally be a multidisciplinary effort. Primary teams often determine the desired drug with intended pharmacodynamic effect. Nephrologists weigh in on clearance or current mode of kidney replacement therapy (Figure 1), and alongside clinical pharmacists, who regularly appreciate pharmacokinetic-pharmacodynamic (PK/PD) indices, determine drug dosing. Twenty-four-hour clinical pharmacy support that is knowledgeable regarding dynamic changes in kidney function and modes of kidney replacement therapy is not prevalent. Thus, it is paramount that nephrologists are informed regarding PK/PD concepts and targets. Comprehensive kidney care cannot be myopic and cast drug dosing as tangential territory owned by clinical pharmacy. The complexity of dose determination necessitates specific and regular input communicated into plans. In particular, nephrologists must take special attention when beginning kidney replacement therapy or changing mode of therapy (Figure 1).

Dosing nomograms are popular and practical mechanisms for guiding drug dosing [16, 17]. The main drawback is that limited variables (weight, kidney function, modality of kidney replacement therapy) are used to determine dosing. More recently, software programs have been developed that can incorporate a multitude of variables into complex modeling (linear regression, Bayesian prediction, artificial intelligence) for achieving PK/PD targets [18-20]. Initial dosing recommendations compiled for various blood purification methods were rooted in limited data [17], and due to updates in kidney replacement therapy (equipment, filters, prescriptions), growing literature and frequent updates are likely necessary [21].

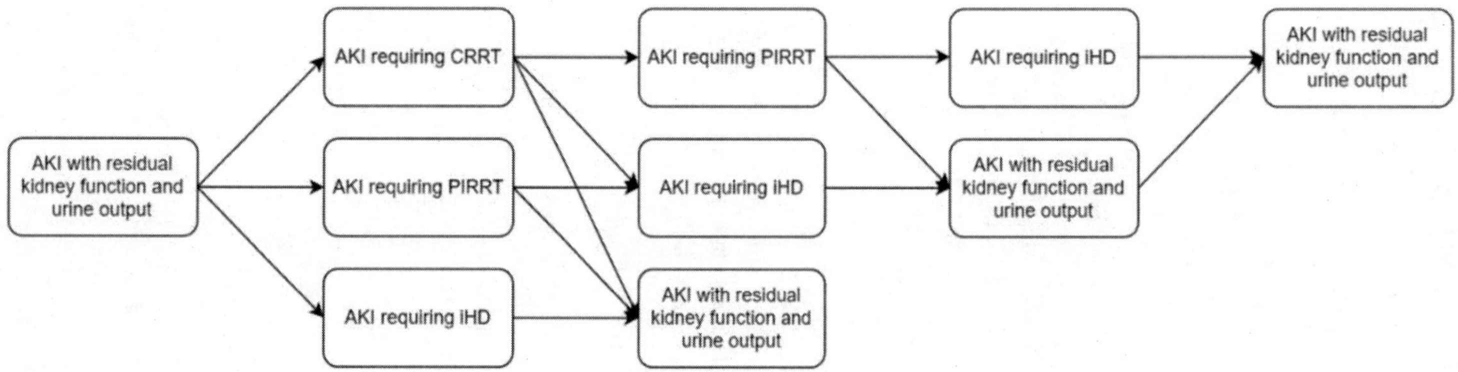

CRRT – Continuous Renal Replacement Therapy; PIRRT – Prolonged Intermittent Renal Replacement Therapy; iHD – intermittent hemodialysis.

Figure 1. Potential Kidney Therapy Transitions during Critical Illness Warranting Medication Dose Adjustments.

Hemodialysis

As alluded to above, drug dosing in AKI requiring hemodialysis (AKI-HD) is largely extrapolated from studies in patients with ESKD. However, many of these studies were performed on more outdated dialyzers that did not use the more commonly used synthetic/semisynthetic materials or high-flux membranes. Unfortunately, these few older studies in patients with ESKD have not been revisited with newer equipment. As a result, confidence in dosing in AKI-HD, a clinical scenario that is not equivalent due to differences in non-renal elimination, is wanting.

As with before, assessment of clinical characteristics, clearance, and drug properties is necessary prior to estimating dosing, and in AKI-HD, clearance is dictated by dialysis prescription. A simple, but not perfectly precise method for assessing clearance of drugs from hemodialysis can be calculated from measurements of drug concentration at two sampling sites: the inlet limb of the dialyzer ($I_{[drug]}$) and the limb exiting from the dialyzer back to the patient ($E_{[drug]}$). Depending on if concentrations are drawn from plasma or whole blood, clearance can be determined by plasma flow (Q_p) or blood flow (Q_b) multiplied by the ratio of the difference in the two concentrations over the drug concentration from the inlet limb: $Q_{p \text{ or } b} * (I_{[drug]}-E_{[drug]})/ I_{[drug]}$. In patients receiving large volume removal, the exiting concentration would be falsely high. Thus, more precise estimations can be achieved from dividing the total quantity of drug in dialysate by the area under the curve through the time of therapy, derived from several concentrations from the inlet limb [13, 22]. Unfortunately, regular application outside of coordinated studies is impractical due to limited access to laboratories capable of determining such concentrations in a timely manner.

Critical drugs that experience drug clearance due to dialysis usually warrant dosing post-HD therapy. Typical recommendations assume thrice/weekly intermittent HD. Consequently, supplemental dosing is necessary in hospitalized patients who often receive more frequent dialysis as a part of supportive care.

Peritoneal Dialysis

In clinical scenarios where other modes of therapy are unavailable, impractical, or simply less desirable, urgent-start peritoneal dialysis has recently attracted more attention for use in AKI [23]. Urea clearance attributed to the majority of peritoneal dialysis prescriptions is often quoted as being equivalent to ~10 ml/min. Antibiotics would be estimated to have lower clearance, as they are larger than urea. With the need for kidney replacement therapy, the assumption of very limited residual kidney function is reasonable. Thus, one can conclude that drug dosing regimens for creatinine clearance <15 ml/min are clinically applicable.

Intraperitoneal antibiotics are preferred for peritonitis as they can achieve rapid intraperitoneal therapeutic drug level. The International Society for Peritoneal Dialysis provides detailed recommendations for both continuous administration or intermittent administration with one dwell in continuous ambulatory peritoneal dialysis or the long dwell in automatic peritoneal dialysis [24].

Prolonged Intermittent Renal Replacement Therapy (PIRRT)

Prolonged intermittent renal replacement therapy (PIRRT) largely consists of sustained low efficiency dialysis (SLED) and curtailed versions of continuous veno-venous hemofiltration (CVVH) and continuous veno-venous hemodialysis (CVVHD), sometimes referred to as accelerated veno-venous hemofiltration (AVVH) and SHIFT, respectively.

SLED has a longer history of use, and for that reason has some limited real-world data that governs the dosing of few commonly employed drugs such as vancomycin. However, these studies are quite dated and the variability of prescription (duration, blood flow, dialysate flow, filter size, etc.) among institutions, and even individual providers, employing SLED generates inconsistent clearance. When asked about dosing of commonly used antibiotics in the ICU, 69 surveyed pharmacists with experience dosing antibiotics in ICU patients on renal replacement therapy provided a wide-ranging array of responses [25]. Depending on the antibiotic in question, dosing recommendations varied by 4 to as high as 12-fold, highlighting a need to avoid medications with narrow therapeutic indices unless accompanied by therapeutic drug monitoring.

Real-world data governing drug dosing during PIRRT not performed via SLED is almost non-existent. Existing guidance is derived from Monte-Carlo simulations of 5000 patients [26-29] utilizing body weights and pharmacokinetic parameters from a prior observational study of 100 patients [30]. Assuming 40 liters of therapeutic fluid per session (4 liters/hour x 10 hours or 5 liters/hour x 8 hours), Mueller and colleagues have provided estimates for dosing of common antibiotics that serve as the best available guidance until more real-world data is generated (26-29). Importantly, certain medications like fluoroquinolones for treating gram negatives are recommended against due to difficulty maintaining within therapeutic index(31). Based on the above in silico studies, doses of ciprofloxacin and levofloxacin needed to treat *Pseudomonas aeruginosa* far exceed FDA-approved doses. Other drugs, such as daptomycin and newer drugs, have no enlightening studies or data to inform dosing. Thus, providers of kidney care should be aware of which medications are not compatible with various forms of PIRRT.

Regardless of the chosen therapy, practitioners of PIRRT encounter common problems related to the extended periods of limited clearance when not on therapy, and substantial clearance while on therapy. As a result, confidence is lacking regarding the ability to maintain medications within their therapeutic index for adequate periods of time. Secondly, hospitals usually have set times for drug dosing depending on the parameter associated with the drug order (i.e., BID, every 12 hours; TID, every 8 hours). If PIRRT is not employed at set times, coordinating drug dosing with ICU teams and pharmacists can be extremely challenging. PIRRT serves a practical need in avoiding the complications related to continuous therapy in patients that are de-escalating from more critical illness. However, the considerations regarding drug dosing are substantial, and it remains one of the larger obstacles to increasing the adoption of these intermediate modes of ICU kidney replacement therapy.

Continuous Renal Replacement Therapy (CRRT)

While CRRT retains many of the same prescriptive variables noted in intermittent hemodialysis, the therapy does not enjoy the same standardization and quality metrics. As a result, provider preference, facility complexity, and other aspects unrelated to clinical outcomes influence prescription, resulting in substantial variability. First, the modality, whether diffusive, convective, or a hybrid of the two, can affect drug clearance. Medications are larger molecules than urea or creatinine, and convective means of clearance are more effective at producing middle and large solute clearance. Secondly, the therapy fluid dose, and to a lesser extent, prescribed blood flow, is often variable throughout a clinical course and among different clinical scenarios. Additionally, discrepancies between prescribed doses and delivered doses are unpredictable. Lastly, how the proximity of drug administration to the dialysis access impacts clearance is unknown. As a result, critical drugs should ideally be administered through peripheral access when feasible.

Given that the sieving coefficient of creatinine is 1, the therapy fluid dose can easily be described as creatinine clearance in milliliters per minute (mL/min). For example, an effluent dose of 2,000 ml per hour equates to an estimated creatinine clearance of 33.33 ml/min [2,000 ml/hr * (1 h/60 min)]. Because practitioners are concerned with the available free drug that behaves as an active moiety, the quantity of drug bound to protein can be subtracted. Thus, if drug *X* is 20% protein bound, then a practitioner could theoretically consider dosing an antibiotic at 80% of the estimated creatinine clearance. Referring back to the example of an effluent dose of 2,000 ml/hr, drug *X* should be dosed for 80% of this dose (1,600 ml/hr or an estimated creatinine clearance of 26.67 ml/min). Clearance is reliably informed by effluent rate in many key antimicrobials: vancomycin, meropenem, and piperacillin-tazobactam [21, 32]. However, applying creatinine kinetics blindly and universally to drug dosing with CRRT is problematic in many ways. Dosing regimens in CKD are based on creatinine clearance in steady state. Drug elimination in a patient with CKD and a steady state eGFR of 30 ml/min often has more real-world data that supports recommended doses. On the other hand, a critically ill patient experiencing an AKI requiring CRRT with an effluent dose of 1800 ml/hr, which equates to a similar creatinine clearance of 30 ml/min, has demonstrably different clinical characteristics that would affect drug pharmacokinetics. Additionally, while the goal in kidney failure is to supplant kidney function, kidney replacement therapy poorly mimic native kidney clearance.

Because of these numerous variables related to prescription and clinical condition, investigating appropriate dosing is exceedingly difficult and few studies exist. While not universally applicable to all drug categories, critical antibiotics for patients undergoing CRRT were commonly found to be inadequate [33-36]. Studies in critical illness, albeit irrespective of CRRT utilization, have delineated better outcomes with higher target concentrations [37, 38]. Consequently, a trend towards more aggressive antimicrobial dosing, particularly at the earliest stage of a clinical course, has emerged.

AKI requiring CRRT is a common complication of extracorporeal membranous oxygenation (ECMO). Briefly, ECMO induces decreased bioavailability due to extracorporeal sequestration of drugs and pharmacokinetic alterations. Ex-vivo study has suggested that highly protein-bound drugs and those with higher octanol-water partition coefficient are more susceptible to sequestration [39]. Practical understanding of how to determine individual drug dosing is still lacking as understanding of the impact of ECMO, much less the interaction between AKI-CRRT and extracorporeal circuitry, is still in its infancy. Guiding evidence is sparse, but a matched cohort study of the administration of meropenem for patients on ECMO receiving CRRT noted high interindividual variability [40].

Non-Antimicrobial Drug Dosing in Critical Illness Requiring Kidney Replacement Therapy

Many clinical guidelines exist regarding antimicrobial dosing for patients with reduced kidney function or requiring distinct kidney replacement therapies. Antimicrobial therapy garners massive attention and institutions have often developed dosing nomograms, algorithms, or software programs tailored to their facility's available antimicrobials, dosing and infusion strategy, local epidemiology and pattern of antimicrobial susceptibility, and modes of kidney replacement therapy. As a result, this chapter does not extensively review practical antimicrobial dosing in each mode of kidney replacement therapy. Conversely, non-antimicrobial medications are infrequently referenced. Briefly discussed below, are commonly used non-antimicrobial medications in critical care requiring kidney replacement therapy.

Antiarrhythmics

Amiodarone has not been specifically studied in PIRRT or CRRT; however, no dose adjustment is believed to be necessary in AKI requiring any form of kidney replacement therapy.

Anti-Epileptic Drugs

Anti-epileptic drug elimination is poorly studied with real-world data existing largely in the form of case reports [41]. Despite being highly protein bound, dose supplementation after HD may be needed for phenytoin, and thankfully, more readily available drug levels (relative to other anti-epileptic drugs) can assist with dosing efforts. By contrast, levetiracetam experiences limited protein binding and is much more readily removed with reports of sieving coefficients ranging from 0.89 to 1.03 in CVVH [42, 43]. However, levetiracetam has not been cleared in similar manners to other molecules with equivalent sieving coefficients, namely urea or creatinine [43]. While data is limited, a dose reduction based on creatinine clearance attributed to therapy fluid rate or doses used in intermittent HD would likely be insufficient to achieve a target trough values. However, one should note that levetiracetam target trough values are not associated with clinical outcomes as the ability to access therapeutic drug monitoring is rare.

Transplant Immunosuppression

Commonly used agents in transplant recipients – thymoglobulin, basiliximab, belatacept, cyclosporine, tacrolimus, sirolimus, rituximab – are not significantly removed in any kidney replacement therapy. The lone exception, azathioprine, is considered moderately dialyzable as evidenced from 45% of the drug removed over an 8 hour session of HD [44]. With newer high-flux membranes, this removal may be even greater.

Anticoagulation

Among commonly used anticoagulants, direct thrombin inhibitors, which undergo hepatic metabolism, are dialyzable. One report suggests that ~50-60% of dabigatran is removed over 4 hours of HD [45]. Unsurprisingly, dabigatran removal with CRRT has also been described in case reports of patients with life-threatening bleeding [46, 47]. Given its large V_d and some degree of protein binding, rebound increases in dabigatran levels are anticipated after suspension of therapy. Argatroban clearance is increased by 20% with HD [48]. Its clearance in CRRT has been deemed clinically insignificant [49] and is often used as alternative anticoagulation in patients receiving CRRT with heparin-induced thrombocytopenia. Finally, bivalirudin is believed to undergo 25% removal with thrice/weekly HD and require dose adjustment in both PIRRT and CRRT [50].

Conversely, warfarin and factor Xa inhibitors, i.e., apixaban, rivaroxaban, are highly protein bound and not significantly removed with kidney replacement therapy. Heparin is also poorly dialyzed and no supplemental dose or adjustment is recommended in any form of kidney replacement therapy.

Conclusion

AKI is typically part of a dynamic clinical course that makes drug dosing complicated. Future study will hopefully provide more evidence-based dosing guidelines. This expanding knowledge, coupled with the development of forecasting models and evolving kidney replacement therapies, will require frequent updates to our understanding of PK/PD drug profiles. Sole reliance on clinical pharmacy is not adequate to avoid dosing errors and imprecision. The role of the nephrologist in interpreting kidney function and complex replacement therapy clearance is crucial to administering vital medicines.

References

[1] Pickering JW, Frampton CM, Walker RJ, Shaw GM, Endre ZH. Four hour creatinine clearance is better than plasma creatinine for monitoring renal function in critically ill patients. *Crit Care* (London, England). 2012;16(3):R107.

[2] Chen S. Retooling the creatinine clearance equation to estimate kinetic GFR when the plasma creatinine is changing acutely. *J Am Soc Neph: JASN*. 2013;24(6):877-88.

[3] Dewitte A, Joannès-Boyau O, Sidobre C, Fleureau C, Bats ML, Derache P, et al. Kinetic eGFR and Novel AKI Biomarkers to Predict Renal Recovery. *Clin J Am Soc Neph: CJASN*. 2015;10(11):1900-10.

[4] Pianta TJ, Endre ZH, Pickering JW, Buckley NA, Peake PW. Kinetic Estimation of GFR Improves Prediction of Dialysis and Recovery after Kidney Transplantation. *PloS one*. 2015;10(5):e0125669.

[5] O'Sullivan ED, Doyle A. The clinical utility of kinetic glomerular filtration rate. *Clin Kidney J*. 2017;10(2):202-8.

[6] Ronco C, Bellomo R, Kellum JA. Acute kidney injury. *Lancet* (London, England). 2019;394(10212):1949-64.

[7] Göcze I, Jauch D, Götz M, Kennedy P, Jung B, Zeman F, et al. Biomarker-guided Intervention to Prevent Acute Kidney Injury After Major Surgery: The Prospective Randomized BigpAK Study. *Ann Surg*. 2018;267(6):1013-20.

[8] Fiorentino M, Xu Z, Smith A, Singbartl K, Palevsky PM, Chawla LS, et al. Serial Measurement of Cell-cycle Arrest Biomarkers [TIMP-2]•[IGFBP7] and Risk for Progression to Death, Dialysis or Severe Acute Kidney Injury in Patients with Septic Shock. *Am J Respir and Crit Care Med*. 2020;202(9):1262-70.

[9] Udy AA, Roberts JA, Boots RJ, Paterson DL, Lipman J. Augmented renal clearance: implications for antibacterial dosing in the critically ill. *Clin Pharmacokinet*. 2010;49(1):1-16.

[10] Vilay AM, Churchwell MD, Mueller BA. Clinical review: Drug metabolism and nonrenal clearance in acute kidney injury. *Crit Care* (London, England). 2008;12(6):235.

[11] Yeung CK, Shen DD, Thummel KE, Himmelfarb J. Effects of chronic kidney disease and uremia on hepatic drug metabolism and transport. *Kidney Int*. 2014;85(3):522-8.

[12] Nolin TD, Appiah K, Kendrick SA, Le P, McMonagle E, Himmelfarb J. Hemodialysis acutely improves hepatic CYP3A4 metabolic activity. *J Am Soc Neph : JASN*. 2006;17(9):2363-7.

[13] Matzke GR, Aronoff GR, Atkinson AJ, Jr., Bennett WM, Decker BS, Eckardt KU, et al. Drug dosing consideration in patients with acute and chronic kidney disease-a clinical update from Kidney Disease: Improving Global Outcomes (KDIGO). *Kidney Int*. 2011;80(11):1122-37.

[14] Roberts JA, Lipman J. Pharmacokinetic issues for antibiotics in the critically ill patient. *Crit Care Med*. 2009;37(3):840-51; quiz 59.

[15] Macias WL, Mueller BA, Scarim SK. Vancomycin pharmacokinetics in acute renal failure: preservation of nonrenal clearance. *Clin Pharmacol Ther*. 1991;50(6):688-94.

[16] Chai MG, Cotta MO, Abdul-Aziz MH, Roberts JA. What Are the Current Approaches to Optimising Antimicrobial Dosing in the Intensive Care Unit? *Pharmaceutics*. 2020;12(7).

[17] Heintz BH, Matzke GR, Dager WE. Antimicrobial dosing concepts and recommendations for critically ill adult patients receiving continuous renal replacement therapy or intermittent hemodialysis. *Pharmacotherapy*. 2009;29(5):562-77.

[18] Mohan M, Batty KT, Cooper JA, Wojnar-Horton RE, Ilett KF. Comparison of gentamicin dose estimates derived from manual calculations, the Australian 'Therapeutic Guidelines: Antibiotic' nomogram and the SeBA-GEN and DoseCalc software programs. *Br J Clin Pharmacol*. 2004;58(5):521-7.

[19] Donagher J, Martin JH, Barras MA. Individualised medicine: why we need Bayesian dosing. *Internal medicine journal.* 2017;47(5):593-600.

[20] Avent ML, Rogers BA. Optimising antimicrobial therapy through the use of Bayesian dosing programs. *Int J Clin Pharmacol.* 2019;41(5):1121-30.

[21] Hoff BM, Maker JH, Dager WE, Heintz BH. Antibiotic Dosing for Critically Ill Adult Patients Receiving Intermittent Hemodialysis, Prolonged Intermittent Renal Replacement Therapy, and Continuous Renal Replacement Therapy: An Update. *Ann Pharmacolther.* 2020;54(1):43-55.

[22] Lee CS, Marbury TC. Drug therapy in patients undergoing haemodialysis. Clinical pharmacokinetic considerations. *Clin Pharmacokinet.* 1984;9(1):42-66.

[23] Sourial MY, Sourial MH, Dalsan R, Graham J, Ross M, Chen W, et al. Urgent Peritoneal Dialysis in Patients With COVID-19 and Acute Kidney Injury: A Single-Center Experience in a Time of Crisis in the United States. *Am J Kidney Dis.* 2020;76(3):401-6.

[24] Li PK, Szeto CC, Piraino B, de Arteaga J, Fan S, Figueiredo AE, et al. ISPD Peritonitis Recommendations: 2016 Update on Prevention and Treatment. *Perit Dial Int.* 2016;36(5):481-508.

[25] Mei JP, Ali-Moghaddam A, Mueller BA. Survey of pharmacists' antibiotic dosing recommendations for sustained low-efficiency dialysis. *Int J Clin Pharmacol.* 2016;38(1):127-34.

[26] Gharibian KN, Mueller BA. Fluconazole dosing predictions in critically-ill patients receiving prolonged intermittent renal replacement therapy: a Monte Carlo simulation approach. *Clin Nephrol* . 2016;86(7):43-50.

[27] Lewis SJ, Kays MB, Mueller BA. Use of Monte Carlo Simulations to Determine Optimal Carbapenem Dosing in Critically Ill Patients Receiving Prolonged Intermittent Renal Replacement Therapy. *J Clin Pharmacol.* 2016;56(10):1277-87.

[28] Jang SM, Gharibian KN, Lewis SJ, Fissell WH, Tolwani AJ, Mueller BA. A Monte Carlo Simulation Approach for Beta-Lactam Dosing in Critically Ill Patients Receiving Prolonged Intermittent Renal Replacement Therapy. *J Clin Pharmacol.* 2018;58(10):1254-65.

[29] Lewis SJ, Mueller BA. Development of a vancomycin dosing approach for critically ill patients receiving hybrid hemodialysis using Monte Carlo simulation. *SAGE open medicine.* 2018;6:2050312118773257.

[30] Gashti CN, Salcedo S, Robinson V, Rodby RA. Accelerated venovenous hemofiltration: early technical and clinical experience. *Am J Kidney Dis.* 2008;51(5):804-10.

[31] Lewis SJ, Chaijamorn W, Shaw AR, Mueller BA. In silico trials using Monte Carlo simulation to evaluate ciprofloxacin and levofloxacin dosing in critically ill patients receiving prolonged intermittent renal replacement therapy. *Renal Replace Ther.* 2016;2(1):45.

[32] Jamal JA, Udy AA, Lipman J, Roberts JA. The impact of variation in renal replacement therapy settings on piperacillin, meropenem, and vancomycin drug clearance in the critically ill: an analysis of published literature and dosing regimens*. *Crit Care Med.* 2014;42(7):1640-50.

[33] Seyler L, Cotton F, Taccone FS, De Backer D, Macours P, Vincent JL, et al. Recommended β-lactam regimens are inadequate in septic patients treated with continuous renal replacement therapy. *Crit Care.* 2011;15(3):R137.

[34] Lewis SJ, Mueller BA. Antibiotic dosing in critically ill patients receiving CRRT: underdosing is overprevalent. *Semin Dial.* 2014;27(5):441-5.

[35] Burger R, Guidi M, Calpini V, Lamoth F, Decosterd L, Robatel C, et al. Effect of renal clearance and continuous renal replacement therapy on appropriateness of recommended meropenem dosing regimens in critically ill patients with susceptible life-threatening infections. *J Antimicrob Chemother*. 2018;73(12):3413-22.

[36] Wilson FP, Berns JS. Vancomycin levels are frequently subtherapeutic during continuous venovenous hemodialysis (CVVHD). *Clin Nephrol.* 2012;77(4):329-31.

[37] Roberts JA, Paul SK, Akova M, Bassetti M, De Waele JJ, Dimopoulos G, et al. DALI: defining antibiotic levels in intensive care unit patients: are current β-lactam antibiotic doses sufficient for critically ill patients? *Clin Infec Dis.* 2014;58(8):1072-83.

[38] McKinnon PS, Paladino JA, Schentag JJ. Evaluation of area under the inhibitory curve (AUIC) and time above the minimum inhibitory concentration (T>MIC) as predictors of outcome for cefepime and ceftazidime in serious bacterial infections. *Inj J Antimicrob Agents*. 2008;31(4):345-51.

[39] Cheng V, Abdul-Aziz MH, Roberts JA, Shekar K. Overcoming barriers to optimal drug dosing during ECMO in critically ill adult patients. *Expert Opin Drug Metab Toxicol.* 2019;15(2):103-12.

[40] Shekar K, Fraser JF, Taccone FS, Welch S, Wallis SC, Mullany DV, et al. The combined effects of extracorporeal membrane oxygenation and renal replacement therapy on meropenem pharmacokinetics: a matched cohort study. *Crit Care*. 2014;18(6):565.

[41] Mahmoud SH. Antiepileptic Drug Removal by Continuous Renal Replacement Therapy: A Review of the Literature. *Clin Drug Investig.* 2017;37(1):7-23.

[42] Kalaria SN, Armahizer M, McCarthy P, Badjatia N, Gobburu JV, Gopalakrishnan M. A Practice-Based, Clinical Pharmacokinetic Study to Inform Levetiracetam Dosing in Critically Ill Patients Undergoing Continuous Venovenous Hemofiltration (PADRE-01). *Clin Transl Sci*. 2020;13(5):950-9.

[43] Van Matre ET, Mueller SW, Fish DN, MacLaren R, Cava LF, Neumann RT, et al. Levetiracetam Pharmacokinetics in a Patient with Intracranial Hemorrhage Undergoing Continuous Veno-Venous Hemofiltration. *Am J Med Case Rep.* 2017;18:458-62.

[44] Schusziarra V, Ziekursch V, Schlamp R, Siemensen HC. Pharmacokinetics of azathioprine under haemodialysis. *Int J Pharmacol Biopharm.* 1976;14(4):298-302.

[45] Khadzhynov D, Wagner F, Formella S, Wiegert E, Moschetti V, Slowinski T, et al. Effective elimination of dabigatran by haemodialysis. A phase I single-centre study in patients with end-stage renal disease. *Thromb haemost.* 2013;109(4):596-605.

[46] Parli SE, Thompson Bastin ML, Lewis DA. Use of Continuous Renal Replacement Therapy for Removal of Dabigatran in a Patient in Need of Emergent Surgery. *Case Rep Crit Care.* 2016;2016:9692568.

[47] Vitale C, Berutti S, Montaruli B, Cosseddu D, Sivera P, Verdecchia C, et al. [The effects of continuous renal replacement therapy (CRRT) and intermittent haemodialysis (IHD) in the treatment of dabigatran overdose. Case report. *G Ital Nephrol.* 2014;31(2):gin/31.2.13.

[48] Murray PT, Reddy BV, Grossman EJ, Hammes MS, Trevino S, Ferrell J, et al. A prospective comparison of three argatroban treatment regimens during hemodialysis in end-stage renal disease. *Kidney Int.* 2004;66(6):2446-53.

[49] Tang IY, Cox DS, Patel K, Reddy BV, Nahlik L, Trevino S, et al. Argatroban and renal replacement therapy in patients with heparin-induced thrombocytopenia. *Ann Pharmacother.* 2005;39(2):231-6.

[50] Tsu LV, Dager WE. Bivalirudin dosing adjustments for reduced renal function with or without hemodialysis in the management of heparin-induced thrombocytopenia. *Ann Pharmacothe*. 2011;45(10):1185-92.

In: Issues in Kidney Disease – Acute Kidney Injury
Editors: S. Z. Fadem and A. Arslan Yousuf Awan ISBN: 978-1-68507-002-1

Chapter 18

ACUTE KIDNEY INJURY IN PREGNANCY

Sayna Norouzi[1,*], MD, James Yoon[1], MD, Amir Abdi Pour[1], MD and Silvi Shah[2], MD, MS, FACP, FASN, FAST
[1]Loma Linda University Medical Center, Loma Linda, CA, USA
[2]University of Cincinnati, Cincinnati, OH, USA

ABSTRACT

Acute Kidney Injury (AKI) in pregnancy can complicate the pregnancy course and is considered one of the most serious complications. The differential diagnosis of AKI in pregnancy is very broad and needs a meticulous assessment. Timing of AKI in pregnancy can be a very helpful parameter in order to categorize etiologies of AKI in pregnancy. In this chapter, we are going to discuss epidemiology, prognosis, etiologies and treatment options for AKI in pregnancy.

Keywords: AKI, pregnancy, preeclampsia

INTRODUCTION

During pregnancy, kidneys undergo significant changes, both anatomic and physiologic. Kidney size increases by approximately 1 to 1.5 cm as a result of increased kidney weight and dilatation of the urinary collecting system. Physiologic changes happen due to hemodynamic changes (increased cardiac output, plasma volume expansion, and systemic vasodilation) during pregnancy. These changes result in an increase in the glomerular filtration rate (GFR) by approximately 50% in the first trimester; hence, there is a decrease in blood urea nitrogen (BUN) to less than 13 and serum creatinine (Cr) to 0.4-0.5 mg/dl [1].

Acute kidney injury (AKI) remains one of the most serious complications of pregnancy. In underdeveloped nations, septic abortion and preeclampsia are considered the most common

* Corresponding Author's E-mail: Sayna.nrz@gmail.com.

causes of AKI during pregnancy. A recent study showed an increase in pregnancy related AKI in recent years. This study looked at the 48,316,430 maternal hospitalization from 2005-2015; of them 0.07% were complicated by AKI. Interestingly, the data showed an increase in AKI rate in 2015 when compared with AKI incidence rate in 2005 (3.5/10,000 in 2005 vs 11.8/10,000 in 2015) [2].

AKI in pregnancy has been linked to adverse maternal and fetal outcomes. Based on a study of pregnancy patients from Canada who developed AKI and required dialysis, 4.3% died, and 3.9% remained on dialysis for up to 4 months post-delivery. The mortality rate among these patients was significantly higher when compared to pregnant patients without AKI (0.01%) [3]. However, a more recent study showed higher odds of miscarriage (aOR, 1.64; 95% CI, 1.3 to 2.07) and mortality (aOR, 1.53; 95% CI, 1.25 to 1.88) amongst patients with pregnancy related AKI [2].

Unfortunately, once AKI is severe enough to require dialysis during pregnancy, the chance of full recovery decreases. Review of research indicates that maternal outcomes for patients who develop AKI depend on available health care resources. An Indian study shows that 18.3% of pregnancy-related AKI patients required dialysis, and of those, 9% remained on dialysis for up to 6 months after delivery [3]. Based on a recent study, the rate of AKI amongst hospitalized pregnant patients was around 0.08%; it also showed that the risk of developing AKI is higher in African Americans, patients with diabetes, and Native Americans when compared to non-diabetic white pregnant hospitalized patients. Requiring hospitalization for a pregnancy related AKI is associated with higher mortality rate and cardiovascular events [5].

Pregnancy-related AKI can be suspected once the BUN is higher than 13 or the serum creatinine level becomes higher than 0.7-0.8 mg/dL; however, there is no standardized criteria for pregnancy related AKI [1, 4]. The gold standard to measure GFR during pregnancy is still the 24-hour creatinine clearance. However, adequate 24-hour urinary collection during pregnancy can be hindered due to urinary retention. Cystatin C accuracy in GFR calculation has not been well studied during pregnancy; in addition, there are studies suggesting that cystatin C may be released by the placenta as well, which can interfere with precise GFR calculation [6].

Pregnancy-related AKI can be secondary to multiple etiologies. Diagnosis of pregnancy-related AKI underlying etiology is time sensitive, as a timely and accurate detection and intervention is crucial in this setting. Usually, AKI occurs in patients experiencing other symptoms such as hypertension or hypotension, proteinuria, or recent health events (sepsis, abortion, or low intake).

Conditions such as preeclampsia and HELLP syndrome (hemolysis, elevated liver enzymes, low platelet count) should always be part of differential diagnoses. Severe AKI has been seen only in 1% of patients with preeclampsia and is considered a rare complication in this setting; however, AKI is more common in patients suffering from HELLP syndrome and has been seen in up to 15% of those patients.

Etiologies of AKI could be divided based on the trimester. During the first trimester, volume depletion secondary to hyperemesis gravidarum or hemodynamic changes due to septic abortions and early miscarriages can be more common.

As we move towards the second and third trimesters, differentials such as preeclampsia, HELLP syndrome, acute fatty liver of pregnancy (AFLP), thrombotic thrombocytopenic purpura (TTP), abruption placentae, cortical necrosis, and urinary retention due to gravid uterus would be much more common. Many of these conditions such as AFLP, HELLP syndrome, and preeclampsia may have overlapping symptoms and laboratory findings that can make the diagnosis challenging [1, 3, 4].

Atypical hemolytic uremic syndrome (aHUS) usually occurs near term or postpartum. Infectious etiologies causing hemodynamic changes, such as acute pyelonephritis, can happen almost any time during pregnancy [1].

Diagnosing pregnancy-related AKI requires an extensive workup and a broad differential diagnosis should be considered as well. Another way to narrow down the etiologies of pregnancy-related AKI is to categorize it into the three major groups of prerenal, intrarenal and postrenal. This chapter will further discuss the etiologies of pregnancy-related AKI and available treatment options in detail.

Table 1. Differential based on timing within the gestational period

First Trimester	Second/Third Trimester	Peripartum/Postpartum
Hyperemesis gravidarum Septic abortions/early miscarriages	Abruptio placentae AFLP Cortical necrosis Gravid uterus HELLP syndrome Preeclampsia TTP Uterine hemorrhage.	Atypical HUS NSAID use Puerperal sepsis
Can happen anytime during pregnancy: Acute postinfectious glomerulonephritis, lupus nephritis, acute pyelonephritis, dehydration, calculus of urinary tract		

AFLP: Acute Fatty Liver of Pregnancy, TTP: Thrombotic Thrombocytopenic Purpura. HELLP: Hemolysis, Elevated Liver enzymes, Low Platelet count, HUS: Hemolytic Uremic Syndrome.

The timing of some conditions might overlap between the end of one trimester and beginning of another and this table is just an estimation of timing.

Table 2. Differential based on three major groups: prerenal, intrarenal, and post-renal

Pre-renal	Intra renal	Post-renal
Abruptio placentae Hyperemesis gravidarum Puerperal sepsis Uterine hemorrhage	Acute postinfectious glomerulonephritis AFLP Cortical necrosis HELLP TTP Lupus nephritis	Calculus of urinary tract Gravid uterus

AFLP: Acute Fatty Liver of Pregnancy, TTP: Thrombotic Thrombocytopenic Purpura. HELLP: Hemolysis, Elevated Liver enzymes, Low Platelet count, HUS: Hemolytic Uremic Syndrome.

DIAGNOSIS

Preeclampsia/HELLP Syndrome, AFLP, and TTP/aHUS

Timely and accurate diagnosis of the cause of AKI is required to implement the proper therapies. A special emphasis is placed on differentiating preeclampsia/HELLP, AFLP, and TTP/aHUS since features may overlap, more than one process may be present, and management differs based on etiology.

Preeclampsia

Preeclampsia typically occurs in the late second and third trimester. The most frequently presenting symptom in severe preeclampsia is epigastric or right upper quadrant pain but other symptoms including nausea, vomiting, headache, visual disturbances, and sudden onset of edema can be seen as well.

Some of the serious maternal complications of preeclampsia includes HELLP (20%), DIC (10-20%), pulmonary edema (2-5%), and placental abruption (1-2%) [7]. Overt AKI is a rare complication of preeclampsia (1%) but is more frequently seen with HELLP (7-15%) [8, 9].

Revised ISSHP guidelines from 2014 defines preeclampsia as the following [10]:

Hypertension developing after 20 weeks of gestation combined with one or more of the following new-onset conditions:

1. Proteinuria (spot urine protein/creatinine >= 0.3 mg/mg) or >= 300 mg/day or at least 2+ on dipstick testing
2. Other maternal organ dysfunction
   a) Kidney impairment (serum creatinine >= 1.1 mg/dl)
   b) Liver involvement (elevated transaminases at least 2x upper limit +/- right upper quadrant or epigastric abdominal pain
   c) Neurological complications (including eclampsia, altered mental status, blindness, stroke, hyperreflexia with clonus, severe headaches accompanied by hyperreflexia, and persistent visual scotomata)
   d) Hematologic complications (thrombocytopenia [plt count below 150 * 10^9/l], DIC, hemolysis
3. Uteroplacental dysfunction
   a) Fetal growth restriction

Preeclampsia with HELLP Syndrome

Hemolysis, elevated liver enzymes, and low platelet count (HELLP) syndrome is now widely considered a variant of preeclampsia in which hepatic dysfunction and microangiopathic hemolytic anemia with thrombocytopenia predominate. HELLP affects women most commonly in the third trimester but may present in the second trimester or early postpartum period as well. The clinical presentation of HELLP can be very similar to that of preeclampsia (epigastric or right upper quadrant, nausea, vomiting, headache) but maternal complications of hepatic capsular hematoma and retinal detachment have also been reported [11].

The diagnosis of HELLP is based on the following laboratory criteria [12]:

1. The presence of microangiopathic hemolytic anemia as evidenced by schistocytes in blood smear, serum total bilirubin >= 1.2 mg/dl, LDH > 600 U/L, and low haptoglobin.
2. Increased liver transaminases and in particular, aspartate transaminase (ALT) > 70 U/L.
3. Thrombocytopenia, defined by platelet count <100 x 10^9/l.

Acute Fatty Liver of Pregnancy

Acute fatty liver of pregnancy (AFLP) occurs in the third trimester. It is characterized by sudden onset of acute liver failure with coagulopathy, and if left untreated progresses to fulminant liver failure. Early symptoms include fatigue, nausea, vomiting, abdominal pain, and fever. With progression, patients develop jaundice and hepatic encephalopathy.

AFLP can only made once viral hepatitis and biliary obstruction have been excluded. Laboratory findings reveal increased hepatic transaminases, increased alkaline phosphatase and bilirubin, coagulopathy (low fibrinogen, prolonged prothrombin time, depressed antithrombin III, and thrombocytopenia), hypoglycemia, and leukocytosis. Abdominal ascites may be present. A liver biopsy is not necessary to make a diagnosis and may be contraindicated due to the presence of coagulopathy. Hypertension is not a key feature in AFLP, though it may be present.

Thrombotic Thrombocytopenic Purpura

Thrombotic thrombocytopenic purpura affects women at any time during pregnancy. Clinical features are microangiopathic hemolytic anemia, severe thrombocytopenia, neurological symptoms, and fever. Diagnosis is made by serological testing demonstrating ADAMTS013 activity <10%. Hypertension is not a key feature of TTP or aHUS.

Atypical HUS

In contrast to TTP, aHUS occurs mainly in the first six months postpartum. aHUS have similar clinical features like TTP, but presents with more severe kidney dysfunction, and less neurological manifestations. Diagnosis is made with genetic testing for the complement cascade gene mutation.

Key Differentiating Features between Preeclampsia/ HELLP, AFLP, and TTP/aHUS

Key differentiating characteristics:

1. Hypertension:
   - Preeclampsia/HELLP > AFLP >> TTP/aHUS
2. Microangiopathic hemolytic anemia and thrombocytopenia:
   - TTP/aHUS >> HELLP >> AFLP
3. Coagulopathy and liver dysfunction:
   - AFLP ~ HELLP >> TTP/aHUS

OTHER ETIOLOGIES

Hyperemesis Gravidarum

Hyperemesis gravidarum causing AKI occurs most commonly in the first trimester of pregnancy. Patients present with severe and persistent nausea and vomiting leading to weight loss (exceeding 5% of pre-pregnancy body weight), hypokalemia, and metabolic alkalosis. Hemoconcentration, ketonuria, mild elevation of aminotransferases, and mild hyperthyroidism may also be seen.

Acute Cortical Necrosis

Clinical history often very useful in revealing the cause of acute cortical necrosis. Acute cortical necrosis can occur due to septic abortions typically early in pregnancy (before 20 weeks gestation), or from peripartum obstetrical complications such as placenta abruption, sepsis, amniotic emboli, and retained product of conception. Ultrasonography or computed tomography (CT) scan shows hypoechoic or hypodense areas in the renal cortex.

Acute Pyelonephritis

Gestational pyelonephritis is a serious condition associated with premature labor, IUGR, sepsis, and AKI. The patient presents with fever, chills, nausea and vomiting, flank pain, and costovertebral angle tenderness. Laboratory assessment will reveal peripheral leukocytosis, and urinalysis showing pyuria and bacteriuria +/- hematuria and WBC casts. The computed tomography scan may show normal kidney morphology, swelling in affected areas of the kidney, perinephric fat stranding (nonspecific), or perinephric abscess.

Urinary Tract Obstruction from Gravid Uterus

Obstruction occurs late in pregnancy due to the large uterus compressing the ureters. Physiologic hydronephrosis becomes more pronounced as pregnancy progresses, which makes differentiating from true obstruction difficult.

Diagnostic Testing

Workup of AKI in pregnancy requires a systematic approach guided by clinical suspicion in a timely manner. The differential must include both syndromes specific to pregnancy, as well as etiologies that affect the general population.

Physiologic changes in pregnancy may manifest in a shift in normal lab values. Due to increased GFR and plasma volume, serum creatinine typically decreases to 0.4-0.5 mg/dL. Therefore, a mild AKI may not be identified when pre-pregnancy or early pregnancy baseline values are unknown. Likewise, up to 300 mg/day of protein excretion may be a result of physiologic changes in pregnancy.

Diagnostic Testing

Pregnancy associated AKI

1. Urinalysis with microscopy, urine culture
2. Quantification of protein excretion: 24-hour collection or spot protein-to-creatinine ratio
3. Evaluation for microangiopathic hemolysis and thrombocytopenia: Complete blood count withperipheral blood smear
4. Evaluation for renal and liver function: Complete metabolic panel including serum aspartate aminotransferase (AST) and alanine aminotransferase (ALT), total bilirubin level, alkaline phosphatase, and prothrombin time test (PT/INR)
5. Total, direct, and indirect bilirubin, haptoglobin, lactate dehydrogenase
6. If evidence of MAHA and thrombocytopenia present, ADAMTS-13 and complement cascade gene mutation genetic test
7. Renal ultrasound

Non-Pregnancy Associated AKI

1. Urinary findings consistent with glomerulonephritis: Antinuclear antibody, complement C3, complement C4, total complement CH50, antineutrophil cytoplasmic antibody, double-stranded DNA antibody, etc.

Table 5. Diagnostic criteria of AKI according to RIFLE, AKIN, and KDIGO

The current diagnostic criteria of AKI are as follows:

1. RIFLE:
    1. Risk: SCr increase 1.5x or GFR decrease 25%; UOP < 0.5 ml/kg/h for 6 hrs
    2. Injury: SCr increase 2x or GFR decrease 50%; UOP < 0.5 ml/kg/h for 12 hrs
    3. Failure: SCr increase 3x or GFR decrease >= 75% or SCr>= 4 mg/dl (acute rise of >= 0.5 mg/dl); UOP < 0.3 ml/kg/h for 24 hrs or anuria for 12 hrs
    4. Loss: Persistent AKI = complete loss of renal function >4 weeks
    5. ESRD: End-stage kidney disease >3 months
2. AKIN:
    1. Defined by sudden decrease (in 48 hrs) of renal function: SCr of at least 0.3mg/dl or 1.5x of baseline; or by decrease UOP <0.5 ml/kg/h for more than 6 hrs
        1. Stage 1: SCr increase 0.3 or UOP < 0.5 ml/kg/h for 6 hrs
        2. Stage 2: SCr increase 2-3x baseline or UOP < 0.5 ml/kg/hr for 12 hrs
        3. Stage 3: SCr increase >3x or SCr>= 4 ml/dl with SCr increase at least >= 0.5 mg/dl or UOP < 0.3 ml/kg/h for 24 hrs or anuria for 12 hrs
3. KDIGO
    1. SCr increase by >= 0.3 mg/dl within 48 hrs or
    2. SCr increase to >= 1.5x baseline known or presumed to have occurred within the prior 7 days or
    3. Urine volume <0.5 ml/kg/h for 6 hrs
        1. Stage 1: 1.5-1.9x baseline or >0.3 mg/dl; UO < 0.5 ml/kg/h for 6-12 hrs
        2. Stage 2: 2.0-2.9x baseline; UO < 0.5 ml/kg/h for >12 hrs
        3. Stage 3: 3.0x baseline or increase of SCr to 4.0 mg/dl OR initiation of RRT, or in patients <18 years a decrease in eGFR to <35 ml/min per 1.73 m^2; UO < 0.3 ml/kg/h for >24 hrs OR anuria for >12 hrs

Different Diagnostic Criteria of AKI

While conventional criteria to define AKI (RIFLE, AKIN, KDIGO) has shown predictive value for in-hospital mortality compared to non-AKI patients, these methods have not yet been validated in pregnant women [13]. Therefore, there is no agreed-upon definition of AKI in pregnancy. However, many have suggested starting an investigation in women with serum creatinine >1 mg/dl or an increase of 0.5 mg/dl above baseline within 48 hours, particularly in the setting of oliguria or anuria.

Indications for Kidney Biopsy

Although pregnancy does not increase the risks of kidney biopsy above that of the general population when performed in patients with well-controlled blood pressure and normal coagulation indices, the clinical indication should be carefully reviewed when planning to biopsy during pregnancy. Kidney biopsy can be considered when sudden deterioration of renal function occurs before 32 weeks gestation with no obvious cause. The etiology may be a rapidly progressive glomerulonephritis that may respond to aggressive treatment with pulsed steroids, immunosuppressive therapy, and/or plasma exchange when diagnosed early. If AKI persists despite resolution of thrombocytopenia and hemolysis, a renal biopsy for confirmation of diagnosis and for prognosis is indicated. Finally, renal biopsy is recommended for symptomatic nephrotic syndrome before 32 weeks gestation to identify optimal therapy because the combination of pregnancy and nephrotic syndrome places the patient in a highly thrombogenic state. A renal biopsy is usually not performed after 32 weeks as the risk outweighs the benefit of establishing a diagnosis so late in pregnancy [14].

TREATMENT

PE/HELLP Syndrome

Delivery is the only definitive treatment for preeclampsia and HELLP syndrome. The timing of delivery should be based on optimizing fetal outcomes while minimizing maternal risks. After the hypertension and preeclampsia interventional trial at near term (HYPITAT) trials, there is consensus that women with preeclampsia before 37 weeks can be managed expectantly in hopes of further fetal growth and maturation [15, 16]. However, indications for prompt delivery include the following: progressive maternal organ dysfunction, inability to control BP, failure of fetal growth or concern about fetal status, and gestational age beyond 37 weeks [12].

AFLP

Early diagnosis, supportive care, and prompt and urgent delivery are the mainstay treatment of AFLP. Without prompt delivery, AFLP progresses to fulminant liver failure and death. Administration of glucose to achieve glycemic control, correction of coagulopathy with blood products, and a low protein diet and lactulose for hepatic encephalopathy treats the metabolic dysregulation seen in AFLP. Spontaneous kidney recovery typically follows delivery but may require temporary kidney replacement therapy.

TTP/aHUS

The first line treatment of TTP is plasmapheresis with fresh frozen plasma as the replacement fluid to remove circulating ADAMTS-13 antibodies and to replenish the deficient ADAMTS-13 protease. High dose corticosteroids and other immunosuppressive agents can be considered for severe or refractory TTP.

The monoclonal humanized IgG antibody eculizumab is first line therapy for aHUS. Response to therapy is determined by the normalization of platelet count and lactate dehydrogenase level, with at least a 25% improvement in serum creatinine. If possible, platelet transfusions should be avoided due to the increased risk of microvascular thrombosis in the setting of TMA (Thrombotic Microangiopathy) syndromes.

Hyperemesis Gravidarum

Isotonic intravenous fluids will correct the volume depletion, underlying acid-base, and electrolyte abnormalities. Women should try to become aware of and avoid environmental triggers and foods that may exacerbate nausea and vomiting. Pyridoxine-doxylamine succinate, diphenhydramine, meclizine, prochlorperazine, metoclopramide, ondansetron, and glucocorticoids may be used as antiemetics. Controversies about a potential small increase in risk of congenital abnormalities before 10 weeks gestation should be discussed for ondansetron. Glucocorticoids should be used after the first trimester.

Pyelonephritis

Women with pyelonephritis in pregnancy should be hospitalized for parenteral antibiotics. Cephalosporins and penicillins are generally safe and effective in pregnancy. Therapy should be continued for 14 days after the patient has become afebrile. Suppressive therapy with a low-dose antibiotic should be continued until 4-6 weeks postpartum [17].

Need for Dialysis and Outcomes

The indications for dialysis for AKI in pregnancy are similar to that of the general population. Symptoms of uremia (encephalopathy, asterixis, and pericarditis), hyperkalemia, metabolic acidosis, and volume overload refractory to initial medical therapy warrant prompt initiation of dialysis.

Based on a large 15-year study of deliveries in Ontario, Canada, the incidence of pregnancy related AKI requiring dialysis is low (cumulative incidence of 1 per 10,000). AKI requiring dialysis is nearly four times more likely in women with a major medical complication during pregnancy such as preeclampsia, thrombotic microangiopathy, pregnancy-related liver disease, sepsis, postpartum hemorrhage, etc. The mortality rate of women with AKI requiring dialysis was 4.3%, compared to 0.01% in women without kidney injury. Of women who survived, 3.9% remained dependent on chronic dialysis after 90 days postpartum [18].

References

[1] Gilbert SJ, Weiner DE, Gipson DS, Perazella MA, Tonelli M, *National Kidney Foundation. National Kidney Foundation's primer on kidney diseases*. Sixth edition. ed. Philadelphia, PA: Elsevier/Saunders; 2014. xvii, 646 pages

[2] Beers K, Wen HH, Saha A, Chauhan K, Dave M, Coca S, et al. Racial and Ethnic Disparities in Pregnancy-Related Acute Kidney Injury. *Kidney360.* 2020;1(3):169-78.

[3] Jim B, Garovic VD. Acute Kidney Injury in Pregnancy. *Semin Nephrol.* 2017;37(4):378-385.

[4] Gonzalez Suarez ML, Kattah A, Grande JP, Garovic V. Renal Disorders in Pregnancy: core Curriculum 2019. *Am J Kidney Dis*. 2019;73(1):119-130.

[5] Shah S, Meganathan K, Christianson AL, Harrison K, Leonard AC, Thakar CV. Pregnancy-Related Acute Kidney Injury in the United States: Clinical Outcomes and Health Care Utilization. *Am J Nephrol.* 2020;51(3):216-226.

[6] Mussap M, Noto A. Renal disorders in pregnancy. *J Lab Precis Med.* 2020;5.

[7] Prakash J, Ganiger VC. Acute kidney injury in pregnancy-specific disorders. *Indian J Nephrol.* 2017;27(4):258-270.

[8] Kuklina EV, Ayala C, Callaghan WM. Hypertensive disorders and severe obstetric morbidity in the United States. *Obstet Gynecol.* 2009;113(6):1299-1306.

[9] Sibai BM, Ramadan MK, Usta I, Salama M, Mercer BM, Friedman SA. Maternal morbidity and mortality in 442 pregnancies with hemolysis, elevated liver enzymes, and low platelets (HELLP syndrome). *Am J Obstet Gynecol.* 1993;169(4):1000-1006.

[10] Claramonte Nieto M, Meler Barrabes E, Garcia Martínez S, Gutiérrez Prat M, Serra Zantop B. Impact of aging on obstetric outcomes: defining advanced maternal age in Barcelona. *BMC Pregnancy Childbirth.* 2019;19(1):342.

[11] Gul A, Aslan H, Cebeci A, Polat I, Ulusoy S, Ceylan Y. Maternal and fetal outcomes in HELLP syndrome complicated with acute renal failure. *Ren Fail.* 2004;26(5):557-562. d

[12] Brown MA. CHAPTER 43 - Pregnancy with Preexisting Kidney Disease. In: Floege J, Johnson RJ, Feehally J, eds. *Comprehensive Clinical Nephrology.* 4th ed. Philadelphia: Mosby; 2010:516-526.

[13] Luo X, Jiang L, Du B, Wen Y, Wang M, Xi X; Beijing Acute Kidney Injury Trial (BAKIT) workgroup. A comparison of different diagnostic criteria of acute kidney injury in critically ill patients. *Crit Care.* 2014;18(4):R144. d

[14] Lindheimer MD, Davison JM. Renal biopsy during pregnancy: 'to b . . . or not to b . . .?'. *Br J Obstet Gynaecol.* 1987;94(10):932-934.

[15] Koopmans CM, Bijlenga D, Groen H, et al; HYPITAT study group. Induction of labour versus expectant monitoring for gestational hypertension or mild pre-eclampsia after 36 weeks' gestation (HYPITAT): a multicentre, open-label randomised controlled trial. *Lancet.* 2009;374(9694):979-988.

[16] van Baaren G-J, Broekhuijsen K, van Pampus MG, et al; HYPITAT-II Study Group. An economic analysis of immediate delivery and expectant monitoring in women with hypertensive disorders of pregnancy, between 34 and 37 weeks of gestation (HYPITAT-II). *BJOG.* 2017;124(3):453-461.

[17] Jolley JA, Wing DA. Pyelonephritis in pregnancy: an update on treatment options for optimal outcomes. *Drugs.* 2010;70(13):1643-1655.

[18] Hildebrand AM, Liu K, Shariff SZ, et al. Characteristics and Outcomes of AKI Treated with Dialysis during Pregnancy and the Postpartum Period. *J Am Soc Nephrol.* 2015;26(12):3085-3091.

In: Issues in Kidney Disease – Acute Kidney Injury
Editors: S. Z. Fadem and A. Arslan Yousuf Awan

ISBN: 978-1-68507-002-1

Chapter 19

ACUTE KIDNEY INJURY AFTER KIDNEY TRANSPLANTATION

Amna Ilahe[1,3], MD, Amanda Condon[2], Van N. Ngo[2] and Irfan A. Agha[1,2,*], MD

[1]Dallas Renal Group, PA, Dallas, TX, USA
[2]Medical City Dallas Transplant Institute, Dallas, TX, USA
[3]Methodist Dallas Medical Center Transplant Center, Dallas, TX, USA

ABSTRACT

Acute Kidney Injury (AKI) is commonly encountered in patients with kidney transplantation. The post-transplant milieu introduces several variables that portend unique risks making the allograft vulnerable to AKI. Some of these variables, like the predisposition to alloimmune injury or vascular anastomotic catastrophes, may lead to damage or even loss of the allograft in short order.

The clinical scenarios precipitating AKI after transplant differ somewhat based on the time distance from the transplant surgery itself. This allows us to develop a nuanced clinical approach to the diagnosis and management of commonly encountered AKI syndromes in this difficult patient population. The salient risk profile a day after transplant surgery is very different from the predisposing factors encountered six months after transplant. But at any stage, a delay in diagnosis and management of AKI in these patients may lead to potentially irreversible damage. Therefore, each instance of AKI in a kidney transplant recipient must be investigated expeditiously, thoroughly, and systematically to correctly identify the cause and arrive at the appropriate intervention.

Keywords: acute kidney injury, acute renal failure, kidney transplantation, Delayed Graft Function, acute rejection

* Corresponding Author's E-mail: iagha@dallasrenalgroup.com.

INTRODUCTION

From the time an allograft is harvested from a donor and placed into a recipient, it faces a hostile mechanical, metabolic, and immune environment. This makes it uniquely vulnerable to various forms of injury and, in many cases, this manifests as an acute kidney injury.

AKI after renal transplantation is therefore quite commonly encountered after kidney transplantation [1]. Events transpiring in the initial days after transplantation cast long shadows on eventual allograft function and longevity [2]. Therefore, AKI after transplantation requires thorough analysis and quick action to protect the precious allograft.

Given the peculiar circumstances that must be navigated in a kidney transplant recipient, it is most useful to break down evaluation of AKI and management outlines based on proximity to the transplant event itself. These arbitrary time frames are devised to conceptualize the various factors operative in driving kidney injury after transplant, and a fair bit of overlap may be observed.

AKI IN THE FIRST 48 HOURS

AKI is not uncommon in the first 24-48 hours after transplantation, and each instance must be navigated as an emergent situation. Mostly, this injury is driven by rapidly correctable variables but, in rare instances, vascular anastomotic complications that threaten the allograft can occur and must always be suspected and excluded. The cost of failure to appreciate such complications in a timely fashion may deny the patient benefit of the very narrow window that exists for any impactful therapeutic intervention.

Precise definition of AKI in this time window may be tricky. Traditionally, kidney function (and dysfunction) has been defined by assessing two complementary aspects: urine output and clearance markers.

In the immediate postoperative environment, the creatinine level may fluctuate based on many factors. These include pre-transplant residual function, the proximity of the last dialysis treatment to the transplant event, as well as the degree of renal function recovery after transplantation. As an example, if the patient were dialyzed right before transplant, the creatinine may creep up some after transplant, but this increase may just reflect equilibration after dialysis and may not reflect an AKI per se.

Similarly, the urine output may vary widely based on many factors. At times, a seemingly reasonable urine output may be deceptive – a patient undergoing preemptive transplantation may retain decent urine output due to preserved native kidney urine output, masking allograft oliguria after transplant. Therefore, each of these variables must be interpreted carefully with astute clinical and laboratory correlation to correctly appreciate the situation.

The most proximate factor alerting the clinician to AKI in the immediate postoperative period is decrease in urine flow, and an approach to such an event is outlined in Figure 1. The first step is to carefully assess hemodynamics and volume status. At the same time, it must be ensured that the Foley catheter is draining adequately and is not kinked or clotted. Should restoration of the volume not correct the issue, a diuretic challenge may be indicated. If this is not successful, one must worry about a renal issue (delayed graft function or DGF, arterial, or venous thrombosis) as well as issues with the ureteroneocystostomy (leaks or obstruction). A quick bedside kidney ultrasound with dopplers helps settle many of these issues expeditiously with a high degree of sensitivity.

Should the evaluation reveal adequate volume status, functional foley catheter, patent anastomosis, and absence of leaks, one must settle with a diagnosis of DGF.

HYPOVOLEMIA

Volume depletion commonly leads to oliguria and AKI soon after transplant. Volume depletion is multifactorial. The patients may have been dialyzed and ultrafiltered right before surgery. It is our practice to leave patients slightly above their "dry weight" should they need dialysis in the immediate pre-operative period. Hemodynamic shifts during surgery, as well as intra-operative bleeding with suboptimal resuscitation, may contribute. Use of intraoperative lymphocyte depletion agents (Thymoglobulin, Campath) may on occasion lead to cytokine release, capillary leak, and hypotension. Many centers dose high dose loop diuretics after surgery to promote urine flow. This may at times lead to an exaggerated response with resultant hypovolemia.

Judiciously dosed fluid boluses of isotonic saline followed by an adjustment of the fluid replacement rate should correct hypovolemia and restore urine flow. Attention must be diverted to other possibilities should hypovolemia persist despite appropriate fluid resuscitation.

Bleeding

Bleeding is usually encountered in the immediate postoperative period. Significant bleeding may cause signs of hypovolemia and shock. Urine output may not be a good indicator of the volume status in many cases this early after transplant as the allograft function may not have established. Apart from signs of volume depletion, examination may reveal an obvious bulge or severe tenderness over the transplanted kidney. Should there be a drain in the surgical bed, diagnosis is straightforward. Severe bleeding causing hemorrhagic shock may necessitate re-exploration, control, and evacuation of hematoma.

Less severe cases of bleeding can be stabilized conservatively and are usually self-limiting. One must ensure the resulting hematoma is not compressing the allograft parenchyma or ureter. In the latter scenario, it can cause obstructive kidney injury. These hematomas may need to be drained either surgically in the operation room or percutaneously by the interventional radiology service.

Acute Arterial or Venous Thrombosis

Transplant renal artery or vein thrombosis is a rare but catastrophic complication and requires expedient action. The window of opportunity to salvage an allograft after such an event is narrow.

Some clinical scenarios may prompt a higher index of suspicion for transplant renal artery thrombosis. For example, difficult arterial or venous anastomoses due to technical issues, or the presence of multiple donor arteries requiring multiple anastomoses, may alert the transplant team to a higher risk for this serious complication.

Hyper-coagulable states (antiphospholipid syndrome, factor V Leiden mutation, etc.) predispose to transplant renal arterial or venous thrombosis [3]. Transplant renal vein thrombosis occurs more frequently in patients with DGF [4]. Perinephric hematomas or fluid collections may compress the transplant vessels and lead to thrombotic complications.

The usual presentation is of oliguria despite adequate volume status and may be attended by pain over the allograft. The diagnosis is usually picked up on bedside transplant kidney ultrasound with Doppler examination [5] and represents a surgical emergency. In equivocal cases, when the ultrasound does not provide clarity, a radionuclide scan can be performed. However, it is of crucial importance not to delay action waiting for confirmatory tests should the clinical suspicion be strong. In such cases, urgent re-exploration must be considered. In extreme cases of transplant renal vein thrombosis, one may encounter allograft rupture.

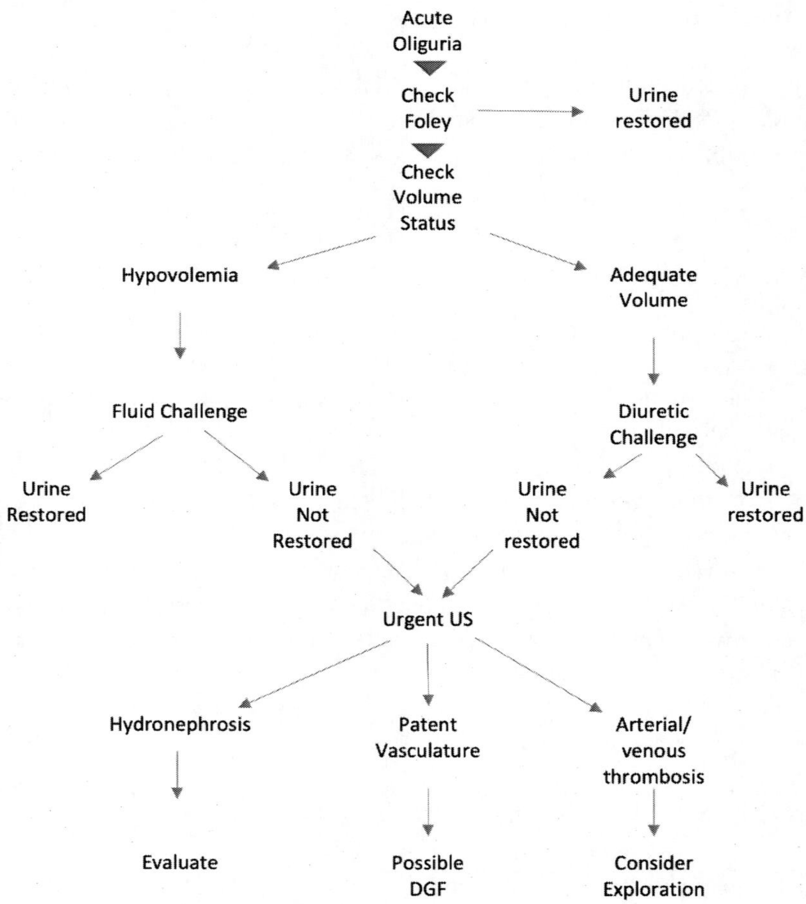

Figure 1. AKI in the immediate post-operative period – a simplified approach.

An Aside on Delayed Graft Function

Delayed Graft Function (DGF) is a complicated, multifactorial AKI process peculiar to kidney transplantation. Though variously defined, a widely accepted version is allograft dysfunction necessitating dialysis within the first week after transplant [6]. This definition pegs DGF to the peri-transplant environment and separates it from events happening later in the post-transplant course.

DGF is not uncommon – incidence of DGF is about 30.8% in recipients of deceased donors in the United States [7]. This predictably increases with more challenging allografts. For example, DGF in kidneys donated after cardiac death may be as high as 45—55% [8]. As a corollary, DGF is uncommon after living donor transplantation. These differences in incidence shed some light on the underlying pathobiological mechanisms of DGF. This sentinel peri-transplant phenomenon is an extremely complicated process and established DGF leads to significantly increased death censored graft loss [2].

Factors related to the donor, the preservation time, as well as dynamics and factors related to the recipient all impact graft function. Donor age, sex (higher incidence for females), and high terminal creatinine affect DGF. Length of cold ischemia time, warm ischemia time (especially in donation after cardiac-death scenarios), preservation solution, and use of pulsatile perfusion may affect graft function. Recipient factors that place the allograft at a disadvantage like dialysis vintage, diabetes, hypertension, obesity, and small for size organs all impact DGF rates [9-11].

DGF is initiated by ischemic injury sustained during the organ harvest process. Deprived of oxygen, the tubular epithelial cells deplete existing adenosine triphosphate (ATP), which is converted into adenosine monophosphate (AMP). Sustained hypoxia leads to further breakdown of AMP to adenine nucleotides, which readily diffuse out of the cells, making re-synthesis of AMP and ATP after re-perfusion difficult [12]. Breakdown of AMP also generates hypoxanthine, which is converted to xanthine by xanthine-oxidase generating hydrogen peroxide and superoxide, leading to oxidant injury. The cytosolic calcium levels increase as the endoplasmic reticulum is unable to sequester it and cellular extrusion of calcium is paralyzed. Increased cytosolic calcium activates key enzymes that disrupt the cellular cytoskeleton.

Ischemia also affects the vascular endothelial cells. Ischemic stress to the kidney during the harvesting process leads to release of various damage-associated molecular patterns (DAMPs) like hypomethylated deoxyribonucelotide acid (DNA), High Mobility Group Box 1 (HMGB1), heat shock proteins, etc. [13, 14] by the vascular endothelial cells. These DAMPs signal through toll-like receptors (TLRs) and upregulate the cellular inflammasome resulting in an inflammatory milieu. Inflammatory cells including polymorphonuclear cells, the monocyte-macrophage system, and lymphocytes are trafficked in. The complement system has emerged as an important mediator of this inflammatory response. The sublethal membrane attack complex (sMAC) damages target membranes while C5a and C3a fragments, potent anaphylatoxins, are important in recruitment of the inflammatory response [12]. This cross-talk may also explain the higher incidence of cellular rejection in patients with DGF [2].

As a result of these ischemic and inflammatory injuries, the tubular epithelial cells suffer cytoskeletal disruption. At the same time, apoptosis and necrosis related cell programs are invoked. At the earliest stages, this may take the form of loss of cell polarity and integrity of the brush border. With higher degrees of injuries, the tubular cells die and full-blown acute tubular necrosis (ATN) sets in [12].

Some of these mechanistic insights have been utilized in an attempt to decrease the incidence and severity of ischemia/reperfusion injury (IRI). Cold preservation and machine pulsatile perfusion have been used to mitigate DGF [15, 16]. Preservation solutions like University of Wisconsin Solution contain adenosine and allopurinol as additives. Adenosine is thought to support re-synthesis of intracellular ATP during reperfusion. Allopurinol prevents conversion of hypoxanthine to xanthine thereby decreasing the generation of reactive oxygen species. Both are thought to be helpful in mitigating ischemia-reperfusion injury [12, 17, 18].

There is no specific therapy for DGF. Like ATN, it must run its course. However, as noted above, DGF is associated with a higher risk of acute rejection [2]. Immunosuppression must be carefully monitored to adequately deny alloimmune activity while avoiding drug related toxicity. Persistent DGF, especially more than 7-10 days, merits an allograft biopsy to exclude co-existent rejection.

AKI in the First Few Weeks after Transplant

Once the critical first and second days after transplant are negotiated, the patient is usually transferred out of the intensive care setting and the recovery process begins in earnest. A persistent decline in creatinine as steady urine flow establishes signifies improving allograft function. The Foley catheter is removed at the post-operative day 3 to 5, based on center practices and preferences. Most uncomplicated kidney transplant recipients are discharged from the hospital around the fifth post-operative day.

This sequence is disrupted should the kidney function not improve or should it deteriorate after initial improvement. This is the time when alloimmune risk to the allograft may manifest as rejection. Some glomerular diseases (e.g., hemolytic uremic syndrome due to factor H deficiency or anti-glomerular basement membrane or anti-GBM disease) may recur early and lead to AKI.

Careful analysis of the clinical and laboratory data is imperative to assess for this and proceed to biopsy to exclude this potentially organ threatening complication. A simplified approach to AKI in the first few weeks after transplantation is presented in Figure 2.

In the first few weeks after transplant, the patient remains quite susceptible to hemodynamic shifts. As allograft function improves, the excess water and salt accumulated pre-transplant as well as during the salt loading experienced in the immediate post-transplant period are mobilized. Blood pressure improves and the antihypertensive regimen needs to be repeatedly adjusted to avoid hypotension and to maintain adequate perfusion of the allograft. Should the effective perfusion pressure not be adequate, the allograft function may deteriorate. This, if identified and controlled early, is readily reversible. However, persistent hypotension may lead to renal ischemic injury as well as other obvious deleterious consequences.

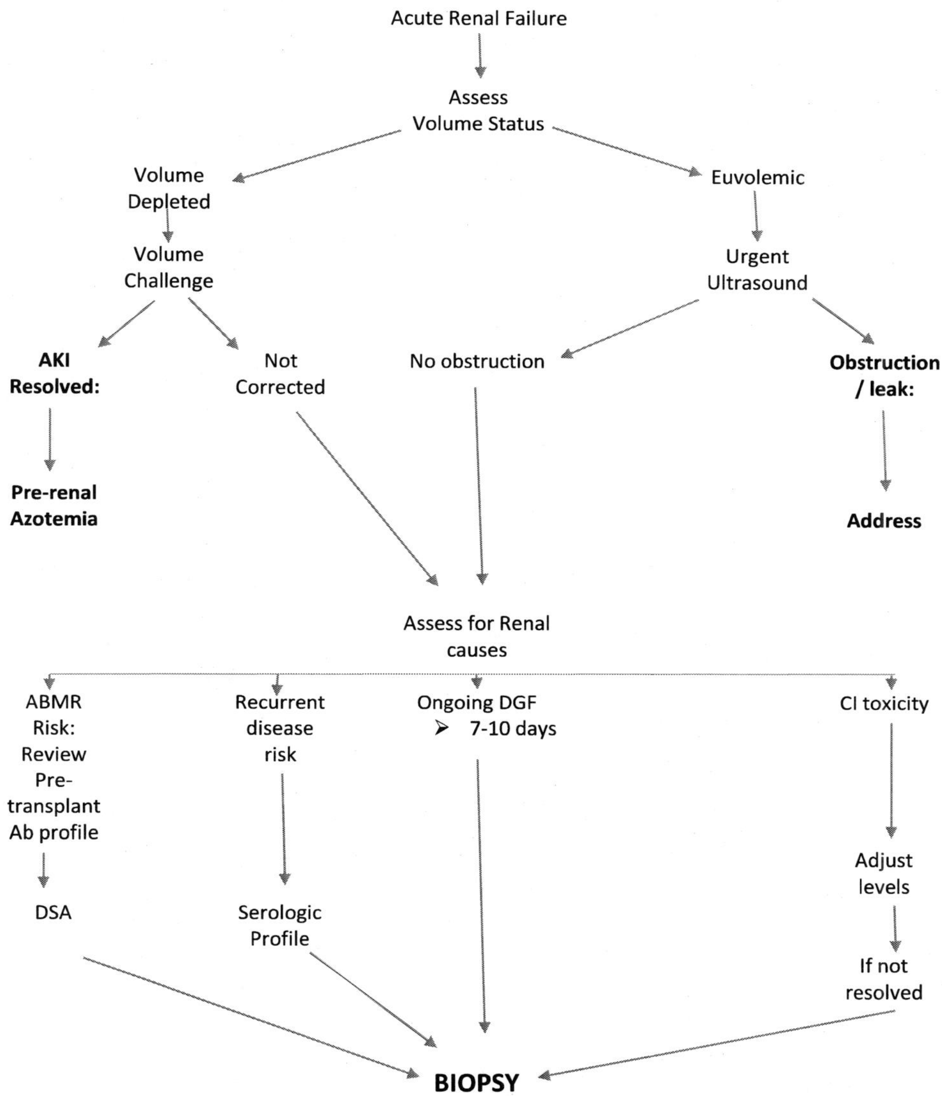

Figure 2. AKI in the First Few Weeks after Transplant.

An Aside on Calcineurin Inhibitor Use and Toxicity

Calcineurin Inhibitors (CNI) form the backbone of immunosuppression for more than 90% of transplants occurring in the US [19]. Most programs introduce CNIs within the first 48 hours of transplantation. Levels are driven to the desired therapeutic range within a few days, optimally prior to discharge. CNI- induced nephrotoxicity is an established adverse effect of cyclosporine and tacrolimus and can manifest as acute or chronic nephrotoxicity.

Acute nephrotoxicity has been associated with high systemic CNI exposure in the immediate post-transplantation phase [20, 21]. Acute nephrotoxicity is less common in the current era of transplantation due to advances in induction immunosuppression and multimodal maintenance immunosuppression, which has allowed for the reduction of target troughs of CNIs. However, understanding the mechanisms and identification of CNI-induced acute nephrotoxicity is important for optimal patient management.

Both cyclosporine and tacrolimus have narrow therapeutic indexes necessitating therapeutic drug monitoring to avoid toxicity and ensure efficacy. CNIs demonstrate high intra- and interpatient pharmacokinetic variability due to many factors that influence absorption, distribution, metabolism, and elimination. The absorption of cyclosporine and tacrolimus within the gastrointestinal tract is incomplete and variable and can be influenced by food consumption, gastrointestinal motility impairment, and diarrhea.

Genetic polymorphisms within the Cytochrome P450 3A5 (CYP3A5) system have been shown to significantly alter metabolism of tacrolimus causing slow or rapid metabolism of tacrolimus [22]. The CYP3A5*1 polymorphism that causes rapid metabolism of tacrolimus is more common in African American (45-80%), Asian (15-35%), and Hispanic (13-26%) individuals [23]. Patients who are rapid metabolizers of tacrolimus are exposed to higher peak plasma concentrations (C_{max}) and experience increased rates of adverse effects. Higher tacrolimus dose requirements have been associated with chronic CNI-associated nephrotoxicity and overall worse transplant outcomes [23].

Use of CYP3A4 inhibitors (like verapamil or ketoconazole) to spare CNI dose has been utilized by some programs, but it is not recommended due to the risk of supratherapeutic troughs as well as the possibility of introducing other drug interactions into a patient's medication regimen.

A new formulation of once-daily extended-release tacrolimus (LCPT) was designed to delay the absorption of tacrolimus along the gastrointestinal tract, eliminating the variability of increased absorptions by rapid metabolizers. Patients can achieve the same therapeutic trough concentrations while lowering the peak plasma concentration of tacrolimus. Although current data do not describe an improvement in CNI-induced acute nephrotoxicity with the use of LCPT, it may reduce utilization of CYP3A4 inhibitors, which are commonly used in this patient population and often result in supratherapeutic CNI troughs.

Acute CNI nephrotoxicity often manifests as increased serum creatinine and hyperkalemia, which resolve after dose reduction or discontinuation of CNI. The exact mechanisms by which CNIs induce nephrotoxicity are not fully understood. The majority of what is known is derived from animal models evaluating the effects of varying doses of cyclosporine or tacrolimus on renal physiology. Acute nephrotoxicity due to CNIs has been linked to acute arteriolopathy, which includes vasoconstriction of the afferent and efferent renal arteriole, activation of the renin-angiotensin-aldosterone system (RAAS), and a reduction in factors associated with vasodilation such as prostacyclin and nitric oxide [24, 25]. The ultimate effect of this vasoconstriction results in a reduction of renal blood flow and decrease in the glomerular filtration rate (GFR).

CNI-dependent vasoconstriction is concentration-dependent, reversible, and believed to not confer any long-term complications if remedied with appropriate dose reductions. This is especially important when considering the impact vasoconstriction and reduced glomerular filtration can have on a recovering allograft in the first few weeks after transplantation. Given this risk of arteriolar vasoconstriction and decreased GFR with acute toxicity of CNIs, delayed introduction of CNIs in patients at risk for or having sustained DGF has been theorized. The idea was to keep CNIs off and allow better perfusion of the allograft and promote recovery [26]. However, in recent practice, a delay in initiation of CNIs has not translated into a quicker resolution of DGF [27]. Indeed, there is a higher risk of breakthrough rejection as institution of appropriately robust immunosuppression is being delayed. Therefore, this strategy has fallen out of favor. It is not appropriate to delay CNI administration during the allograft recovery period, especially if the patient has not received depleting antibody as induction, elevating risk of breakthrough rejection. Use of depleting antibodies (like Thymoglobulin or Campath) may widen the window or provide some cover to modulate tacrolimus levels [28, 29].

In the modern era of immunosuppression, the availability of several agents has provided more options and the possibility of individualizing immunosuppression. Though acute calcineurin toxicity is largely reversible, long-term exposure in certain patients may not be optimal. Similarly, at times, calcineurin inhibitors may lead to endothelial toxicity resulting in a thrombotic microangiopathy [30]. In such circumstances, calcineurin inhibitors may need to be avoided altogether or substituted with alternate agents.

The mammalian target of rapamycin (mTOR) inhibitors (sirolimus, everolimus) emerged as potential alternate anchors of immunosuppression. The ELITE-Symphony trial attempted to test this theory by comparing low-dose tacrolimus, low- and standard-dose cyclosporine, and low-dose sirolimus in renal transplant recipients. Though the DGF rates were lower in the sirolimus arm compared to tacrolimus, the acute rejection rates, patient and allograft survival were better in the tacrolimus arm. Tacrolimus also demonstrated a better profile when it came to treatment failure [31]. The risk of acute rejection and delayed wound healing issues with sirolimus have made it relatively unattractive as a frontline immunosuppression agent.

Belatacept is a co-stimulation blocking agent that has emerged as a useful maintenance immunosuppression agent [32, 33]. It is frequently utilized to minimize or avoid nephrotoxic effects of CNIs where necessary. It has also been successfully used in cases where thrombotic microangiopathy was suspected to be a complication of CNI exposure [34].

Acute Rejection in the First Few Weeks after Transplantation

In the modern era of transplantation, there has been a steady decline in the incidence of acute rejection in the first year after transplantation and presently hovers just below 8% [19]. This is welcome news, but acute rejection remains a risk that needs to be carefully assessed and stratified in every transplant recipient.

Ever since cross matches became mainstream after the seminal work of Paul Terasaki [35], and subsequent refinements in technique as well as increasing sophistication in understanding and detecting donor specific antibodies, hyperacute rejection has become exceedingly rare. Similarly, with refinements in immunosuppression, the incidence of acute cellular or antibody-mediated rejection in the first few weeks after transplantation remain quite low.

Early Cell-Mediated Rejection

Cell-mediated rejection (CMR) early after transplant is likely through direct antigen presentation (presentation of alloantigen by donor derived passenger antigen presenting cells in the context of MHC Class II molecules to recipient CD4 T Helper cells). This can potentially happen days to weeks after transplantation but in today's robust immunosuppression milieu (Over 90% patients receive induction immunosuppression – 70% with depleting antibodies and 20% interleukin 2 receptor antagonist) the incidence of early T cell mediated rejection (TCMR) remains rather low.

As noted above, DGF engages the innate immune system with cross-talk with the adaptive immune response. There is a higher incidence of acute cellular rejection noted in patients who have suffered DGF but overall, it is relatively unusual to find CMR this early after transplantation. A high index of suspicion must nevertheless be kept in patients with prolonged DGF. A surveillance biopsy is performed in patients with DGF who fail to improve in 7-10 days. Obviously, in patients who demonstrate deterioration of allograft function in which obvious pre- and post-renal causes have been excluded, a biopsy must be obtained.

Acute TCMR is characterized by infiltration of the interstitium by T-lymphocytes and cells of the monocyte–macrophage lineage. The T cells infiltrate into the interstitium by traversing the allograft microcirculation and are of the CD4 and CD8 phenotypes as well as effector T memory cells. These T cells elaborate several cytokines, most notably interferon gamma which further upregulates several genes including several chemokines as well as human leukocyte antigen (HLA) class I and class II molecules, promoting further signaling and inflammation [36].

Table 1. Banff Classification of T Cell-Mediated Rejection (adapted from reference 37)

Feature	**0**	**1**	**2**	**3**
Interstitial Inflammation in unscarred cortical parenchyma (i)	None or <10%	10-25%	26-50%	50%
Mononuclear cells in tubules -Tubilitis (t)	None or a single focus of tubulitis only	Foci with 1-4 cells/tubular cross section	Foci with 5-10 cells/tubular cross section	Foci >10 cells/tubular cross section OR >2 ares of TBM destruction + i ≥ 2 and t2 elsewhere
Vasculitis (v)	No arteritis	Mild – moderate Intimal arteritis in at least one arterial cross section	Severe Intimal Arteritis > 25% lumen lost in at least one arterial cross section	Transmural arteritis and/or arterial fibrinoid change
TCMR Grades				
Borderline	t > 0 BUT i ≤1 and v=0			
IA	t 2 AND i ≥ 2			
IB	t 3 and i ≥ 2			
IIA	V1 regardless of scores for t and i			
IIIA	V2 regardless of scores for t and i			
IIIB	V3 regardless of scores for t and i			

TBM: tubular basement membrane.

This accumulation of monocytes, macrophages, and T cells in the interstitium is a major component of the TCMR and is appreciated as the "i" score in the Banff Scheme (see Table 1). As TCMR progresses, the epithelium begins to de-differentiate and eventually the basement membrane is injured allowing the T cells to infiltrate the tubules. This is identified as tubulitis – the "t" score of the Banff Scheme.

Acute cellular rejection is diagnosed based on histopathological criteria. The various features taken into consideration and the stages of acute TCMR are summarized in Table 1 above.

The management paradigm of cell-mediated rejection has not changed much through the decades. Most centers would initiate therapy with high dose steroids and, in higher grades of rejection, add lymphocyte depleting agents like thymoglobulin. Response to therapy and eventual outcomes of pure TCMR are favorable [38] further emphasizing early recognition and appropriate therapy.

Early Antibody-Mediated Rejection

As noted above, refinements in antibody detection and cross match techniques have rendered hyperacute and early antibody-mediated rejection (AMR) uncommon. However, we are transplanting more complicated patients, many of whom are sensitized and may harbor small amounts of HLA antibodies directed towards the donor. These antibodies may not be enough to affect a meaningful change on cross match testing but after transplantation, may launch a memory (anamnestic) response against donor antigens of interest. Also, centers transplanting patients requiring HLA antibody desensitization or ABO antibody reduction assume a higher risk of antibody-mediated rejection.

It is instructive here to review generation of HLA antibodies and the mechanisms that lead to early active ABMR. B cells are produced in the bone marrow and undergo scrutiny to delete autoreactive cells. After this program of central tolerance is complete, B cells travel to the secondary lymphoid organs. On exposure to antigen-presenting cells, some of the follicular B cells are activated, enter the germinal center reaction, and eventually develop memory B cells and plasmablasts. They also generate a specific phenotype of plasma cells called long-lived plasma cells (LLPC, CD19-, CD38+ and CD138 hi). These travel back to the bone marrow and can survive in the bone marrow niche for decades. This is illustrated in Figure 3.

After exposure to HLA antigens (by way of pregnancy, blood transfusions, or previous transplantation, for example), the B cells of interest experience follicular reaction and generate plasma cells as well as memory B cells. The plasma cells produce steady antibody for long periods of time. It is this antibody that we pick during the pre-transplant workup. If present in significant amounts, these antibodies may impact cross match results, rendering the transplant high risk and mandating further evaluation and consideration.

At times, these antibodies are present in smaller amounts, not sufficient to impact cross match results. However, should there be a good quantity of memory B cells present as well, then upon exposure to antigen of interest (in case an organ with the mismatched antigen of interest is transplanted) these memory cells can mount a robust and rapid antibody generation response that may lead to early active ABMR.

An antibody-mediated rejection through such a mechanism is usually a pure antibody-mediated rejection phenotype and manifests within the first few weeks after transplant. The HLA antibodies target the glomerular and peritubular capillary endothelium setting up intense microvascular inflammation. In most cases, these antibodies are efficient at fixing complement, which manifests as marked C4d positivity on immunofluorescence. The severe peritubular capillary inflammation may lead to tubular ischemia that may manifest as ATN. In severe cases, marked endothelial damage may present as a thrombotic microangiopathy.

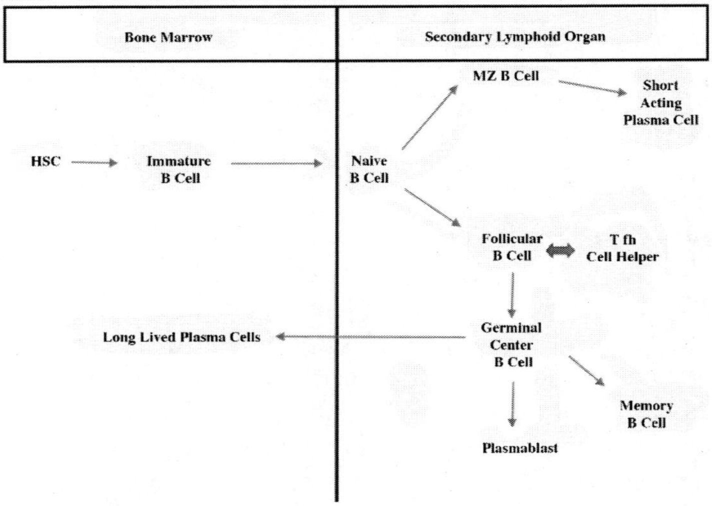

HSC: Hematopoietic Stem cell.
MZ: Marginal Zone.
Tfh: T follicular help cell.

Figure 3. Origins of antibody producing cells.

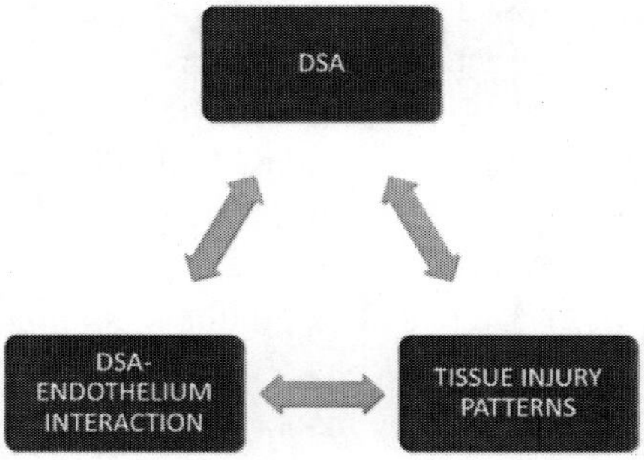

Figure 4. Cardinal features of ABMR diagnosis.

Thus, the operative paradigm of early active ABMR is generation of antibody from a pre-existing repertoire of memory B cells, rapid escalation of the antibody response, interaction of the antibody with donor glomerular and peritubular capillary endothelia and damage thereof leading to various characteristic morphological patterns and allograft dysfunction. The Banff Scheme captures on these concepts, with the diagnostic formulation hinging on three cardinal features of donor-specific alloantibody (DSA), evidence of interaction of the DSA with the endothelium and generation of specific injury patterns, as illustrated in Figure 4. The Banff categorization of Active ABMR is presented in Table 2.

Table 2. Banff Classification of Active Antibody Mediated Rejection (adapted from reference 37)

Feature	0	1	2	3
Glomerulitis "g" Score	None	<25%	26-75%	75%
Peritubular capillaritis "ptc" Score	<3 leukocytes	At least 1 leukocyte in ≥10 cortical PTCs With 3-4 leukocytes in most severely involved PTC	At least 1 leukocyte in ≥10 cortical PTCs With 5-10 leukocytes in most severely involved PTC	At least 1 leukocyte in ≥10 cortical PTCs With >10 leukocytes in most severely involved PTC
C4d Score	No C4d	Minimal (>0 but <10% of PTC and medullary vasa recta)	Focal (10-50% of PTC and medullary vasa recta)	Diffuse (>50% of PTC and medullary vasa recta)

DIAGNOSIS OF ACTIVE ABMR
No Criterion of Chronicity
+
At least 1 criterion each from Groups 1,2 and 3

Group 1	**Group 2**	**Group 3**
g>0	C4d >1	DSA
Ptc >0	Mvi (g+ptc >1)	C4d >1
TMA	Expression of gene transcripts associated with AMR	Expression of gene transcripts associated with AMR
ATN		

The management of early active ABMR hinges around three cardinal principles: removal of circulating antibody, targeting antibody producing cells and endothelial protection, as illustrated in Table 3:

Table 3. Management options for early active ABMR

Treatment of early Active ABMR
Removal of Antibody • Plasmapheresis • IVIG
Reducing Antibody producing Cells • Steroids • Antibodies targeting CD20 • Proteosome inhibitors • Anti CD 38 antibody
Endothelial Protection • Anti-Complement Factor 5 agents

Most programs initiate therapy for treatment of early active ABMR with a combination of 3-5 sessions of plasmapheresis and low dose IVIG (100 mg/kg after each session). Some programs elect to use high dose IVIG alone or in combination with plasmapheresis and rituximab depending on the severity of the rejection phenotype (39).

Memory B cells as well as early plasmablasts express CD20 and antibodies to CD 20 (e.g., Rituximab) are used to target these cells. As the plasmablasts mature into plasma cells, they lose CD20 and gain CD38. Plasma cells are susceptible to proteosome inhibition (Bortezomib, carfilzomib) as well as the anti CD38 antibody Daratumumab. Resistant cases are supported with terminal complement blockade using agents like eculizumab to protect the endothelium from complement-mediated damage.

If treated appropriately and aggressively, the early acute ABMR phenotype responds better to therapy than its more chronic counterparts.

Obstructive Complications in the First Few Weeks

Ureteral Leaks

Ureteral leaks happen within the first few days after a transplant. The usual source is the ureteroneocystostomy. Many transplant surgeons deploy indwelling ureteral stents to protect against mechanical stress on the ureter and to ensure patency should there be edema at the anastomosis. These stents are removed a few weeks after transplant.

The diagnosis is not difficult if there is a drain in place. Analysis of drain fluid for creatinine will reveal a much higher creatinine level compared to blood. If a drain is not in place, the leak may reveal itself as a peri-transplant fluid collection. A cystogram or radionuclide scan will reveal the diagnosis. Needle aspiration of the fluid will confirm high creatinine levels.

Most leaks can be treated conservatively by prolonged bladder drainage with a Foley catheter, a maneuver to keep pressures low around the ureteroneocystostomy to allow healing. Should there be an associated obstruction, deployment of a percutaneous nephrostomy tube to divert urine may become necessary. Leaks that do not heal with conservative measures would require surgical revision and reimplantation of the ureter or creation of a ureteroureterostomy utilizing the native ureter.

Ureteral Stenosis

Ureteral obstruction is seen in up to 10% of transplants [40] and usually occurs within the first few weeks after transplant.

In most cases, ureteric obstruction is a result of ureteric ischemia. The ureter is supplied by small branches from the renal artery. The distal ureter may be at a disadvantage from a blood supply standpoint and, in most cases, it is the distal ureter near the ureteroneocystostomy that is affected by this ischemic damage [40]. In some cases, a tight anti-reflux tunnel at the ureteroneocystostomy as well as pressure from a fluid collection or hematoma may lead to ureteric obstruction.

Ureteric obstruction results in hydronephrosis and AKI. It is readily picked up in most cases by bedside ultrasonography. CT Scans offer greater detail by helping localize the site of obstruction as well as better definition of perinephric collections if a urinoma or a hematoma with ureteric compression is being evaluated, for example.

Once the diagnosis of ureteric obstruction is established, the usual first step is to resolve any obstructive injury by urinary diversion utilizing a percutaneous nephrostomy tube. Once this is in place and the AKI has resolved, the interventionalist may attempt an anterograde nephrostogram. If able, he or she would float or deploy a ureteral stent in anterograde fashion [40, 41].

In many cases, this resolves the issue. Recurrent obstruction after stent removal may warrant a reassessment of the situation and consideration for surgical revision and possible reimplantation or creation of a ureteroureterostomy.

Lymphoceles

A lymphocele is a fluid collection between the kidney allograft and the bladder [42]. Lymphoceles result from extravasation of lymph from lymphatics transected during dissection in the recipient and from the hilum of the donor kidney. Most lymphoceles are asymptomatic and require no intervention.

At times, lymphoceles may become symptomatic because of size or location. Increasing size may lead to discomfort, distention, and/or unilateral edema because of ipsilateral venous compression. Pressure on the ureter may lead to hydronephrosis and AKI. In such circumstances, the lymphocele can be drained percutaneously and, in many cases, resolves thereafter. Should the lymphocele recur, become loculated, or appear at a site making percutaneous drainage difficult, it can be treated by surgical marsupialization into the peritoneal cavity either laparoscopically or by an open procedure [48].

AKI after the First Month

The tumultuous period of rapid changes that follow the transplant surgery begins to calm down into a steady routine by the end of the first month. By this time, the patients have largely recovered from the surgery and, in many cases, the indwelling stents have been removed, allograft function has stabilized, and the drug regimens are subject to less variability.

The kidney remains under significant alloimmune threat as well as open to other injuries. Certain nephrotropic opportunistic infections become relevant in this time frame. Just as before, any AKI must be assessed carefully, methodically, and systematically. Figure 6 covers a basic approach to AKI in a kidney transplant patient after the first month.

The Alloimmune Risk – Rejection after the First Few Months of Transplant

The biology of the alloimmune mechanisms start shifting after the first few months. In the initial months, rejection processes are driven either by pre-existing memory cells or through allorecognition by the direct pathway (antigen presentation by passenger donor antigen presenting cells, in the donor APC HLA II molecules, to the recipients CD4 T cells and B cells.) This leads to immune activation and generation of an immune response.

This mechanism is quite steadily exhausted as the donor antigen presenting cells (APCs) are depleted. Antigen presentation now proceeds in a more traditional process dubbed indirect antigen presentation. The recipient APCs pick up donor antigens, process them and present them to recipient T Cells in the context of HLA II molecules. They interact with B cells as well. Thus, a traditional immune response is generated.

It is quite evident that the most effective way to thwart such activity is by maintaining immunosuppression at appropriately therapeutic levels. Indeed, emergence of de-novo donor specific antibodies as well as precipitation of frank rejection after the first few months of transplantation is directly related to underimmunosuppression, either prescriptive or due to non-adherence [43].

The phenotype of these rejections is different as well. The rejections that are seen in later months are much more likely to be mixed AMRs and CMRs, though pure CMRs and AMRs may still be seen. The AMRs are less likely to have C4d (compared to the early acute cohorts) and their response to therapy is not as good [44]. They are much more likely to slide into chronic ABMR. Consequently, these allografts are much more likely to have significantly decreased survival.

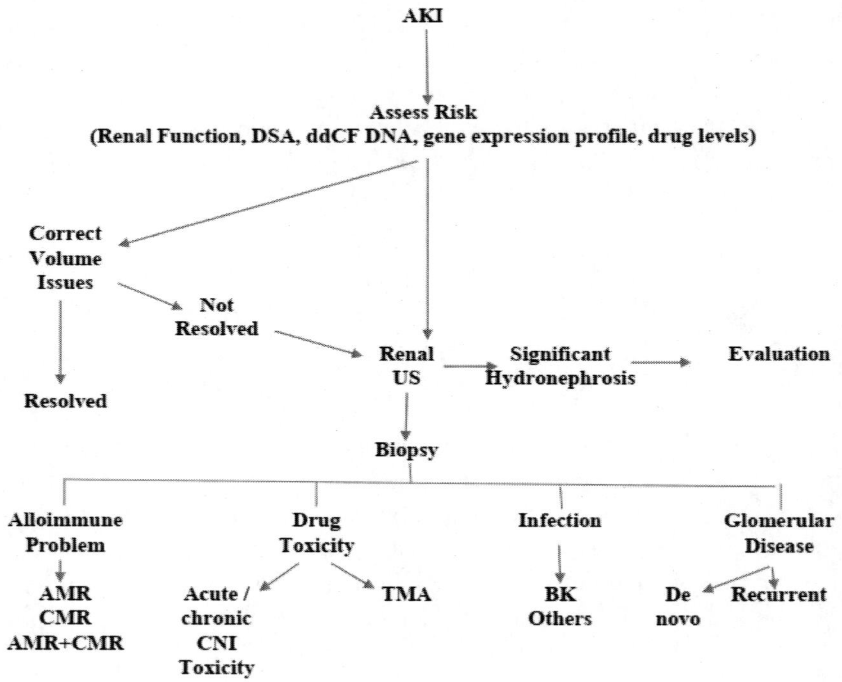

DSA: Donor specific antibodies.
AMR Antibody mediated Rejection.
CMR: Cell mediated rejection.
CNI calcineurin Inhibitor.
TMA: Thrombotic Microangiopathy.
ddCF DNA: Donor derived cell free DNA.

Figure 6. AKI after the first month of transplantation.

It is because of these uncertainties that the need for better monitoring of allograft health and function is highlighted.

Traditionally, proteinuria and serum creatinine have been used as the main benchmarks of allograft health and then tested for DSAs and performed biopsies (surveillance or for cause) to adjudicate deterioration. Proteinuria and creatinine are insensitive markers when it comes to screening for alloimmune activity – there may be significant active inflammation in the kidney without proteinuria or elevated creatinine. DSAs can be unpredictable. The gold standard, allograft biopsy is an invasive procedure with its attendant complications and costs.

In recent years, new tools have become available to help monitor allograft health. Measurement of gene expression profiles to help detect sub clinical rejection (45) as well as detection of donor-derived cell-free DNA (dd-cfDNA) (46) for allograft injury have been tested clinically and are being utilized by various transplant centers. They are being used either as surveillance tests, for cause when the creatinine is already up or post treatment surveillance once an acute rejection has been treated. These are exciting new developments and will add to the non-invasive repertoire of tests to draw up an immunological map of a particular patient's alloimmune risk.

Thus, when a patient's creatinine is elevated, a negative dd-cfDNA test has an extremely high negative predictive value for acute rejection (46). On the other hand, if the dd-cfDNA value is elevated, that may suggest allograft injury and may help the argument to proceed to a biopsy sooner rather than later.

An Aside on BK Nephropathy

Over the past two decades, the BK virus has emerged as an important pathogen, quite specifically targeting patients who have received kidney transplants. It is a double stranded DNA virus that belongs to Polyomaviridae family. It is a ubiquitous virus, and a large majority of children are exposed to it in their early childhood. The prevalence of circulating antibody to the BK virus increases from 50% at age 3 to almost 100% at age 10-11 with a subsequent decline to 67% by age 35 [47]. The primary infection is either completely asymptomatic or takes the form of a mild respiratory illness. Upon resolution of the primary infection, the virus resides in the kidney in a latent state. The body's immune mechanisms are quite adept at keeping the virus restricted to this latency. However, in states of immunosuppression, the virus may start replicating again. This virological reactivation may be seen in conditions like diabetes, pregnancy and even with aging. However, this results in an inconsequential viruria.

In patients with kidney transplantation, the degree of immunosuppression is significantly more pronounced. Heavy viruria leads to virema and sustained viremia may precipitate nephropathy. Though the virus was first described in 1971, it really did not assume significance as a pathogen until the last years of the last millennium. Contemporaneously, tacrolimus and mycophenolate mofetil had emerged as newer, more effective and more robustly immunosuppressive drugs. This led to the insight that the virus was very immune sensitive, a fact displayed in a large prospective trial [48]. The impact of reduction of immunosuppression on viral kinetics was studied as well.

Soon thereafter, a few principles were defined when dealing with the BK virus in kidney transplant patients:

- The virus was strongly associated with the degree of immunosuppression afforded to the patient.
- Viruria predated viremia in almost all cases, and nephropathy followed a period of sustained viremia.

- The negative predictive value of a negative BK PCR in the blood was extremely high [49], enough to exclude the diagnosis of BK nephropathy.
- It also emerged that early detection and proactive management by reducing immunosuppression exposure led to clearance of viremia and avoided nephropathy in many cases.
- On the other hand, if viremia were allowed to fester, nephropathy could precipitate. Further inaction could lead to progression of nephropathy and irreversible damage to the allograft.

These principles have become the backbone of management of BK infection in kidney transplant patients. Many programs have set up surveillance programs by screening the urine or blood to identify patients at risk for BK nephropathy and then take evasive action for those thought to be at high risk, usually patients with sustained high-level viremia.

In patients not being screened, often the first indicator of BK nephropathy is an elevated creatinine level. The diagnosis is confirmed by sending molecular studies for the virus and by performing an allograft biopsy. This importance of early detection, and especially detection before nephropathy has set in and causes allograft dysfunction, is highlighted in the study of the histopathologic classification systems for BK nephropathy. The Banff working group for Polyoma Nephropathy presented one such classification system in 2018 – BK nephropathy was placed in Class I, II or III with rising degrees of tubular viral effect and chronic inflammatory changes. There is a direct correlation of histopathological class of BK nephropathy at diagnosis with outcomes – patients placed in Class I at diagnosis experienced an average increase in their creatinine levels of 0.4 mg/dl over the next 2 years while those placed in class III at diagnosis suffered an average increase of 4.8 mg/dl; half of the patients placed in class III at diagnosis lost their allografts [50].

Thus, in a way, diagnosis of BK nephropathy in the setting of AKI represents a failure to anticipate and pre-empt this outcome. Consideration, however, must be given to BK nephropathy in every case of AKI after the first 1-2 month of transplantation.

Despite several attempts, no antiviral agents have been clearly found to be of conclusive or decisive benefit in BK nephropathy. The cornerstone of therapy remains reduction of immunosuppression. In some cases, passive immunity by way of intravenous immunoglobulin may be of some benefit.

Glomerulonephritis in the Allograft

Glomerular disease is a common cause of chronic kidney disease in the native kidneys. Many of these diseases can recur in an allograft. Alternatively, a glomerulonephritis can occur de novo. Different glomerular disease processes have different propensities to manifest in the allograft. Their biological behavior is also affected as these processes are now operating in a milieu of immunosuppression.

Many glomerular diseases, especially diseases of the podocyte (Focal Segmental Glomerulosclerosis, Minimal Change Disease and Membranous Nephropathy) initially present as nephrotic syndrome and if left untreated, lead to progressive attrition of the allograft and eventual graft failure. These typically do not present with an AKI, though at times due to massive proteinuria an ATN may result.

On the other hand, there are many classes of glomerular disease, as well as diseases of the endothelium and basement membrane, that can and do present as AKI, as summarized in Table 4.

Systemic Lupus Erythematosus (SLE) and IgA nephropathy (also known as Berger's disease) are classic examples of diseases driven by antigen-antibody complexes. Recurrence after transplantation is not uncommon, but in the modern era of immunosuppression, is largely restricted to sub-clinical or mildly clinical disease. In some cases, more aggressive forms of disease, including crescentic phenotypes and rapidly progressive renal failure, may be seen. This remains a relatively uncommon phenomenon [51, 52]. Recurrence of antineutrophil cytoplasmic antibody (ANCA) driven vasculitis is seen in about 17% of cases, but allograft loss is seen in only 7% due to the recurrence [53].

Anti-glomerular basement membrane antibody disease (anti-GBM) can recur early and lead to an AKI. This is seen in patients who are transplanted with high levels of circulating anti GBM antibody. It is therefore recommended to ensure the anti-GBM antibody levels have dropped to appropriately low levels prior to undertaking transplantation.

Diseases of complement dysregulation may frequently recur in the allograft. These are highly polymorphic disorders but do tend to recur in the allograft frequently. The recurrence may be early or late and depending on the disease process may lead to slowly progressive allograft dysfunction or a more abrupt loss of GFR, qualifying their consideration in the spectrum of AKI. Disorders of alternate complement pathway regulation centered around deficiency of Factor H and Factor I, for instance, may lead to early complement-mediated hemolytic uremic syndrome, thrombotic microangiopathy, and AKI. Untreated, this may lead to graft loss. On the other hand, some forms of C3 glomerulopathy may demonstrate a subacute course taking years to destroy the allograft.

Table 4. Glomerulonephritis after Transplantation

Disease category	Usual Presentation	AKI
Podocytopathies (MCD, FSGS, MN)	Progressive proteinuria Nephrotic Syndrome	Unusual. May have an ATN with florid onset of nephrotic syndrome
ICGN IgA Nephropathy SLE	Isolated Hematuria Hematuria and proteinuria CKD AKI Hematuria and proteinuria CKD AKI	Not common but may present with proliferative / crescentic disease and AKI Not common but may present with proliferative / crescentic disease and AKI
AAV	Hematuria and proteinuria Progressive CKD AKI	Not common but may present with crescentic disease and AKI
Complement Mediated Disease cHUS C3GN	TMA and MAHA Proteinuria Hematuria and proteinuria Progressive CKD AKI	Common May be seen.
Anti GBM Disease	AKI	High risk if pre-transplant anti GBM levels high.

Conclusion

AKI is not an uncommon event after kidney transplantation. Depending on the cause, AKI may have significantly short and long-term effects on allograft survival. Many such causes, if not identified early and treated effectively, can lead to irreversible damage to the allograft.

It is therefore important to develop a methodological approach to each episode of AKI. Careful appreciation of the timeframe in which the injury is manifesting itself, informing a considered meticulous approach is essential to correctly identifying and managing AKI after transplantation.

Kidney transplant patients require management by an effective team comprising transplant nephrologists and surgeons, radiologists with expertise in imaging kidney allografts, transplant infectious disease specialists, pathologists with expertise in interpreting kidney allograft biopsies, and transplant pharmacists. A comprehensive approach to care delivered by a multidisciplinary team is the optimal way to care for these complicated patients. AKI in a kidney transplant patient should be considered an emergent crisis requiring consideration and participation by every member of this team to ensure timely, accurate, and effective management.

Conflict of Interest

Author	Potential Conflict	Relevant
Irfan A Agha, MD	Consultancy / Advisory Board with CareDx, AstraZenica, Cara Pharmaceuticals, Aurinia, GSK.	No
Amna Ilahe, MD	None	
Amanda Condon, PharmD	None	
Van Ngo, MD	None	

References

[1] Rahamimov R, van Dijk TY, Molcho M, Vahav I, Mor E, Ben Dor N, Goldman S, Rozen-Zvi B. Acute Kidney Injury and Long-Term Risk for Cardiovascular Events in Patients after Kidney Transplantation. *Kidney Blood Press Res.* 2019;44(5):1149-1157.

[2] Lim WH, Johnson DW, Teixeira-Pinto A, Wong G. Association Between Duration of Delayed Graft Function, Acute Rejection, and Allograft Outcome After Deceased Donor Kidney Transplantation. *Transplantation*. 2019;103(2):412-419.

[3] Arache W, Bahadi A, Kabbaj DE. Thromboses des artères rénales révélant un syndrome des anticorps antiphospholipides [Renal artery thrombosis revealing antiphospholipid antibody syndrome]. *Pan Afr Med J.* 2018;31:150. French.

[4] Bakir N, Sluiter WJ, Ploeg RJ, van Son WJ, Tegzess AM. Primary renal graft thrombosis. *Nephrol Dial Transplant*. 1996;11(1):140-7.

[5] Cai S, Ouyang YS, Li JC, Dai Q, Tan L, Xia Y, Xu ZH, Li HJ, Jiang YX. Evaluation of acute renal artery thrombosis or embolism with color Doppler sonography. *Clin Imaging*. 2008;32(5):367-71.

[6] Yarlagadda SG, Coca SG, Garg AX, Doshi M, Poggio E, Marcus RJ, Parikh CR. Marked variation in the definition and diagnosis of delayed graft function: a systematic review. *Nephrol Dial Transplant*. 2008;23(9):2995-3003.

[7] Wang CJ, Wetmore JB, Israni AK. Old versus new: Progress in reaching the goals of the new kidney allocation system. *Hum Immunol*. 2017;78(1):9-15.

[8] Zens TJ, Danobeitia JS, Leverson G, Chlebeck PJ, Zitur LJ, Redfield RR, D'Alessandro AM, Odorico S, Kaufman DB, Fernandez LA. The impact of kidney donor profile index on delayed graft function and transplant outcomes: A single-center analysis. *Clin Transplant*. 2018;32(3):e13190.

[9] Irish WD, Ilsley JN, Schnitzler MA, Feng S, Brennan DC. A risk prediction model for delayed graft function in the current era of deceased donor renal transplantation. *Am J Transplant*. 2010;10(10):2279-86.

[10] Doshi MD, Garg N, Reese PP, Parikh CR. Recipient risk factors associated with delayed graft function: a paired kidney analysis. *Transplantation*. 2011;91(6):666-71.

[11] Meier-Kriesche HU, Arndorfer JA, Kaplan B. The impact of body mass index on renal transplant outcomes: a significant independent risk factor for graft failure and patient death. *Transplantation*. 2002;73(1):70-4.

[12] Devarajan P. Update on mechanisms of ischemic acute kidney injury. *J Am Soc Nephrol*. 2006; 17(6):1503-20.

[13] Mannon RB. Delayed Graft Function: The AKI of Kidney Transplantation. *Nephron*. 2018;140(2):94-98.

[14] Siedlecki A, Irish W, Brennan DC. Delayed graft function in the kidney transplant. *Am J Transplant*. 2011;(11):2279-96.

[15] Belzer FO, Southard JH. Principles of solid-organ preservation by cold storage. *Transplantation*. 1988;45(4):673-6.

[16] Wight JP, Chilcott JB, Holmes MW, Brewer N. Pulsatile machine perfusion vs. cold storage of kidneys for transplantation: a rapid and systematic review. *Clin Transplant*. 200;17(4):293-307.

[17] Mangino MJ, Ametani M, Szabó C, Southard JH. Poly(ADP-ribose) polymerase and renal hypothermic preservation injury. *Am J Physiol Renal Physiol*. 2004;286(5): F838-47.

[18] Agarwal A, Murdock P, Fridell JA. Comparison of histidine-tryptophan ketoglutarate solution and University of Wisconsin solution in prolonged cold preservation of kidney allografts. *Transplantation*. 2006;81(3):480-2.

[19] Hart A, Smith JM, Skeans MA, Gustafson SK, Wilk AR, Castro S, Foutz J, Wainright JL, Snyder JJ, Kasiske BL, Israni AK. OPTN/SRTR 2018 Annual Data Report: Kidney. *Am J Transplant*. 2020;20 Suppl s1:20-130.

[20] Nankivell BJ, Borrows RJ, Fung CL, O'Connell PJ, Chapman JR, Allen RD. Calcineurin inhibitor nephrotoxicity: longitudinal assessment by protocol histology. *Transplantation*. 2004 Aug 27;78(4):557-65.

[21] Haas M, Sonnenday CJ, Cicone JS, Rabb H, Montgomery RA. Isometric tubular epithelial vacuolization in renal allograft biopsy specimens of patients receiving low-dose intravenous immunoglobulin for a positive crossmatch. *Transplantation*. 2004;78(4):549-56.

[22] Prograf. Package insert. *Astellas Pharma US*, Inc; 2012.

[23] Trofe-Clark J, Brennan DC, West-Thielke P, Milone MC, Lim MA, Neubauer R, Nigro V, Bloom RD. Results of ASERTAA, a Randomized Prospective Crossover Pharmacogenetic Study of Immediate-Release Versus Extended-Release Tacrolimus in African American Kidney Transplant Recipients. *Am J Kidney Dis*. 2018;71(3): 315-326.

[24] Lanese DM, Conger JD. Effects of endothelin receptor antagonist on cyclosporine-induced vasoconstriction in isolated rat renal arterioles. *J Clin Invest*. 1993;91 (5):2144-9.

[25] Lamas S. Cellular mechanisms of vascular injury mediated by calcineurin inhibitors. *Kidney Int*. 2005;68(2):898-907.

[26] Novick AC, Hwei HH, Steinmuller D, Streem SB, Cunningham RJ, Steinhilber D, Goormastic M, Buszta C. Detrimental effect of cyclosporine on initial function of cadaver renal allografts following extended preservation. Results of a randomized prospective study. *Transplantation*. 1986;42(2):154-8.

[27] Andrés A, Budde K, Clavien PA, Becker T, Kessler M, Pisarski P, Fornara P, Burmeister D, Hené RJ, Cassuto-Viguier E; SENIOR Study Team. A randomized trial comparing renal function in older kidney transplant patients following delayed versus immediate tacrolimus administration. *Transplantation*. 2009;88(9):1101-8.

[28] Liu Y, Liu H, Shen Y, Chen Y, Cheng Y. Delayed Initiation of Tacrolimus Is Safe and Effective in Renal Transplant Recipients With Delayed and Slow Graft Function. *Transplant Proc*. 2018;50(8):2368-2370.

[29] Hill P, Cross NB, Barnett AN, Palmer SC, Webster AC. Polyclonal and monoclonal antibodies for induction therapy in kidney transplant recipients. *Cochrane Database Syst Rev*. 2017;1(1):CD004759.

[30] Fortin MC, Raymond MA, Madore F, Fugère JA, Pâquet M, St-Louis G, Hébert MJ. Increased risk of thrombotic microangiopathy in patients receiving a cyclosporin-sirolimus combination. *Am J Transplant*. 2004;4(6):946-52.

[31] Ekberg H, Tedesco-Silva H, Demirbas A, Vítko S, Nashan B, Gürkan A, Margreiter R, Hugo C, Grinyó JM, Frei U, Vanrenterghem Y, Daloze P, Halloran PF; ELITE-Symphony Study. Reduced exposure to calcineurin inhibitors in renal transplantation. *N Engl J Med*. 2007;357(25):2562-75.

[32] Vincenti F, Charpentier B, Vanrenterghem Y, Rostaing L, Bresnahan B, Darji P, Massari P, Mondragon-Ramirez GA, Agarwal M, Di Russo G, Lin CS, Garg P, Larsen CP. A phase III study of belatacept-based immunosuppression regimens versus cyclosporine in renal transplant recipients (BENEFIT study). *Am J Transplant*. 2010;10(3):535-46.

[33] Vincenti F, Rostaing L, Grinyo J, Rice K, Steinberg S, Gaite L, Moal MC, Mondragon-Ramirez GA, Kothari J, Polinsky MS, Meier-Kriesche HU, Munier S, Larsen CP. Belatacept and Long-Term Outcomes in Kidney Transplantation. *N Engl J Med*. 2016 Jan 28;374(4):333-43. Erratum in: *N Engl J Med*. 2016;374(7):698.

[34] Cicora F, Paz M, Mos F, Roberti J. Use of belatacept as alternative immunosuppression in three renal transplant patients with de novo drug-induced thrombotic microangiopathy. *Case Rep Med*. 2013;2013:260254.

[35] Patel R, Terasaki PI. Significance of the positive crossmatch test in kidney transplantation. *N Engl J Med*. 1969;280(14):735-9.

[36] Halloran PF. T cell-mediated rejection of kidney transplants: a personal viewpoint. *Am J Transplant*. 2010;10(5):1126-34.

[37] Loupy A, Haas M, Solez K, Racusen L, Glotz D, Seron D, Nankivell BJ, Colvin RB, Afrouzian M, Akalin E, Alachkar N, Bagnasco S, Becker JU, Cornell L, Drachenberg C, Dragun D, de Kort H, Gibson IW, Kraus ES, Lefaucheur C, Legendre C, Liapis H, Muthukumar T, Nickeleit V, Orandi B, Park W, Rabant M, Randhawa P, Reed EF, Roufosse C, Seshan SV, Sis B, Singh HK, Schinstock C, Tambur A, Zeevi A, Mengel M. The Banff 2015 Kidney Meeting Report: Current Challenges in Rejection Classification and Prospects for Adopting Molecular Pathology. *Am J Transplant.* 2017;17(1):28-41.

[38] Famulski KS, Einecke G, Sis B, Mengel M, Hidalgo LG, Kaplan B, Halloran PF. Defining the canonical form of T-cell-mediated rejection in human kidney transplants. *Am J Transplant*. 2010;10(4):810-20.

[39] Jordan SC, Reinsmoen N, Peng A, Lai CH, Cao K, Villicana R, Toyoda M, Kahwaji J, Vo AA. Advances in diagnosing and managing antibody-mediated rejection. *Pediatr Nephrol.* 2010;25(10):2035-45; quiz 2045-8.

[40] Kumar S, Ameli-Renani S, Hakim A, Jeon JH, Shrivastava S, Patel U. Ureteral obstruction following renal transplantation: causes, diagnosis and management. *Br J Radiol.* 2014;87(1044):20140169.

[41] Sandhu C, Patel U. Renal transplantation dysfunction: the role of interventional radiology. *Clin Radiol*. 2002;57(9):772-83.

[42] Haberal M, Boyvat F, Akdur A, Kırnap M, Özçelik Ü, Yarbuğ Karakayalı F. Surgical Complications After Kidney Transplantation. *Exp Clin Transplant*. 2016;14(6): 587-595.

[43] Jordan SC, Vo AA. Donor-specific antibodies in allograft recipients: etiology, impact and therapeutic approaches. *Curr Opin Organ Transplant*. 2014;19(6):591-7.

[44] Schinstock CA, Mannon RB, Budde K, Chong AS, Haas M, Knechtle S, Lefaucheur C, Montgomery RA, Nickerson P, Tullius SG, Ahn C, Askar M, Crespo M, Chadban SJ, Feng S, Jordan SC, Man K, Mengel M, Morris RE, O'Doherty I, Ozdemir BH, Seron D, Tambur AR, Tanabe K, Taupin JL, O'Connell PJ. Recommended Treatment for Antibody-mediated Rejection After Kidney *Transplantation*: The 2019 Expert Consensus From the Transplantion Society Working Group. *Transplantation.* 2020;104(5):911-922.

[45] Friedewald JJ, Kurian SM, Heilman RL, Whisenant TC, Poggio ED, Marsh C, Baliga P, Odim J, Brown MM, Ikle DN, Armstrong BD, Charette JI, Brietigam SS, Sustento-Reodica N, Zhao L, Kandpal M, Salomon DR, Abecassis MM; Clinical Trials in Organ Transplantation 08 (CTOT-08). Development and clinical validity of a novel blood-based molecular biomarker for subclinical acute rejection following kidney transplant. *Am J Transplant*. 2019;19(1):98-109.

[46] Bloom RD, Bromberg JS, Poggio ED, Bunnapradist S, Langone AJ, Sood P, Matas AJ, Mehta S, Mannon RB, Sharfuddin A, Fischbach B, Narayanan M, Jordan SC, Cohen D, Weir MR, Hiller D, Prasad P, Woodward RN, Grskovic M, Sninsky JJ, Yee JP, Brennan DC; Circulating Donor-Derived Cell-Free DNA in Blood for Diagnosing Active Rejection in Kidney Transplant Recipients (DART) Study Investigators. Cell-Free DNA and Active Rejection in Kidney Allografts. *J Am Soc Nephrol*. 2017;28(7):2221-2232.

[47] Shah KV, Daniel RW, Warszawski RM. High prevalence of antibodies to BK virus, an SV40-related papovavirus, in residents of Maryland. *J Infect Dis*. 1973;128(6):784-7.

[48] Brennan DC, Agha I, Bohl DL, Schnitzler MA, Hardinger KL, Lockwood M, Torrence S, Schuessler R, Roby T, Gaudreault-Keener M, Storch GA. Incidence of BK with

tacrolimus versus cyclosporine and impact of preemptive immunosuppression reduction. *Am J Transplant*. 2005;(3):582-94.

[49] Nickeleit V, Klimkait T, Binet IF, Dalquen P, Del Zenero V, Thiel G, Mihatsch MJ, Hirsch HH. Testing for polyomavirus type BK DNA in plasma to identify renal-allograft recipients with viral nephropathy. *N Engl J Med*. 2000;342(18):1309-15.

[50] Nickeleit V, Singh HK, Randhawa P, Drachenberg CB, Bhatnagar R, Bracamonte E, Chang A, Chon WJ, Dadhania D, Davis VG, Hopfer H, Mihatsch MJ, Papadimitriou JC, Schaub S, Stokes MB, Tungekar MF, Seshan SV; Banff Working Group on Polyomavirus Nephropathy. The Banff Working Group Classification of Definitive Polyomavirus Nephropathy: Morphologic Definitions and Clinical Correlations. *J Am Soc Nephrol*. 2018;29(2):680-693.

[51] Norby GE, Strøm EH, Midtvedt K, Hartmann A, Gilboe IM, Leivestad T, Stenstrøm J, Holdaas H. Recurrent lupus nephritis after kidney transplantation: a surveillance biopsy study. *Ann Rheum Dis*. 2010;69(8):1484-7.

[52] Goral S, Ynares C, Shappell SB, Snyder S, Feurer ID, Kazancioglu R, Fogo AB, Helderman JH. Recurrent lupus nephritis in renal transplant recipients revisited: it is not rare. *Transplantation*. 2003;75(5):651-6.

[53] Moroni G, Belingheri M, Frontini G, Tamborini F, Messa P. Immunoglobulin A Nephropathy. Recurrence after Renal Transplantation. *Front Immunol*. 2019;10:1332.

INDEX

A

B

C

D

E

F

G

H

I

J

K

L

M

N

O

P

Q

R

S

T

U

V

W